Reproductive Tract Infections

Reproductive Tract Infections

Editor: Christian Ball

AMERICAN
MEDICAL PUBLISHERS
www.americanmedicalpublishers.com

AMERICAN
MEDICAL PUBLISHERS
www.americanmedicalpublishers.com

Cataloging-in-Publication Data

Reproductive tract infections / edited by Christian Ball.
p. cm.
Includes bibliographical references and index.
ISBN 978-1-63927-232-7
1. Generative organs--Infections. 2. Generative organs, Female--Infections. 3. Generative organs--Diseases.
4. Urinary tract infections. I. Ball, Christian.
RC877 .R47 2022
616.65--dc23

American Medical Publishers,
41 Flatbush Avenue,
1st Floor, New York,
NY 11217, USA

ISBN 978-1-63927-232-7 (Hardback)

Contents

Preface

The infections that affect the reproductive tract are known as reproductive tract infections. It affects different reproductive parts in males and females. In males, it affects urethra, testicles and penis. Whereas, in females, it infects the upper reproductive tract which includes fallopian tubes, ovary and uterus, and lower reproductive tract including vagina, cervix and vulva. There are three main types of reproductive infections - endogenous infections, iatrogenic infections and sexually transmitted infections. The endogenous infections arise from an infectious agent previously present within the body. Sexually transmitted infections are spread by sexual activities. Each infection has its symptoms and may be caused by a bacterium, fungus, virus or other organisms. Some reproductive tract infections such as AIDS and herpes are non-curable. They can cause impotence, ectopic pregnancy, premature ejaculation and dysmenorrhea. This book contains some path-breaking studies in the field of reproductive tract infections. It strives to provide a fair idea about such infections and to help develop a better understanding of their diagnosis and management. This book will serve as a valuable source of reference for graduate and post graduate students.

This book is a comprehensive compilation of works of different researchers from varied parts of the world. It includes valuable experiences of the researchers with the sole objective of providing the readers (learners) with a proper knowledge of the concerned field. This book will be beneficial in evoking inspiration and enhancing the knowledge of the interested readers.

In the end, I would like to extend my heartiest thanks to the authors who worked with great determination on their chapters. I also appreciate the publisher's support in the course of the book. I would also like to deeply acknowledge my family who stood by me as a source of inspiration during the project.

Editor

1

Young male sex workers are at high risk for sexually transmitted infections, a cross-sectional study from Dutch STI clinics, the Netherlands, 2006–2012

N. Fournet[1,2*], F. D. H. Koedijk[1,3], A. P. van Leeuwen[4], M. S. van Rooijen[4], M. A. B. van der Sande[1,5] and M. G. van Veen[4]

Abstract

Background: Male sex workers (MSW) are particularly exposed to sexually transmitted infections (STI) including HIV. In the Netherlands, data about STI among MSW are scarce. We estimated chlamydia, gonorrhoea, syphilis and HIV diagnoses among MSW attending STI clinics and determined associated factors to guide prevention policies.

Methods: Using 2006–2012 cross-sectional national surveillance data from Dutch STI clinics, we calculated the proportion of consultations with a positive test for any of three bacterial STI or HIV among MSW. Associated factors were determined by using Poisson logistic regression with robust variance.

Results: We identified 3,053 consultations involving MSW, of which 18.1 % included at least one positive bacterial STI test and 2.5 % a positive HIV test. Factors associated with bacterial STI and/or HIV diagnoses were respectively age groups < 35 y.o. and self-reporting homo- or bisexual preferences (aRR = 1.6; 95 % CI: 1.3–2.1), and age group 25–34 y.o. (aRR = 2.7; 95 % CI: 1.2–6.5) and self-reporting homo- or bisexual preferences (aRR = 24.4; 95 % CI: 3.4–176.9). Newly diagnosed and pre-existing HIV infection were associated with an increased risk for bacterial STI (aRR = 2.7, 95 % CI: 1.7–2.6 and aRR = 2.1, 95 % CI: 2.2–3.4 respectively). MSW with no history of HIV screening were more likely to be tested positive for HIV compared to those with a previous HIV-negative test (aRR = 2.6, 95 % CI: 1.6–4.3).

Conclusion: Health promotion activities should target MSW who are young, homo- or bisexual, those who are HIV-infected or who have never been tested for HIV, to increase early diagnosis, prevention and treatment.

Keywords: Sexually transmitted infections, Sex workers, Public health surveillance, Male, HIV, Risk factors

Background

Sex workers are at high risk for contracting sexually transmitted infections (STI) including human immunodeficiency virus (HIV) [1–3]. In Europe, the majority of sex workers are women whereas male sex workers (MSW) represent an estimated 7 % of the sex workers population [4]. Studies about risk for acquiring bacterial STI and HIV among MSW are limited but suggest a high risk among this population, even higher than among female sex workers (FSW) [5, 6].

A European HIV/AIDS survey reported a high prevalence of HIV among non-injecting drug-using (IDU) MSW (up to 12 % in Spain) compared to less than 1 % among non-IDU FSW [7]. Studies in Belgium [6] and Australia [3] reported that almost one-third of MSW had one or more STI. These higher prevalences of STI and HIV among MSW than among FSW can be explained by differences in sexual behaviours and characteristics. Indeed, more than 85 % of MSW have sex with men [3, 5, 8–10]. Men who have sex with men (MSM) have been reported to more frequently engage in unsafe sex practices [10] and to have higher prevalences of STI and HIV compared to

* Correspondence: nellyfournet@yahoo.fr
[1]Epidemiology and Surveillance Unit, Centre for Infectious Diseases Control, National Institute for Public Health and the Environment (RIVM), P.O. Box 1, 3720 BA Bilthoven, The Netherlands
[2]European Programme for Intervention Epidemiology Training (EPIET), European Centre for Disease Prevention and Control (ECDC), Stockholm, Sweden
Full list of author information is available at the end of the article

heterosexual men [11–14]. Furthermore, the male sex work industry seems markedly different from the female sex work sector. It is less organised and MSW tend to hide their commercial sexual practices [5, 15]. In a study on MSW attending genitourinary clinics in the United Kingdom in 2011, MSW more frequently attended clinics and were significantly more likely to be diagnosed with a bacterial STI or with HIV than other male attendees [16]. Additional studies suggest that MSW are difficult to reach by education and intervention programmes [5, 15].

In the majority of European countries, sex work is prohibited, although largely tolerated. In the Netherlands, however, voluntary adult prostitution is recognised as a legal occupation. In 2000, a national law was passed to allow, regulate, and control prostitution in which adult sex workers are voluntarily engaged. In 2004, a study reported an estimated 25,000 sex workers in the country, 90 % being women, 5 % men and 5 % transgender [17]. Due to the high mobility of sex workers, absolute numbers could be underestimated.

In the Netherlands, many studies about STI among high risk groups concerned MSM [11, 13, 18–20], FSW, and transgender sex workers [21], but so far none focused on men, including MSM, involved in the sex work industry. Therefore, a sound understanding of MSW characteristics is needed to develop comprehensive sexual health promotion programmes targeting this group.

The first objective of this study was to assess the percentage of consultations with at least one positive bacterial (chlamydia, gonorrhoea, syphilis) STI or HIV test among MSW who attended STI clinics in the Netherlands between 2006 and 2012. The second objective was to determine factors associated with bacterial STI and HIV diagnoses among MSW to guide targeted prevention programmes.

Method

Setting

In the Netherlands, 26 STI clinics — mostly within the Public Health Services — are distributed across the country and provide anonymous free-of-charge STI/HIV testing and treatment of STI for high risk groups. High risk groups encompass people matching one or more of the following criteria: reporting STI-related symptoms, notified or referred for STI testing, aged below 25 years, MSM, involved in sex work, originated from HIV endemic area, reporting three or more sexual partners in the previous six months or reporting a partner from one of these high risk groups.

At STI clinics all attendees are anonymously tested for chlamydia, gonorrhoea, and syphilis even if the individual do not present symptoms or complaints. Diagnoses are carried out locally in STI clinics-affiliated laboratories in accordance with standard procedures [14]. Chlamydia diagnosis is performed in all laboratories by using nucleic acid amplified test (NAAT) on urine sample or urethral swab. *Neisseria gonorrhoea* diagnosis methods vary between laboratories: culture is primarily performed in symptomatic attendees whereas NAAT is primarily performed in asymptomatic attendees. Syphilis testing is done using *Treponema pallidum* hemagglutination assay (TPHA) [14]. Since 2010, a national opt-out policy for HIV testing is implemented and HIV tests are routinely performed at each visit unless the patient refuses by using previously described methods [22, 23]. Dutch guidelines for MSW recommend to test for STI and HIV every 3 months [24]. Since 2004, demographic, behavioural and clinical information are recorded by physician or nurse in an online registration surveillance database and reported to the Centre for Infectious Diseases Control at the National Institute for Public Health and the Environment (RIVM).

Registration in STI clinics has been harmonised in 2006, therefore, the 2006–2012 period was selected to allow comparable data between the 26 STI clinics.

Ethical approval for the study was not necessary following Dutch law as the study used anonymous patient data collected for routine surveillance [25].

Study design

We conducted a cross-sectional study using all consultations of MSW registered in the online RIVM registration database from 2006 to 2012. Because of the anonymous nature of this surveillance database, identification of repeated consultations for a defined individual was not possible. Consequently, the unit of analysis was a consultation for which a test for bacterial STI or HIV was performed.

Study population

We defined a MSW as a man who reports the exchange of sex for money or other valuable goods, such as drugs, and who has been involved in sex work (legally or not) at least once in the six months prior to consultation at the STI clinic.

Outcomes

For each consultation, two clinical outcomes were analysed separately:

- positive test result for bacterial STI (chlamydia, gonorrhoea, and/or syphilis) and
- positive test result for HIV

We determined the proportion of consultations with at least one positive test result for either a bacterial STI or HIV among MSW.

Data collection and statistical analysis

For each STI clinic visit, data recorded in the national database included year and area of origin, gender, self-defined sexual preference (hetero-, homo- or bisexual), injecting drug use in the past six months (yes/no), bacterial (chlamydia, gonorrhoea or syphilis) STI in the past two years (yes/no), previous HIV test (no test/positive test/negative test) and clinical outcomes. Age groups 15–24 years, 25–34 years and ≥35 years were analysed and sexual preferences were analysed in two categories: homo/bisexual.

Descriptive analyses were performed for demographic, behavioural, and clinical data. Trends between 2006 and 2012 were determined using the Cochran-Armitage trend test.

Analyses were conducted using SAS 9.3 (SAS Institute Inc., Cary, North Carolina, USA).

Factors associated with a positive test result for either a bacterial STI or for HIV among MSW were determined by using a Poisson logistic regression model with robust variance. Variables associated with the outcomes in univariate analysis (p-value < 0.20) were included in a multivariate model and variables with a p-value greater than 0.05 were eliminated step-by-step, controlling for confounding at each step. Interaction effects were tested in the final model. Results of univariate and multivariate statistical analyses were expressed as adjusted risk ratios (aRR) with Wald 95 % confidence intervals.

For bacterial STI outcome, we studied the association with HIV status considering the following three modalities collected during consultation: negative HIV test/new positive HIV diagnosis/known HIV infection. For new HIV diagnosis outcome, the information about previous HIV tests (yes/no) and co-infection with a bacterial STI (yes/no) diagnosed at the current consultation were included.

Table 1 Characteristics of MSW attending STI clinics in the Netherlands, 2006–2012

	MSW ($N = 3,053$)	
	Number[a]	%
Age group		
15–24 years	789	26
25–34 years	1,252	41
≥ 35 years	1,011	33
Country/Area of origin		
The Netherlands	1,511	50
Eastern Europe	620	20
Other European countries	134	4
Latin America	437	14
Sub-Saharan Africa	40	1
Asia	57	2
Turkey/Morocca	127	4
Other or unknown	124	4
Self-defined sexual preference		
Heterosexual	855	28
Homo/bisexual	2,183	72
Intravenous drug user in the past 6 months		
No	2,919	98
Yes	64	2
Previous bacterial STI[b] in the past 2 years		
No	2,208	84
Yes	429	16
Previous HIV test		
No	648	22
Yes	2,345	78
HIV result among MSW previously tested		
Positive test	207	9
Negative test	2,138	91

[a]Missing data: 1 for age, 3 for Country/area of origin, 15 for self-defined sexual preference, 70 for intravenous drug use, 416 for previous bacterial STI, 60 for previous HIV test

[b]Chlamydia, gonorrhoea and/or syphilis

Results

Characteristics of MSW

Of the 33,719 consultations in Dutch STI clinics involving sex workers between 2006 and 2012, 90.5 % involved FSW, 9.1 % involved MSW and 0.4 % involved transgender. Among the 3,053 consultations involving MSW, median age was 30 years (interquartile range: 24–38 years) and 50 % were from the Netherlands (Table 1). Homo- or bisexual preference, history of bacterial STI in the past two years, and injecting drug use in the past 6 months were respectively reported in 72, 16 and 2 % of consultations involving MSW. History of previous HIV testing was reported in 78 % of consultations involving MSW and a positive HIV test result was reported in 9 % of previously tested MSW.

Percentage of consultations with a positive bacterial STI or HIV test

Between 2006 and 2012, the number of consultations among MSW attending STI clinics for bacterial STI and HIV testing respectively rose from 270 to 663 and from 196 to 599.

The percentage of positive bacterial STI tests increased from 15.2 % in 2006 to 21.1 % in 2010, remained stable until 2011, and dropped to 18.3 % in 2012 (Fig. 1). The Cochran-Armitage trend test indicated an increasing trend in the percentage of positive bacterial STI ($p = 0.017$). This trend is primarily related to an increase in chlamydia (from 12.5 to 13.5 % between

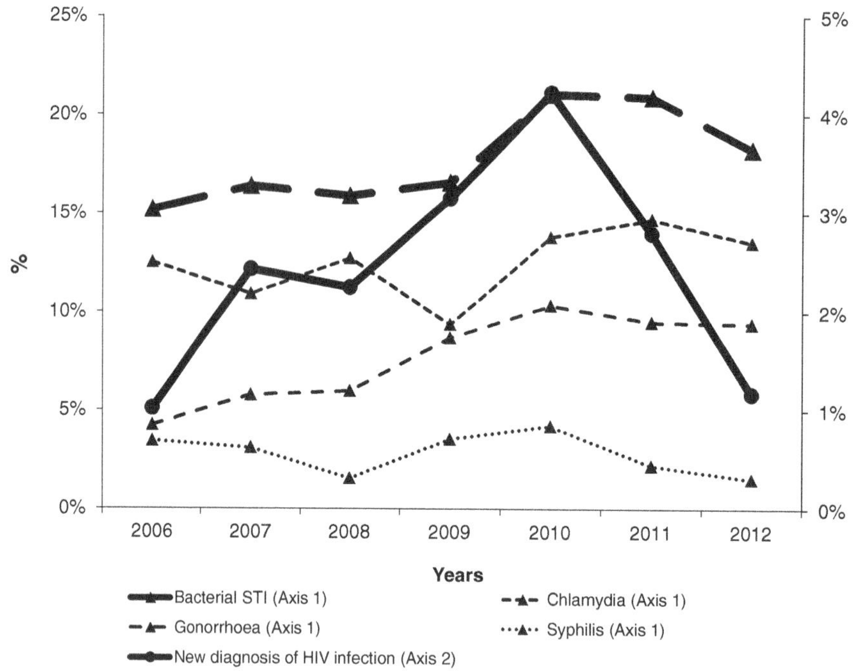

Fig. 1 Percentage of consultations with a positive bacterial STI test or positive HIV test among MSW at STI clinics in the Netherlands, 2006–2012

2006 and 2012) and gonorrhoea (from 4.3 to 9.4 %) diagnoses whereas syphilis remained stable around 3 %. Over the study period, the percentage of positive bacterial STI tests was 18.1 % (95 % CI: 16.7–19.5) among 3,016 consultations involving MSW tested for bacterial STI: one, two (mostly chlamydia and gonorrhoea) and three concurrent STI were respectively confirmed in 15.1, 2.9 and 0.2 % of these consultations. In total, chlamydia was reported in 11.3 % of the consultations, gonorrhoea in 7.5 % and syphilis in 2.6 %.

Between 2006 and 2012, the percentage of positive HIV tests was 2.5 % (95 % CI: 1.9–3.0) among 2,688 consultations involving MSW tested for HIV.

As shown in Fig. 1, the percentage of positive HIV tests over time followed the same trend as those for bacterial STI: it increased from 1.0 % in 2006 to 4.2 % in 2010 then decreased to 1.2 % in 2012, however, this trend was not significant ($p = 0.4$).

Factors associated with a positive bacterial STI test

In the multivariate analysis (Table 2), adjusted on significant variables, compared to MSW older than 35 years, younger MSW were more likely to be diagnosed with a bacterial STI: 2.3 times more for MSW between 15 and 24 years old and 1.4 times more for MSW between 25 and 34 years ($p < 0.001$). MSW who defined themselves as homo-or bisexual had a 62 % increased risk to have a positive bacterial STI test than heterosexual MSW (aRR = 1.62; 95 % CI: 1.27–2.06). Reporting a history of bacterial STI in the past two years was associated with an increased risk of 39 % of having a bacterial STI at the current consultation (aRR = 1.39; 95 % CI: 1.15–1.68). Compared to MSW with a negative HIV test at the current consultation, MSW who had a positive HIV test had a 2.7 higher risk of having a bacterial STI (aRR = 2.71; 95 % CI: 1.68–2.64) and those with a known HIV-positive status had a 2.1 higher risk (aRR = 2.11; 95 % CI: 2.15–3.43).

Factors associated with a positive HIV test

In the multivariate analysis, MSW aged between 25 and 34 years were 2.7 more likely to have a positive HIV test than MSW older than 35 years (aRR = 2.74; 95 % CI: 1.15–6.50). MSW who defined themselves to be homo- or bisexual were 24.4 times more likely to be tested positive for HIV than heterosexual MSW (aRR = 24.41; 95 % CI: 3.37–176.88). MSW who were diagnosed with a bacterial STI had a 384 % increased risk to be also diagnosed with HIV than those who tested negative for bacterial STI (aRR = 4.84; 95 % CI: 2.96–7.90). MSW who were never tested for HIV prior to their consultation were 2.6 times more likely to have a positive HIV test than those who had previously been tested negative for HIV (aRR = 2.59; 95 % CI: 1.56–4.29) (Table 3).

Discussion

Between 2006 and 2012, 18.1 % of consultations at Dutch STI clinics involving MSW resulted in a positive bacterial STI test, and 2.5 % in a positive HIV test. Factors associated with either a positive bacterial STI or

Table 2 Factors associated with at least one positive bacterial STI test for chlamydia, gonorrhoea and/or syphilis in consultations involving MSW ($N = 3,016$) at STI clinics — the Netherlands, 2006–2012

	Diagnosed[a] (*n*)	Tested[a] (*n*)	Percent	Univariate analysis			Multivariate analysis[b]		
				RR	95 % CI	*p* value*	RR adj[c]	95 % CI	*p* value*
Age group						**<.001**			**<.001**
≥ 35 years	119	1 000	11.9	ref			ref		
25–34 years	220	1 238	17.8	1.49	1.21–1.84	**<.001**	1.41	12–1.77	**0.003**
15–24 years	208	777	26.8	2.25	1.84–2.76	**<.001**	2.30	1.83–2.88	**<.001**
Country/Area of origin						0.06			
The Netherlands	245	1 478	16.6	ref					
Eastern Europe	129	618	20.9	1.26	1.04–1.52	0.02			
Other European countries	29	133	21.8	1.32	0.93–1.85	0.12			
Latin America	75	436	17.2	1.04	0.82–1.31	0.76			
Sub-Saharan Africa	4	40	10.0	0.60	0.24–1.54	0.29			
Asia	12	57	21.1	1.27	0.76–2.13	0.36			
Turkey/Morocco	32	127	25.2	1.52	1.10–2.09	0.01			
Other or unknown	21	124	16.9	1.02	0.68–1.53	0.92			
Self-defined sexual preference									
Heterosexual	87	839	10.4	ref			ref		
Homosexual/Bisexual	456	2 162	21.1	2.03	1.64–2.52	**<.001**	**1.62**	**1.27–2.06**	**<.001**
Intravenous drug user in the past 6 months									
No	524	2 886	18.2	ref					
Yes	10	62	16.1	0.89	0.50–1.58	0.69			
Previous bacterial STI[d] in the past 2 years									
No	364	2 181	16.7	ref			ref		
Yes	112	421	26.6	1.59	1.33–1.92	**<.001**	**1.39**	**1.15–1.68**	**0.001**
HIV test result						**<.001**			**<.001**
Negative test	415	2 611	15.9	ref			ref		
Positive test	37	65	56.9	3.58	2.85–4.50	**<.001**	**2.71**	**1.68–2.64**	**<.001**
Known HIV positive	76	205	37.1	2.33	1.91–2.84	**<.001**	**2.11**	**2.15–3.43**	**<.001**

*Bold numbers are significant p value <0.05

[a]509 missing data out of a total of 3,016 consultations in MSW (17 %): 1 for age, 3 for country/area of origin, 15 for self-defined sexual preference, 68 for injecting drug use, 414 for previous bacterial STI, 135 for previous HIV test

[b]Variables included in the multivariate analysis: age group, self-defined sexual preference, previous bacterial STI and HIV test result

[c]Adjusted for age group, self-defined sexual preference, previous bacterial STI and HIV test

[d]Chlamydia, gonorrhoea and/or syphilis

HIV test were young age groups and reporting homo- or bisexual preferences. HIV-positive (new diagnosis or previously known status) MSW were more likely to be diagnosed with a bacterial STI, and those who had never been tested for HIV prior to their consultation were at higher risk for having a positive HIV test than those who previously tested negative.

Limited studies have examined STI and associated risk factors among MSW in the Netherlands. Our results are consistent with other studies performed in Europe among MSW [5, 6, 9] and confirm that MSW are an important population to target for STI control strategies. However, results have to be interpreted and compared with other studies with caution because our data did not allow identification of repeated consultations for a defined individual.

In our study, median age of MSW was 29 years and 33 % were older than 35 years, which is consistent with a study conducted among MSW attendees in STI clinics in the United Kingdom in 2011 [16]. Other studies conducted before 2004 [3, 6, 10] report a lower median age (between 25 and 27). These differences could be explained by changes in MSW characteristics over time. Mean age of MSW visiting STI clinics could have increased over time because MSW could be older or older MSW could visit more often STI clinic.

Our results indicate that the percentage of consultations with either a positive STI or HIV test is significantly

Table 3 Factors associated with a positive HIV test in consultations involving MSW ($N = 2,688$) at STI clinics —the Netherlands, 2006–2012

	Diagnosed[a] (n)	Tested[a] (n)	Percent	Univariate analysis			Multivariate analysis[b]		
				RR	95 % CI	p value*	RR adj[c]	95 % CI	p value*
Age group						**<0.001**			**<0.001**
≥ 35 years	6	859	0.7	ref			ref		
25–34 years	29	1 087	2.7	3.82	1.59–9.16	**0.003**	2.74	1.15–6.50	**0.02**
15–24 years	31	742	4.2	5.98	2.51–14.26	**<0.001**	2.43	0.99–5.92	0.05
Country/Area of origin						0.07			
The Netherlands	24	1 297	1.9	ref					
Eastern Europe	18	587	3.1	1.66	0.91–3.03	0.10			
Other European countries	6	118	5.1	2.75	1.14–6.59	0.02			
Latin America	13	387	3.4	1.82	0.93–3.53	0.08			
Sub-Saharan Africa	2	37	5.4	2.92	0.72–11.91	0.14			
Asia	0	46	0.0	–					
Turkey/Morocco	3	116	2.6	1.40	0.43–4.57	0.58			
Other or unknown	0	97	0.0	–					
Self-defined sexual preference									
Heterosexual	1	793	0.1	ref			ref		
Homosexual/Bisexual	64	1 881	3.4	26.98	3.75–194.21	**<0.001**	24.41	3.37–176.88	**0.002**
Intravenous drug user in the past 6 months									
No	66	2 585	2.6						
Yes	0	52	0.0						
Previous bacterial STI[d] in the past 2 years									
No	51	1 999	2.6	ref					
Yes	12	344	3.5	1.37	0.74–2.54	0.32			
Co-infection with a bacterial STI									
No	28	2 224	1.3	ref			ref		
Yes	37	452	8.2	6.50	4.02–10.51	**<0.001**	4.84	2.96–7.90	**<0.001**
Previous HIV test result									
Negative test	42	2 060	2.0	ref			ref		
No test	21	576	3.6	1.79	1.07–2.99	**0.03**	2.59	1.56–4.29	**<0.001**

*Bold numbers are significant p value <0.05
[a]77 missing data out of a total of 2688 consultations in MSW (3 %): 3 for country/area of origin, 14 for self- defined sexual preference, 51 for injecting drug use, 345 for previous bacterial STI, 12 for STI co-infection, 52 for previous HIV test
[b]Variables included in the multivariate analysis: age group, self- defined sexual preference, co-infection with bacterial STI and previous HIV test result
[c]Adjusted for age group, self- defined sexual preference, co-infection with bacterial STI and previous HIV test result
[d]Chlamydia, gonorrhoea and/or syphilis

higher among younger MSW than among those older than 35 years. In similar studies conducted before 2002 [3, 6, 10], age was not significantly associated with a high risk of STI. Use of safer sexual practices among older MSW might explain these discrepancies over time.

The percentages of consultations with bacterial STI and HIV diagnosis were higher among MSW who defined themselves as homo- or bisexual than among heterosexual. The same result is found among all consultations in STI clinics in the Netherlands between heterosexual males and MSM [26]. Moreover, the percentage of consultations with a positive bacterial STI or HIV test among young MSW who defined themselves as homo- or bisexual (27 and 4 %, respectively for bacterial STI and HIV) is higher than the prevalence reported in 2012 among young MSM (20 %, $p = 0.01$ and 1 %, $p = 0.01$) who visited an STI clinic [26]. In addition, an increased risk for both STI and HIV infection associated with more frequent unsafe sexual practices have also been reported among MSM compared to heterosexuals [12–14], as well as a higher HIV seroprevalence among MSM sex workers [5, 27].

We found a high percentage of consultations with co-infections: HIV seropositivity (newly diagnosed or previously known status) was highly associated with bacterial STI. This result is also consistent with previous studies [12, 28].

In another study implemented in the Netherlands among FSW between 2002 and 2005, HIV prevalence was found to be 1.5 %. With a percentage of positive HIV tests of 2.5 %, our study suggest that MSW are more at risk for HIV than FSW [7].

Our study has several limitations. Firstly, the database does not allow identification of repeated consultations for a defined person. Having repetitive consultations could be an indicator of higher risk of infection if MSW attend the clinic because of persistent risk behaviour or if having symptoms. In a UK study implemented in STI clinics in 2011 [16], MSW had a higher average number of visits than other male attendees and were more likely to be diagnosed with HIV, chlamydia or gonorrhoea and experience reinfections. Moreover, because identification of repeated consultations was not possible, we were not able to calculate incidence which is a more relevant and accurate indicator than the percentage of consultation with positive bacterial or HIV tests.

Secondly, STI clinic used different variable laboratory testing methods and that may have contributed to differences in the detection of STI diagnosis.

Another limitation is that MSW attending STI clinics may not be representative of the overall MSW population in the Netherlands. In addition to STI clinics, STI healthcare in the Netherlands is also provided by general practitioners, HIV treatment centres, and specialised hospital facilities [29]. Furthermore, the most marginalised MSW, those performing illegal business or with an illegal status, may not attend STI clinics or other healthcare providers. Therefore, factors associated with bacterial STI or HIV infection in our study may not be generalizable.

Finally, other factors known to be associated with a higher risk for STI among sex workers, such as sexual practices, condom use, recruitment area, sexual techniques with clients, number of partners, steady or casual partners, etc., were not available in the surveillance database therefore we were not able to investigate more in depth the risk factors associated with both bacterial STI and HIV infection among MSW. Sexual practices and condom use are recorded by some STI clinics but data are not recorded in the national database, which could be improved in the future to allow more in-depth researches.

Conclusion

In conclusion, the high percentage of MSW consultations at Dutch STI clinics with either a positive bacterial STI or HIV test confirms that MSW represent a high risk group for STI infections. MSW, particularly those who have sex with men, are at high risk of contracting STI including HIV and therefore may transmit these infections to their clients or partners. Prevention and intervention activities should particularly target MSW who engage in homo- or bisexual intercourse to stimulate HIV testing, increase early STI diagnoses, ensure early treatment, and therefore interrupt further transmission. In this hard-to-reach population, the Internet could be a useful tool to enhance reach and implementation of actions. Additional studies are needed to investigate other risk factors, identify opportunities for interventions, target MSW populations who do not visit STI clinics and evaluate the impact of interventions measures in this group.

Abbreviations

CI: confident interval; ECDC: European Centre for Disease Prevention and Control; EPIET: European Programme for Intervention Epidemiology Training; HIV: human immunodeficiency virus; MSW: male sex worker; RR: risk ratio; RIVM: National Institute for Public Health and the Environment; STI: sexually transmitted infections; SW: sex worker.

Competing interests

The authors declared that they have no competing interests.

Authors' contributions

FN designed the study, performed the statistical analysis and wrote the manuscript. KFDH and vVMG were involved in the design of the study, supervised the study and revised the manuscript. vRMS and vLAP participated in the design of the study and revised the manuscript. vdSMAB revised the manuscript. All authors were involved in the final manuscript, have commented and approved the final paper.

Acknowledgements

We would like to thank all the STI clinics and Municipal Health Services for their continuing collaboration in collecting data. We would especially like to express our gratitude to Marianne Craanen, Mariska van Huissteden, Sjaak van der Kolk, and Annelies van Dijk from the Prostitutie en Gezondheidscentrum 292 in Amsterdam. We gratefully acknowledge Ioannis Karagiannis (Robert Koch Institut, EPIET) and Yvan Hutin (European Centre for Disease Control, EPIET) for reviewing the manuscript.

Funding

This research received no specific grant from any funding agency in the public, commercial or not-for-profit sectors.

Author details

[1]Epidemiology and Surveillance Unit, Centre for Infectious Diseases Control, National Institute for Public Health and the Environment (RIVM), P.O. Box 1, 3720 BA Bilthoven, The Netherlands. [2]European Programme for Intervention Epidemiology Training (EPIET), European Centre for Disease Prevention and Control (ECDC), Stockholm, Sweden. [3]Public Health Service Twente, Enschede, The Netherlands. [4]Public Health Service Amsterdam, Amsterdam, The Netherlands. [5]Julius Centre for Health Sciences and Primary Care, University Medical Centre Utrecht, Utrecht, The Netherlands.

References

1. Ghys PD, Jenkins C, Pisani E. HIV surveillance among female sex workers. AIDS. 2001;15 Suppl 3:S33–40.
2. Spice W. Management of sex workers and other high-risk groups. Occup Med (Lond). 2007;57(5):322–8.

3. Estcourt CS, Marks C, Rohrsheim R, Johnson AM, Donovan B, Mindel A. HIV, sexually transmitted infections, and risk behaviours in male commercial sex workers in Sydney. Sex Transm Infect. 2000;76(4):294–8.
4. TAMPEP. Sex work in Europe. A mapping of the prostitution scene in 25 European countries; 2009. Retrieved from http://tampep.eu/documents/TAMPEP%202009%20European%20Mapping%20Report.pdf. Accessed 11 Nov 2015.
5. Belza MJ. Risk of HIV infection among male sex workers in Spain. Sex Transm Infect. 2005;81(1):85–8.
6. Leuridan E, Wouters K, Stalpaert M, Van Damme P. Male sex workers in Antwerp, Belgium: a descriptive study. Int J STD AIDS. 2005;16(11):744–8.
7. Eurohiv. HIV/AIDS surveillance in Europe, Mid-year report 2006 (No. 74). Saint-Maurice: Institut de Veille Sanitaire; 2006.
8. Ballester R, Salmeron P, Gil MD, Gimenez C. Sexual behaviors in male sex workers in Spain: modulating factors. J Health Psychol. 2014;19(2):207–17.
9. Ballester R, Salmeron P, Gil MD, Gomez S. Sexual risk behaviors for HIV infection in Spanish male sex workers: differences according to educational level, country of origin and sexual orientation. AIDS Behav. 2012;16(4):960–8.
10. Belza MJ, Llacer A, Mora R, Morales M, Castilla J, de la Fuente L. Sociodemographic characteristics and HIV risk behaviour patterns of male sex workers in Madrid, Spain. AIDS Care. 2001;13(5):677–82.
11. Dukers NH, Fennema HS, van der Snoek EM, Krol A, Geskus RB, Pospiech M, et al. HIV incidence and HIV testing behavior in men who have sex with men: using three incidence sources, The Netherlands, 1984–2005. AIDS. 2007;21(4):491–9.
12. Rieg G, Lewis RJ, Miller LG, Witt MD, Guerrero M, Daar ES. Asymptomatic sexually transmitted infections in HIV-infected men who have sex with men: prevalence, incidence, predictors, and screening strategies. AIDS Patient Care STDS. 2008;22(12):947–54.
13. van Kesteren NM, Hospers HJ, Kok G, van Empelen P. Sexuality and sexual risk behavior in HIV-positive men who have sex with men. Qual Health Res. 2005;15(2):145–68.
14. van Veen MG, Koedijk FD, van der Sande MA. STD coinfections in The Netherlands: specific sexual networks at highest risk. Sex Transm Dis. 2010;37(7):416–22.
15. Mindel A, Estcourt C. Sexual health education for male sex workers. Lancet. 2001;357(9263):1148.
16. Mc Grath-Lone L, Marsh K, Hughes G, Ward H. The sexual health of male sex workers in England: analysis of cross-sectional data from genitourinary medicine clinics. Sex Transm Infect. 2014;90(1):38–40.
17. Brussa L. European network for AIDS & STD prevention among migrant prostitutes, final report No. 6 June 2002-June 2004. Amsterdam: TAMPEP International Foundation; 2004.
18. van Kesteren NM, Hospers HJ, Kok G. Sexual risk behavior among HIV-positive men who have sex with men: a literature review. Patient Educ Couns. 2007;65(1):5–20.
19. Bom RJ, van der Helm JJ, Schim van der Loeff MF, van Rooijen MS, Heijman T, Matser A, et al. Distinct transmission networks of Chlamydia trachomatis in men who have sex with men and heterosexual adults in Amsterdam, The Netherlands. PLoS One. 2013;8(1):e53869.
20. Heymans R, A Matser A, Bruisten SM, Heijman T, Geskus RB, Speksnijder AG, et al. Distinct Neisseria gonorrhoeae transmission networks among men who have sex with men in Amsterdam, The Netherlands. J Infect Dis. 2012;206(4):596–605.
21. van Veen MG, Gotz HM, van Leeuwen PA, Prins M, van de Laar MJ. HIV and sexual risk behavior among commercial sex workers in the Netherlands. Arch Sex Behav. 2010;39(3):714–23.
22. Dukers-Muijrers NH, Niekamp AM, Vergoossen MM, Hoebe CJ. Effectiveness of an opting-out strategy for HIV testing: evaluation of 4 years of standard HIV testing in a STI clinic. Sex Transm Infect. 2009;85(3):226–30.
23. Heijman RL, Stolte IG, Thiesbrummel HF, van Leent E, Coutinho RA, Fennema JS, et al. Opting out increases HIV testing in a large sexually transmitted infections outpatient clinic. Sex Transm Infect. 2009;85(4):249–55.
24. Infectieziektebestrijding LCIR-C. LCI-draaiboek Het soaconsult bij prostituees. 2008.
25. CCMO: Centrale Commisie Mensgebonden Onderzoek [English translation: Central Comitee Human Research]; 2015. http://www.ccmo.nl/nl/uw-onderzoek-wmo-plichtig-of-niet. Accessed 11 Nov 2015.
26. Soetens LC, Koedijk FDH, van den Broek VF, Vriend HJ, Op de Coul ELM, van Aar F, et al. Sexually transmitted infections, including HIV, in the Netherlands in 2012. 2013.
27. Mimiaga MJ, Reisner SL, Tinsley JP, Mayer KH, Safren SA. Street workers and internet escorts: contextual and psychosocial factors surrounding HIV risk behavior among men who engage in sex work with other men. J Urban Health. 2009;86(1):54–66.
28. Zhang X, Wang C, Hengwei W, Li X, Li D, Ruan Y, et al. Risk factors of HIV infection and prevalence of co-infections among men who have sex with men in Beijing, China. AIDS. 2007;21 Suppl 8:S53–57.
29. van den Broek IV, Verheij RA, van Dijk CE, Koedijk FD, van der Sande MA, van Bergen JE. Trends in sexually transmitted infections in the Netherlands, combining surveillance data from general practices and sexually transmitted infection centers. BMC Fam Pract. 2010;11:39.

2

Repeat *Chlamydia trachomatis* testing among heterosexual STI outpatient clinic visitors in the Netherlands

Maartje Visser[1*], Fleur van Aar[1], Femke D. H. Koedijk[2], Carolina J. G. Kampman[2] and Janneke C. M. Heijne[1]

Abstract

Background: Chlamydia infections are common in both men and women, are often asymptomatic and can cause serious complications. Repeat testing in high-risk groups is therefore indicated. In the Netherlands, guidelines on repeat chlamydia testing differ between testing facilities, and knowledge on repeat testing behaviour is limited. Here, we analyse the current repeat testing behaviour of heterosexual STI clinic visitors, and aim to identify groups for which repeat testing advice could be advantageous.

Methods: Longitudinal surveillance data from all Dutch STI outpatient clinics were used, which included all STI clinic consultations carried out among heterosexual men and women between June 2014 and December 2015. Repeat testing was defined as returning to the same STI clinic between 35 days and 12 months after initial consultation. We calculated chlamydia positivity at repeat test stratified by initial test result and time between consultations. Logistic regression analyses were used to identify predictors of repeat testing, and predictors of having a chlamydia positive repeat test.

Results: In total, 140,486 consultations in 75,487 women and 46,286 men were available for analyses. Overall, 15.4% of women and 11.1% of men returned to the STI clinic within the study period. Highest chlamydia positivity at repeat test was seen 3–5 months after initial positive test. Among both women and men, repeat testing was associated with non-Western ethnicity, having had more than two sex partners in the past 6 months, reporting STI symptoms, having a history of STI, and having a chlamydia positive initial test. Among repeat testers, chlamydia positive repeat test was most strongly associated with younger age, followed by a chlamydia positive initial test.

Conclusions: Repeat testing most often resulted in a positive test result among young heterosexuals (<25) and heterosexuals of any age with a chlamydia infection at the initial consultation. Further efforts are needed to determine optimal repeat testing strategies.

Keywords: Chlamydia trachomatis, Sexually transmitted infections, Repeat testing, STI clinic, Public health, The Netherlands

* Correspondence: maartje.visser@rivm.nl
[1]National Institute for Public Health and the Environment, P.O. Box 1, 3720, BA, Bilthoven, the Netherlands
Full list of author information is available at the end of the article

Background

Chlamydia trachomatis (chlamydia) is the most frequently reported bacterial sexually transmitted infection (STI) among heterosexuals [1]. Chlamydia reinfections are also common, with proportions of reinfection of up to 32% in women [2], and 18.3% in men [3]. Chlamydia infections are associated with increased risk of complications such as pelvic inflammatory disease (PID) [4–6]. Repeat testing for chlamydia could identify chlamydia infections at an early stage of infection, thereby possibly reducing the individual risk of complications, and might lead to reduced transmission at the population level [4–6]. Therefore, several countries have established STI care guidelines on repeat testing for heterosexuals [7–10].

Repeat testing guidelines differ between countries with regard to the groups that are targeted, and the advised timing of the repeat test. A mathematical modelling study estimated the risk of a repeat chlamydia infection to be highest 2–5 months after treatment, suggesting a possible window for repeat testing in case of an initial positive test [11]. This is in line with the recommended test interval in most countries for repeat testing after chlamydia infection: the US centre for disease control and prevention recommends men and women to return preferably 3 months after treatment, and at least within 12 months [7]. In Australia, repeat testing at 3 months is recommended [8], and European and UK guidelines recommend repeat testing 3–6 months after treatment for both men and women aged <25 years [9, 10]. Repeat testing after a negative chlamydia test is not explicitly recommended, but annual chlamydia screening is advised in the European and US guidelines for all sexually active men and women aged <25, or women aged <25, respectively [7, 9].

In the Netherlands, guidelines on repeat testing are limited. For men who have sex with men, advice is given to test for STI every 6 or 3 months, depending on risk behaviour [12]. For heterosexuals, guidelines on repeat testing are only established for initial chlamydia positive persons, and differ between testing facilities. In general practitioner guidelines, it is advised to retest patients within 12 months after treatment of an initial infection [13]. STI clinic guidelines recommend repeat testing 4–6 months after treatment [12]. However, while the repeat testing behaviour of MSM has been studied in the past [14, 15], it is not well known to what extend the guidelines for heterosexuals are currently being adhered to. In addition, knowledge on repeat testing among heterosexual STI clinic visitors with an initial negative chlamydia test is limited. Besides initial chlamydia positive attendees, the initial negative attendees are also of interest because Dutch STI clinics are restricted to people at increased risk of STI. Initial negative visitors could therefore still be a potential target group for repeat testing.

Two Dutch studies assessed the uptake of repeat testing after chlamydia infection at STI clinics, with differing results. One study found that 33.4% of all chlamydia positive individuals returned for a repeat test 3–12 months after treatment [16], whereas the other study found 9.2% repeat testing at 5–8 months after treatment among young heterosexuals [17]. However, these studies used regional STI clinic data only, and did not assess repeat testing behaviour and the chlamydia prevalence at repeat consultation among visitors with an initial chlamydia negative test result.

To inform further specification of the Dutch guidelines, and to be able to evaluate them properly in the future, more insight is needed into current chlamydia repeat testing behaviour among Dutch heterosexual STI clinic visitors. In this study, we aimed to describe current repeat testing behaviour and to identify groups for which repeat testing advice could be advantageous. We do this by determining repeat testing uptake and by identifying predictors of repeat testing and predictors of chlamydia positivity at repeat test among heterosexual STI clinic visitors with both an initial negative or an initial positive chlamydia test.

Methods

Study design

This study used Dutch STI clinic surveillance data, containing all consultations from all STI outpatient clinics in the Netherlands. The STI clinic surveillance data contains information on personal characteristics, sexual behaviour, and STI diagnoses of each patient at each consultation. As STI testing at Dutch STI clinics is publicly funded, it is restricted to certain target groups who are considered at high risk for STI based on positivity rates obtained from the STI clinic surveillance data (further referred to as high risk populations) [18]. Heterosexual men and women aged 24 years or younger and MSM are considered at high risk for STI regardless behavioural or other risk factors. Heterosexual men and women aged 25 years and older are allowed to test at the clinics if they report at least one of the following factors: having STI symptoms, being notified by an infected partner, originating from or having a partner from a non-Western area, being a commercial sex worker, having had an STI in the past year, being a victim of sexual violence, or for women having an MSM partner [18].

For this study, we used data from June 1st 2014 to December 31st 2015, as in June 2014 a personal identification number was added to data collection, which enabled linkage of consultations performed on the same individuals at the same STI clinic. We selected consultations of heterosexual men and women who had at least one chlamydia test between June 2014 and December 2015. Individuals who reported having had sex with only the opposite gender in the past 6 months were defined as heterosexuals in this study. Thereby this term does not necessarily reflect the sexual identity of the individual, but rather their self-reported behaviour. Consultations where no chlamydia test was recorded, or that had missing information on chlamydia diagnosis were excluded. STI tests that were not performed at STI clinics, but at other health care settings such as general practitioners or hospitals could not be included, as systematically collected data are not available for these facilities.

The main outcome of interest was repeat testing, which was defined as returning to the STI clinic for a second consultation within 12 months after the initial visit. Individuals were defined as single testers if they had only one STI clinic visit during the study period, or if they returned to the STI clinic after more than 12 months from the initial visit. Although a test of cure (TOC) is generally not recommended in the Netherlands, consultations that were performed within 35 days after the initial consultation were deleted to minimise the risk that possible TOCs were included. Also, the 35 day cut off limits the chance of a repeat test being positive due to residual bacterial material from an already treated chlamydia infection at the initial consultation [19]. Persons with their first consultation within 35 days of the end of the study period (December 31st 2015) were excluded, as they had no opportunity for a repeat test. All analyses were performed using the first two consultations of each individual. Chlamydia positivity was defined as a diagnosed chlamydia infection at any location (urogenital, anorectal, or oral). Chlamydia diagnoses were based on nucleic acid amplification test (NAAT).

Statistical analyses

All analyses were performed for men and women separately because of differences in chlamydia positivity rates and STI clinic visiting behaviour between women and men [18]. First, descriptive analyses were performed. We calculated the time between consecutive consultations of each individual, stratified by the initial test result. We also calculated chlamydia positivity of repeat tests, stratified by time between initial test and repeat test.

Second, we identified predictors of repeat testing using logistic regression analysis, comparing single testers with repeat testers. For this analysis, characteristics from the initial consultation were used, because the initial consultation is the moment when repeat testing advice based on person characteristics can be given. Age was included in three categories; 13–19, 20–24, and 25+, as in the Netherlands persons aged <20 have highest chlamydia positivity rates at STI clinics, and for persons aged >24 different triaging guidelines are in place [18]. Ethnicity was based on country of birth of both the participant and its parents, according to the definitions of Statistics Netherlands [20]. Persons from Western Europe, Northern America, and Australia were considered of Western non-Dutch ethnicity. All other ethnicities were grouped as non-Western, which is the same categorisation as used in triage at the STI clinics. An uncertainty analysis was performed to evaluate whether categorisation of ethnicity into more subgroups would provide different results. All other characteristics were self-reported, except for the chlamydia diagnoses. Some variables could not be included in the logistic regression due to small group sizes, and were only included in descriptive analyses (region of the STI clinic, being HIV positive, being (client of) commercial sex worker, and being a swinger).

Variables were included in multivariable analysis when significant in univariable analysis ($P < 0.1$). If a variable had more than 5% missing values, missings were included in the analysis as a separate category to reduce loss of data. A complete case analysis was performed as uncertainty analysis to evaluate robustness of the model for missing data. The multivariable model was made using backward elimination, using a significance level of 0.05. Because a chlamydia infection at the initial consultation could influence the identified predictors of repeat testing (these people are more likely to receive repeat testing advice), effect modification by chlamydia infection at initial consultation was assessed by adding interaction terms and stratifying analyses. Furthermore, since only 1.5 years of data was available, some people might have had limited opportunity to return for a repeat test within the timeframe of this study. To identify the consequences of this, uncertainty analyses were performed in which only persons with a minimum of 12 months of follow-up time were included.

Last, to assess predictors of having a chlamydia positive repeat test within 1 year after initial consultation, logistic regression analysis was done among the groups of repeat testers. Again, characteristics from the initial consultation and the same methods were used. However, missings were in this model not included as a separate category, as the number of individuals in these groups would become too small for multivariable analysis. The same variables were used as in the previous analysis, with the addition of time between first and repeat test, categorised in ≤6 months and >6 months. An uncertainty analysis was performed using characteristics from the consultation of the repeat test, instead of characteristics from the initial consultation. All analyses were performed using Stata v. 14 (StataCorp, College Station, TX).

Results

Study population

Between June 2014 and December 2015, 152,358 consultations were carried out at the STI clinics in the

Netherlands among 127,650 heterosexual men and women. We excluded 324 consultations because there was missing chlamydia data or no chlamydia test was registered, and 563 consultations because they took place within 35 days of the previous consultation. Five thousand six hundred sixty-five persons were excluded because they did not have more than 35 days of follow-up time. Last, 5320 consultations were excluded because they were performed after the second consultation, leaving 140,486 consultations in 75,487 women and 46,286 men available for analysis. Characteristics at initial consultation stratified for women and men are shown in Additional file 1: Table S1.

Timing and predictors of repeat testing

In total, 15.4% of women and 11.1% of men returned for at least one test within 1 year after the initial consultation (repeat testers), an overall repeat testing rate of 13.7% (Table 1). For STI clinic visitors with an initial chlamydia positive test, 21.1% returned for a repeat test and among visitors with an initial negative test, 12.5% returned for a repeat test. In the uncertainty analysis including only persons with a minimum of 12 months of follow-up time, the overall repeat testing increased to 22.7% among women and 16.7% among men. The median time between first test and repeat test was similar for women (171 days) and men (170 days). Both women and men with a positive initial test returned to the STI clinic for testing sooner compared to individuals with a negative initial test (Additional file 2: Figure S1).

The strongest predictors of repeat testing for men and women were having had more than four sex partners in the past 6 months (adjusted odds ratio [aOR] 2.27 for women and aOR 2.80 for men), and a chlamydia infection at initial consultation (aOR 2.00 for women and aOR 1.85 for men) (Tables 2 and 3). Furthermore, for women, variables predictive for repeat testing were Non-Western ethnicity, use of a condom at last sexual contact, reporting STI symptoms, and having had an STI in the past year. A slightly lower odds of repeat testing was observed for having a high education level, being of western non-Dutch ethnicity, and having received partner notification. Among men, results were comparable except for condom use and partner notification at the initial consultation, which were not associated with repeat testing. In addition, among women, age was not a predictor of repeat testing, but men aged 25 years and older were less likely to be repeat testers compared to 13 to 19 year olds.

Table 1 Testing characteristics of heterosexuals at Dutch STI clinics between June 2014 and December 2015

	Women	Men
Total number of consultations	88,409	52,077
Individuals with N consultations (%)		
1	62,565 (82.9)	40,495 (87.5)
2	12,922 (17.1)	5791 (12.5)
Total number of individuals	75,487	46,286
Individuals with a repeat test within 12 months (overall) (%)	11,612 (15.4)	5157 (11.1)
Repeat testers among initial CT negatives (%)	9136/64,842 (14.1)	3910/39,283 (10.0)
Repeat testers among initial CT positives (%)	2476/10,645 (23.3)	1247/7003 (17.8)
Median time between initial test and repeat test (overall), days (IQR)	171 (111–243)	170 (106–245)
After initial negative test	178 (116–249)	176 (112–252)
After initial positive test	147 (90–218)	147 (90–221)

IQR interquartile range, *CT* Chlamydia

Chlamydia infection at initial consultation was an effect modifier for repeat testing among both women and men. However, none of the directions of effect changed when analyses were stratified (Additional file 3: Table S2). Among both women and men, the effect of number of sex partners and history of STI was slightly weaker among initial chlamydia positives. Among men, the effect of age became stronger among initial chlamydia positives. The uncertainty analysis including persons with a minimum of 12 months of follow-up time, showed that predictors of repeat testing in the logistic regression analysis hardly changed. Only among women, the analysis showed that older women (>25) were less often repeat testers (Additional file 4: Table S3). Uncertainty analyses using complete cases only showed very little differences in the found predictors of repeat testing (compared to the main analyses), indicating that the analyses were also robust to missing values (Additional file 5: Table S4). Analyses including more subgroups for ethnicity did not change the results, and did not reveal a specific non-Western ethnicity group as predictor of repeat testing among women. Among men, Suriname, the Dutch Antilles and Sub-Saharan Africa were associated with more repeat testing in univariable analysis, but numbers in the different subgroups were too low to perform multivariable analysis (Additional file 6: Table S5).

Repeat test positivity and predictors of positive repeat tests

At repeat test, 13.4% of women and 16.7% of men tested positive for chlamydia (compared to 14.1% and 15.1% at initial test). Both for women (Fig. 1a) and men (Fig. 1b), chlamydia positivity at repeat test was higher among individuals with a positive initial test compared to individuals with an initial negative test. Especially between 3 and 5 months after the initial test a clear difference can be seen between people with an initial positive and negative test, as positivity

Table 2 Predictors of repeat testing among heterosexual women at initial consultation, June 2014 to December 2015

	Single testers		Repeat testers		Crude		Adjusted	
	n	%	n	%	OR	95% CI	OR	95% CI
Total	63,875	84.6	11,612	15.4				
Age								
13–19	8543	13.4	1559	13.4	1	–	–	–
20–24	36,471	57.1	6623	57.0	0.99	(0.94–1.05)	–	–
25+	18,861	29.5	3430	29.5	1.00	(0.93–1.06)	–	–
Education level[a]								
Low/medium	17,554	27.5	3201	27.6	1	–	1	–
High	37,118	58.1	5422	46.7	0.80	(0.76–0.84)	0.88	(0.84–0.93)
Ethnicity								
Dutch	47,441	74.4	7906	68.2	1	–	1	–
Western non-Dutch	3718	5.8	613	5.3	0.99	(0.91–1.08)	0.91	(0.83–1.00)
Non-Western	12,650	19.8	3081	26.6	1.46	(1.40–1.53)	1.31	(1.26–1.39)
Number of sex partners in past 6 months								
0–1	21,107	33.7	2461	22.3	1	–	1	–
2–3	29,046	46.4	5162	46.7	1.52	(1.45–1.60)	1.56	(1.48–1.64)
4+	12,471	19.9	3421	31.0	2.35	(2.22–2.49)	2.27	(2.14–2.41)
Condom use at last sexual contact								
No	48,663	78.5	8214	72.6	1	–	1	–
Yes	13,294	21.5	3097	27.4	1.38	(1.32–1.44)	1.10	(1.04–1.15)
Received partner notification								
No	53,816	84.7	9953	86.1	1	–	1	–
Yes	9749	15.3	1610	13.9	0.89	(0.84–0.95)	0.80	(0.75–0.85)
Reported STI symptoms								
No	41,179	64.9	7253	62.8	1	–	1	–
Yes	22,257	35.1	4287	37.2	1.09	(1.05–1.14)	1.08	(1.03–1.12)
History of STI (CT/GO/SY)[a,b]								
No	52,597	82.4	9215	79.4	1	–	1	–
Yes	5072	7.9	1672	14.4	1.88	(1.77–2.00)	1.86	(1.74–1.98)
Chlamydia infection								
No	55,706	87.2	9136	78.7	1	–	1	–
Yes	8169	12.8	2476	21.3	1.85	(1.76–1.94)	2.00	(1.89–2.11)

Abbreviations: *CT* chlamydia, *GO* gonorrhoea, *SY* syphilis
[a]Missing values included in the analysis as a separate category (ORs not shown)
[b]In 2014, history of STI was asked regarding the past 2 years. In 2015 this changed to the past year only

rates of over 25% were found in repeat tests after an initial positive test, while chlamydia positivity of repeat tests after an initial negative test remained constant over time.

Among the repeat testers, being aged >25 years greatly reduced the odds of a chlamydia positive repeat test among both women and men (aOR 0.44 and aOR 0.50, respectively) (Table 4). Furthermore, among women, a chlamydia infection at initial consultation was associated with higher risk for repeat infection, whereas condom use at last sexual contact showed a protective effect. Among men, significant interaction was found between reporting STI symptoms and chlamydia diagnosis; hence, a combined variable was made. For men, having both a chlamydia infection and reporting STI symptoms at initial consultation was associated with increased risk of repeat test positivity (aOR 2.30). Table 5 shows a side by side comparison of predictors of repeat testing and repeat test positivity.

Table 3 Predictors of repeat testing among heterosexual men at initial consultation, June 2014 to December 2015

	Single testers		Repeat testers					
					Crude		Adjusted	
	n	%	n	%	OR	95% CI	OR	95% CI
Total	41,129	88.9	5157	11.1				
Age								
13–19	2596	6.3	299	5.8	1	–	1	–
20–24	19,139	46.5	2582	50.1	1.17	(1.03–1.33)	1.08	(0.94–1.23)
25+	19,394	47.2	2276	44.1	1.02	(0.90–1.16)	0.82	(0.72–0.93)
Education level[a,c]								
Low	12,971	31.5	1516	29.4	1	–	1	–
High	22,363	54.4	2376	46.1	0.91	(0.85–0.97)	0.98	(0.91–1.06)
Ethnicity								
Dutch	26,964	65.6	3006	58.3	1	–	1	–
Western non-Dutch	2524	6.1	322	6.3	1.14	(1.01–1.29)	1.06	(0.93–1.20)
Non-Western	11,602	28.2	1828	35.4	1.41	(1.33–1.50)	1.37	(1.28–1.46)
Number of sex partners in past 6 months								
0–1	8559	21.0	529	10.4	1	–	1	–
2–3	16,191	39.7	1783	34.9	1.78	(1.61–1.97)	1.75	(1.58–1.94)
4+	16,023	39.3	2801	54.8	2.83	(2.57–3.12)	2.80	(2.54–3.09)
Condom use at last sexual contact								
No	29,257	73.8	3720	74.5	1	–	–	–
Yes	10,376	26.2	1273	25.5	0.96	(0.90–1.03)	–	–
Received partner notification								
No	30,763	75.2	3917	76.2	1	–	–	–
Yes	10,155	24.8	1223	23.8	0.95	(0.88–1.01)	–	–
Reported STI symptoms								
No	26,968	65.9	3135	61.1	1	–	1	–
Yes	13,939	34.1	1995	38.9	1.23	(1.16–1.31)	1.10	(1.03–1.17)
History of STI (CT/GO/SY)[a,b]								
No	34,088	82.9	4103	79.6	1	–	1	–
Yes	2610	6.4	721	14.0	2.30	(2.10–2.51)	2.08	(1.90–2.28)
Chlamydia infection								
No	35,373	86.0	3910	75.8	1	–	1	–
Yes	5756	14.0	1247	24.2	1.96	(1.83–2.10)	1.85	(1.72–1.99)

Abbreviations: *CT* chlamydia, *GO* gonorrhoea, *SY* syphilis
[a]Missing values included in the analysis as a separate category (ORs not shown)
[b]In 2014, history of STI was asked regarding the past 2 years. In 2015 this changed to the past year only
[c]Included in the multivariable model due to significance of the 'missing values' category (not shown)

The uncertainty analyses using characteristics from the consultation of the repeat test instead of the initial consultation showed similar results, but receiving partner notification and reporting symptoms also remained in the model, and became the strongest determinants for a positive repeat test (Additional file 7: Table S6). Uncertainty analyses for predictors of having a positive repeat test with persons with a minimum of 12 months follow-up time were not possible due to small sample size.

Discussion

Overall, 15% of heterosexual women and 11% of heterosexual men visiting Dutch STI clinics between June 2014 and December 2015 returned to the same clinic for repeat testing within the study period. The strongest predictors of repeat testing were having had more than four sex partners in the past 6 months and having a chlamydia infection at the initial consultation. Reinfection rates were highest among initial chlamydia positives

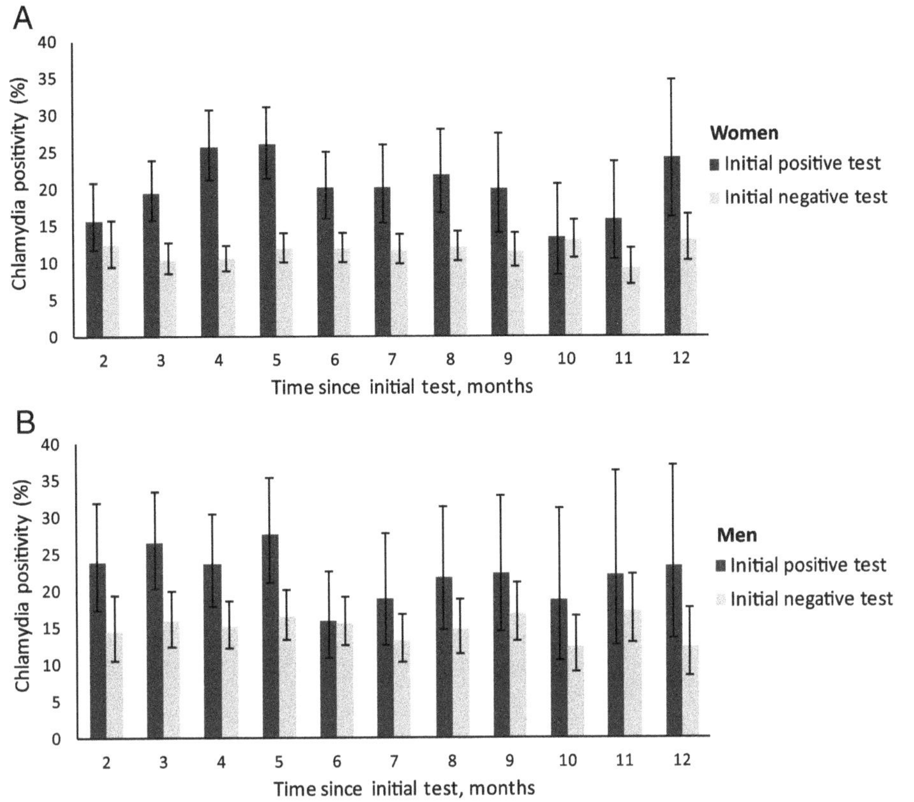

Fig. 1 Chlamydia positivity at repeat test by month after initial test, split by initial test result in heterosexual women (**a**) and men (**b**) testing at STI outpatient clinics in the Netherlands between June 2014 and December 2015. Months were defined as 30 days, and tests performed within 35 days after the initial consultation were not included

at three to 5 months after the initial consultation, with positivity rates over 25%. Chlamydia infection at the initial consultation and young age were strong predictors for having a chlamydia positive repeat test.

This study uses national STI clinic surveillance data, which results in a very large study population, allowing extensive analyses among both initial negative and initial positive visitors. However, there are also limitations to this study. First, linkage of consultations by ID number was only possible for individuals returning to the same STI clinic. Hence, (repeat) tests at other STI clinics or other testing facilities, such as general practitioners or online STI test providers, are not included and this might have resulted in an underestimation of the repeat testing rates. From 2016 onwards, STI clinics ask their attendees if and where they tested for STI in the past year. These new data might provide future insight in repeat testing between STI clinics and from other testing facilities to the STI clinics. Second, as this study used STI clinic surveillance data, only information on individuals who actively returned to the STI clinic was available. The positivity rates in people not returning to the clinics are unknown, which hampers generalisability of our results to all STI clinic visitors. Third, longitudinal data has only been available since June 2014, which resulted in a relative short follow-up time of 1.5 years. Consequently, we have underestimated the percentage of repeat testers as single testers might have returned for a repeat test after the follow-up period, and single testers might have been misclassified if the initial consultation in our data was actually already a repeat test. Uncertainty analyses showed that including only people with a minimum of 12 months follow-up did increase the percentage of repeat testers, but hardly changed the found determinants of repeat testing, indicating that our results were robust for follow-up time. Last, we only included the first two consultations of each individual. As only a small percentage of people had more than two consultations, we expect this exclusion not to have influenced our results.

We found that overall, 13.7% of heterosexuals visiting STI clinics returned for a repeat chlamydia test during our study period, and 20.5% when including only people with a minimum of 1 year follow-up. This is slightly lower than a study among UK genitourinary medicine clinic visitors, where a repeat chlamydia testing incidence of 26 per 100 person years was found [21]. Our study showed that 21.1% returned after an initial positive

Table 4 Predictors of having a chlamydia positive repeat test among repeat testers, using initial STI clinic consultation characteristics[a]

	Crude		Adjusted	
	OR	95% CI	OR	95% CI
Women				
Age				
13–19	1	–	1	–
20–24	0.77	(0.66–0.88)	0.82	(0.70–0.95)
25+	0.38	(0.32–0.45)	0.44	(0.37–0.53)
Condom use at last sexual contact				
No	1	–	1	–
Yes	0.69	(0.60–0.78)	0.83	(0.72–0.95)
Chlamydia infection at initial consultation				
No	1	–	1	–
Yes	2.04	(1.81–2.29)	1.83	(1.62–2.06)
Men				
Age				
13–19	1	–	1	–
20–24	0.77	(0.58–1.02)	0.82	(0.61–1.09)
25+	0.47	(0.35–0.63)	0.50	(0.37–0.66)
Combined variable, reported symptoms and chlamydia infection				
CT negative, no STI symptoms	1	–	1	–
CT negative, reported STI symptoms	1.06	(0.88–1.27)	1.12	(0.93–1.34)
CT positive, no STI symptoms	1.07	(0.84–1.37)	1.00	(0.79–1.28)
CT positive, reported STI symptoms	2.31	(1.89–2.83)	2.30	(1.88–2.82)

[a]Table only includes variables that remained significant in multivariate analysis

test, which was also lower than a study using US laboratory data, where repeat testing was 38% in women and 22% in men after an initial positive test [22]. Our estimate is, however, in the middle of two other regional estimates from the Netherlands (9.2% [17] and 33.4% [16] of repeat tests after an initial positive test). Differences between our study findings and others can be explained by differences in study population, definition of repeat test, and duration of follow-up. Among women, the percentage of repeat testers was higher than among men. This is in line with other Dutch studies on repeat testing [16, 17, 23]. This could be due to the fact that women are known to generally seek health-related information and health care more often than men [24, 25].

Table 5 Comparison of predictors of repeat testing and predictors of having a chlamydia positive repeat test

Characteristics	Associated with repeat testing	Associated with positive repeat test
Chlamydia infection	Yes	Yes
Young age	No	Yes
Non-Western ethnicity	Yes	No
More sex partners	Yes	No

Last, we showed that repeat test positivity rates were highest among initial chlamydia positives between 3 and 5 months after the initial consultation, which is in line with findings from other studies [11, 26] and current repeat testing guidelines after CT infection elsewhere [7–10].

Predictors of repeat testing found in our study were mostly characteristics associated with- or indicative of sexual risk behaviour and risk of STI: higher number of partners, non-Western ethnicity [18, 27], history of STI infection, and chlamydia infection at initial consultation. This might indicate that individuals who are at increased risk are also more motivated to test repeatedly. However, it could also be a consequence of the STI clinic policies, since non-Western ethnicity is a triaging criterion and therefore facilitates admittance to the STI clinic. Strikingly, we did not find young age (<25) to be predictive of repeat testing among women in our main analysis, and only a small effect among men, despite the fact that being aged <25 also is an important triaging criterion. In the uncertainty analyses with persons with a minimum of 12 months follow-up time, women aged >25 were less often repeat testers, which was more in line with the triaging criteria. However, sample sizes were much smaller in the uncertainty analysis, making these results less reliable. Future research using longer time periods is warranted to determine these associations with more certainty.

The strongest predictor for a chlamydia positive repeat test, among repeat testers, was young age. This is in agreement with studies showing that young persons are at increased risk of chlamydia infection [18, 28, 29]. Initial chlamydia infection (women) and initial chlamydia infection combined with symptoms (men) were also strong predictors for having a positive repeat test. Chlamydia infection being a predictor for repeat infection is in line with findings from studies from the UK, US, and Sweden [21, 22, 30]. Our analysis was corrected for several risk behaviour parameters at initial consultation, such as number of partners, but the association between initial and repeat infection might be due to other behavioural or biological factors as well. For example, repeat infections could be a consequence of inadequate partner notification and/or treatment of the partner of the infected index case thereby increasing the probability of reinfection of the index case [31, 32]. Furthermore, treatment failure could also contribute to the association between initial and repeat positive test. In the Netherlands, people tested positive at the urogenital site receive 1 g of azithromycin, whereas those tested positive at the anorectal site receive 7-days (100 mg twice daily) doxycycline [33]. However, treatment failure after urogenital or anorectal infections for chlamydia is possible [34, 35]. For heterosexual men, chlamydia infection was only associated with repeat test positivity if symptoms were also reported. This might indicate that for women and men different mechanisms behind repeat infections are involved. A possible explanation might be that women can be reinfected from the anorectal site to the urogenital site through autoinoculation [36]. At the STI clinics, women are only tested for anorectal infection on indication, which is likely to miss anal infections in women who did not report recent anal intercourse [37]. When women are infected at both anatomic locations, but not tested at the anorectal site, they receive azithromycin, which showed reduced effectiveness for treating anorectal chlamydia infections [35]. This may cause higher rates of repeat infections due to autoinoculation in women, whereas for heterosexual men, autoinoculation is less likely [38].

When comparing the most important predictors of repeat testing with predictors of having a chlamydia positive repeat test among repeat testers, several important findings emerge. First, initial chlamydia infection was associated with both repeat testing and with repeat test positivity. This is an indication that initial positives are indeed at increased risk of repeat infection. It also shows that chlamydia positives are already returning to the STI clinic more often compared to initial chlamydia negatives, following guidelines. However, still only 21% of initial positives were repeat tester. Second, young age (<25) was not associated with repeat testing in the main analysis, and was a strong predictor of a chlamydia infection at repeat test. This indicates that young people may not be returning to the STI clinic more often, even though they are at the highest risk of infection at repeat test compared to the other ages. Therefore, young heterosexual STI clinic visitors could be an important target group for enhancing repeat testing. Third, non-Western ethnicity was associated with repeat testing. However, at repeat test, no difference in chlamydia positivity was seen between persons with non-Western ethnicity compared to persons with Dutch ethnicity. This finding was unexpected, as more STIs are generally found among those with non-Western ethnicity [18, 27]. This might indicate that the selection of persons with non-Western ethnicity that do return to the STI clinics for a repeat test, are not necessarily the ones that are at highest risk of obtaining STIs. Or, vice versa, that those with a Dutch ethnicity returning for a repeated test are the ones with increased risk of STI. The same thing was seen for number of partners; having more partners was associated with repeat testing, but not with positivity at the repeated test. This could also indicate that those returning are not necessarily the ones at highest risk.

Conclusions

Altogether, the results of this study provide an extensive overview of current STI repeat testing behaviour among Dutch heterosexual STI clinic attendees, which can be used as guidance to determine for which groups repeat testing could be most advantageous. Our findings suggest that repeat testing could especially be beneficial for young persons (<25 years) with an initial chlamydia infection. However, interpretation of the results remains challenging due to the use of surveillance data, and since the motivations of people to return (or not return) to the clinic remain unknown. Furthermore, there is little insight into the current practices of STI clinics regarding whether (because of long waiting lists and high workload) and to whom repeat testing advice is given. Gaining insight into current practices is important to identify barriers and attitudes toward repeat testing among health care professionals, which should be taken into account when evaluating the guidelines. More research is needed to determine repeat testing strategies in the Netherlands in terms of (cost) effectiveness, feasibility, and public health impact.

Additional files

Additional file 1: Table S1. Initial consultation characteristics among heterosexuals visiting Dutch STI clinics between June 2014 and December 2015.

Additional file 2: Figure S1. The percentage of repeat tests by month, split by initial chlamydia test result in heterosexual women (A) and men (B) testing at STI outpatient clinics in the Netherlands between June 2014 and December 2015. Months were defined as 30 days and tests performed after 12 months or within 35 days of the initial consultation were not included.

Additional file 3: Table S2. Predictors of repeat testing among heterosexual women at initial STI clinic consultation between June 2014 and December 2015, stratified by chlamydia test result at initial consultation. Predictors of repeat testing among heterosexual men at initial STI clinic consultation between June 2014 and December 2015, stratified by chlamydia test result at initial consultation.

Additional file 4: Table S3. Predictors of repeated testing at initial STI clinic consultation among heterosexual women and men with at least 12 months of follow-up time between June 2014 and December 2015.

Additional file 5: Table S4. Predictors of repeat testing among heterosexual women and men at initial STI clinic consultation between June 2014 and December 2015: results from the original analyses versus complete case analysis.

Additional file 6: Table S5. Predictors of repeat testing among heterosexual women and men at initial STI clinic consultation between June 2014 and December 2015, including multiple ethnicity subgroups.

Additional file 7: Table S6. Determinants of having a chlamydia positive repeat test, using characteristics from repeat test.

Abbreviations

(a)OR: (adjusted) odds ratio; CI: Confidence interval; CT: Chlamydia trachomatis; GO: Gonorrhoea; IQR: Interquartile range; MSM: Men who have sex with men; PID: Pelvic inflammatory disease; STI: Sexually transmitted infection; SY: Syphilis; TOC: Test of cure

Acknowledgements

The authors thank Birgit van Benthem and Marianne van der Sande for their constructive comments on the manuscript.

Funding

No funding was obtained for this study.

Authors' contributions

MV and JH were involved in the design of the study. MV analysed the data and drafted the manuscript. MV, FvA, FK, CK and JH contributed to the interpretation of the results, commented on the manuscript and approved the final version. All authors read and approved the final manuscript.

Consent for publication

Not applicable.

Competing interests

The authors declare that they have no competing interests.

Author details

[1]National Institute for Public Health and the Environment, P.O. Box 1, 3720, BA, Bilthoven, the Netherlands. [2]Public Health Service Twente, postbus 1400, 7500, BK, Enschede, the Netherlands.

References

1. European Centre for Disease Prevention and Control. Sexually transmitted infections in Europe 2013. Stockholm: ECDC; 2015.
2. Hosenfeld CB, Workowski KA, Berman S, Zaidi A, Dyson J, Mosure D, et al. Repeat infection with Chlamydia and gonorrhea among females: a systematic review of the literature. Sex Transm Dis. 2009;36(8):478–89.
3. Fung M, Scott KC, Kent CK, Klausner JD. Chlamydial and gonococcal reinfection among men: a systematic review of data to evaluate the need for retesting. Sex Transm Infect. 2007;83(4):304–9.
4. Lanjouw E, Ouburg S, de Vries HJ, Stary A, Radcliffe K, Unemo M. Background review for the '2015 European guideline on the management of Chlamydia trachomatis infections'. Int J STD AIDS. 2015; doi: 10.1177/0956462415618838.
5. Davies B, Turner KM, Frolund M, Ward H, May MT, Rasmussen S, et al. Risk of reproductive complications following chlamydia testing: a population-based retrospective cohort study in Denmark. Lancet Infect Dis. 2016;16(9):1057–64.
6. Gottlieb SL, Xu F, Brunham RC. Screening and treating Chlamydia trachomatis genital infection to prevent pelvic inflammatory disease: interpretation of findings from randomized controlled trials. Sex Transm Dis. 2013;40(2):97–102.
7. Workowski KA, Bolan GA, Centers for Disease C, Prevention. Sexually transmitted diseases treatment guidelines, 2015. MMWR Recomm Rep. 2015; 64(RR-03):1–137.
8. Australian Sexual Health Alliance: Australian STI management guidelines for use in primary care – chlamydia. (2016). http://www.sti.guidelines.org.au/sexually-transmissible-infections/chlamydia#follow-up. Accessed 6 Sept 2017.
9. Lanjouw E, Ouburg S, de Vries HJ, Stary A, Radcliffe K, Unemo M. 2015 European guideline on the management of Chlamydia trachomatis infections. Int J STD AIDS. 2015; doi: 10.1177/0956462415618837.
10. Nwokolo NC, Dragovic B, Patel S, Tong CY, Barker G, Radcliffe K. 2015 UK national guideline for the management of infection with Chlamydia trachomatis. Int J STD AIDS. 2016;27(4):251–67.
11. Heijne JC, Herzog SA, Althaus CL, Tao G, Kent CK, Low N. Insights into the timing of repeated testing after treatment for Chlamydia trachomatis: data and modelling study. Sex Transm Infect. 2013;89(1):57–62.
12. LCI-RIVM. Consult seksuele gezondheid - deeldraaiboek 6 - Testbeleid. Bilthoven: RIVM: 2017. https://lci.rivm.nl/draaiboeken/consult-seksuele-gezondheid (2016). Accessed 6 Sep 2017.
13. Nederlands Huisartsen Genootschap: NGH standaard M82 soa consult. (2013). https://www.nhg.org/standaarden/samenvatting/het-soa-consult. Accessed 6 Sept 2017.
14. Vriend HJ, Stolte IG, Heijne JC, Heijman T, De Vries HJ, Geskus RB, et al. Repeated STI and HIV testing among HIV-negative men who have sex with men attending a large STI clinic in Amsterdam: a longitudinal study. Sex Transm Infect. 2015;91(4):294–9.
15. Visser M, Heijne JC, Hogewoning AA, van Aar F. Frequency and determinants of consistent STI/HIV testing among men who have sex with men testing at STI outpatient clinics in the Netherlands: a longitudinal study. Sex Transm Infect. 2017;93:396–403.
16. Dukers-Muijrers NH, van Liere GA, Hoebe CJ. Re-screening Chlamydia trachomatis positive subjects: a comparison of practices between an STI clinic, general practitioners and gynaecologists. Sex Transm Infect. 2013;89(1):25–7.
17. Kampman C, Koedijk F, Driessen-Hulshof H, Hautvast J, van den Broek I. Retesting young STI clinic visitors with urogenital Chlamydia trachomatis infection in the Netherlands; response to a text message reminder and reinfection rates: a prospective study with historical controls. Sex Transm Infect. 2016;92(2):124–9.
18. Visser M, van Aar F, van Oeffelen AAM, van den Broek IVF, Op de Coul ELM, Hofstraat SHI, et al. Sexually transmitted infections, including HIV, in the Netherlands in 2016. Bilthoven: National Institute for Public Health and the Environment; 2017.

19. Papp JR, Schachter J, Gaydos CA, Van Der Pol B. Recommendation for the laboratory-based detection of Chlamydia trachomatis and Neisseria gonorrhoeae - 2014. MMWR Recomm Rep. 2014;63(RR02):1–19.
20. Stronks K, Kulu-Glasgow I, Agyemang C. The utility of 'country of birth' for the classification of ethnic groups in health research: the Dutch experience. Ethn Health. 2009;14(3):255–69.
21. Woodhall SC, Atkins JL, Soldan K, Hughes G, Bone A, Gill ON. Repeat genital Chlamydia trachomatis testing rates in young adults in England, 2010. Sex Transm Infect. 2013;89(1):51–6.
22. Hoover KW, Tao G, Nye MB, Body BA. Suboptimal adherence to repeat testing recommendations for men and women with positive Chlamydia tests in the United States, 2008-2010. Clin Infect Dis. 2013;56(1):51–7.
23. Gotz HM, Wolfers ME, Luijendijk A, van den Broek IV. Retesting for genital Chlamydia trachomatis among visitors of a sexually transmitted infections clinic: randomized intervention trial of home- versus clinic-based recall. BMC Infect Dis. 2013;13:239.
24. Ek S. Gender differences in health information behaviour: a Finnish population-based survey. Health Promot Int. 2015;30(3):736–45.
25. Thompson AE, Anisimowicz Y, Miedema B, Hogg W, Wodchis WP, Aubrey-Bassler K. The influence of gender and other patient characteristics on health care-seeking behaviour: a QUALICOPC study. BMC Fam Pract. 2016;17:38.
26. Stephens N, Coleman D, Shaw K, O'Sullivan M, McGregor A, Cooley L, et al. Chlamydia retesting and retest positivity rates: results from a state-wide laboratory data linkage study in Tasmania, 2012?13. Sex Health. 2017; doi: 10.1071/SH16137.
27. Haasnoot A, Koedijk FD. Op de Coul EL, Gotz HM, van der Sande MA, van den Broek IV, et al. comparing two definitions of ethnicity for identifying young persons at risk for chlamydia. Epidemiol Infect. 2012;140(5):951–8.
28. Velicko I, Ploner A, Sparen P, Marions L, Herrmann B, Kuhlmann-Berenzon S. Sexual and testing behaviour associated with Chlamydia trachomatis infection: a cohort study in an STI clinic in Sweden. BMJ Open. 2016;6(8):e011312.
29. Harder E, Thomsen LT, Frederiksen K, Munk C, Iftner T, van den Brule A, et al. Risk factors for incident and redetected Chlamydia trachomatis infection in women: results of a population-based cohort study. Sex Transm Dis. 2016;43(2):113–9.
30. Nielsen A, Marrone G, De Costa A. Chlamydia trachomatis among youth - testing behaviour and incidence of repeat testing in Stockholm County, Sweden 2010-2012. PLoS One. 2016;11(9):e0163597.
31. Low N, Heijne JC, Herzog SA, Althaus CL. Reinfection by untreated partners of people treated for Chlamydia trachomatis and Neisseria gonorrhoeae: mathematical modelling study. Sex Transm Infect. 2014;90(3):254–6.
32. Golden MR, Whittington WL, Handsfield HH, Hughes JP, Stamm WE, Hogben M, et al. Effect of expedited treatment of sex partners on recurrent or persistent gonorrhea or chlamydial infection. N Engl J Med. 2005;352(7):676–85.
33. LCI-RIVM. Chlamydia trachomatis en lymfogranuloma venereum richtlijn. (2013). https://lci.rivm.nl/richtlijnen/chlamydia-trachomatis-en-lymfogranuloma-venereum#index_Profylaxe%2D-Behandeling. Accessed 6 Sept 2017.
34. Kong FY, Tabrizi SN, Law M, Vodstrcil LA, Chen M, Fairley CK, et al. Azithromycin versus doxycycline for the treatment of genital chlamydia infection: a meta-analysis of randomized controlled trials. Clin Infect Dis. 2014;59(2):193–205.
35. Kong FY, Tabrizi SN, Fairley CK, Vodstrcil LA, Huston WM, Chen M, et al. The efficacy of azithromycin and doxycycline for the treatment of rectal chlamydia infection: a systematic review and meta-analysis. J Antimicrob Chemother. 2015;70(5):1290–7.
36. Heijne JC, van Liere GA, Hoebe CJ, Bogaards JA, van Benthem BH, Dukers-Muijrers NH. What explains anorectal chlamydia infection in women? Implications of a mathematical model for test and treatment strategies. Sex Transm Infect. 2016; doi: 10.1136/sextrans-2016-052786.
37. van Liere GA, Hoebe CJ, Wolffs PF, Dukers-Muijrers NH. High co-occurrence of anorectal chlamydia with urogenital chlamydia in women visiting an STI clinic revealed by routine universal testing in an observational study; a recommendation towards a better anorectal chlamydia control in women. BMC Infect Dis. 2014;14:274.
38. Rank RG, Yeruva L. Hidden in plain sight: chlamydial gastrointestinal infection and its relevance to persistence in human genital infection. Infect Immun. 2014;82(4):1362–71.

3

Combination with antimicrobial peptide lyses improves loop-mediated isothermal amplification based method for *Chlamydia trachomatis* detection directly in urine sample

Jekaterina Jevtuševskaja[1*], Julia Uusna[1,2], Liis Andresen[1], Katrin Krõlov[1], Made Laanpere[3], Tiia Grellier[1], Indrek Tulp[2,4] and Ülo Langel[1,5]

Abstract

Background: *Chlamydia trachomatis* is an obligate intracellular human pathogen and is the most common cause of sexually transmitted diseases affecting both men and women. The pathogen can cause prostatitis and epididymitis in men. In women, cervicitis, pelvic inflammatory disease, ectopic pregnancy and acute or chronic pelvic pain are frequent complications. More than half of *C. trachomatis*-positive patients have minimal or no symptoms, providing an ongoing reservoir for the infection. The lack of sensitive large-scale applicable point- of- care (POC) tests for *C. trachomatis* detection makes it difficult to diagnose chlamydia infection efficiently in resource-limited environments.

Methods: A rapid and sensitive assay based on loop-mediated isothermal amplification method (LAMP) was combined with antimicrobial peptide lysis, which is able to detect at least 7 *C. trachomatis* pathogens per reaction directly from urine samples.

Results: Our study comprising 91 first-void urine samples showed that specificity of the assay is 100 % and sensitivity 73 % when using antimicrobial peptide lysis mix. Additionally we demonstrate that our assay does not give any cross-reactivity with 30 pathogen's DNA potentially present in the urine samples. Furthermore, the assay's novel approach does not require purification or extraction of DNA from clinical sample prior to amplification, so the need for specialized equipment is eliminated.

Conclusions: The whole procedure is significantly less laborious, less time-consuming and consequently less expensive for early detection and identification of infectious disease. *C. trachomatis* specific LAMP assay is relatively simple to perform and could therefore be applied in numerous POC settings.

Keywords: Loop-mediated isothermal amplification, Point-of-care assay, *Chlamydia trachomatis*, Pathogen detection in crude urine, Diagnostics of sexually transmitted diseases

* Correspondence: iriss@ut.ee
[1]University of Tartu, Institute of Technology Laboratory of Molecular Biotechnology, Nooruse 1, Tartu 50411, Estonia
Full list of author information is available at the end of the article

Background

Chlamydia trachomatis is a widespread sexually transmitted obligatory intracellular human pathogen, most often prevalent in adolescents and young adults of age 15–25 who have new or multiple sexual partners. The pathogen can also be passed from an infected mother to her baby during vaginal childbirth [1]. In men *Chlamydia trachomatis* usually cause prostatitis and epididymitis and is mostly symptomatic causing a mild to moderate, clear to white urethral discharge, burning sensation during urination or dysuria [2]. Patients infected with this pathogen have often minimal or no symptoms which impede the diagnosis. So it is very important to identify *C. trachomatis* in the early stage of infection and start immediate treatment as soon as possible to prevent the development of further long-term complications and decrease the chance of getting other infections such as *N. gonorrhoeae* or *Human immunodeficiency virus* [3].

The current gold standards for *Chlamydia trachomatis* clinical diagnostics is widely used PCR-based techniques (Abbot Real Time CT/NG assay; Roche Cobas Amplicor CT/NG assay eg) which is highly specific (amplify the specific DNA region of the multicopy cryptic plasmid) and sensitive but is time- consuming, requires complicated and expensive laboratory apparatus and need to prior extraction of genetic material from the sample. As an alternative different simple easy-to-use immunnoassay-based POC tests for detection *Chlamydia trachomatis* have been developed to reduce operating time, high-dependency, postoperative care time, numbers of outpatient clinic visits and ensure optimal use of professional time. In spite of the fact that most enzymatic POC tests have a high specificity up to 99 % they all have alarmingly poor sensitivity 0–30 % depending on test in comparison to nucleic acid amplification based techniques [4–9]. Limited sensitivity is a critical barrier to effective treatment and control of infectious diseases suggesting that there is still clear need for more sensitive and cost effective *C. trachomatis* diagnostic platforms.

As an alternative to the PCR based diagnostics, different nucleic acid amplification assays were developed allowing detection of pathogens in laboratories with a limited resources and POC settings. Although, novel nucleic acid amplification based tests are highly sensitive (91–100 %) [10, 11] they are susceptible to various biological components present in the sample, and thus do not allow the detection of pathogenic targets directly from crude extracts [12, 13]. Normally, unprocessed urine requires DNA extraction prior to amplification [14, 15] therefore several pathogen cell lysate preparation techniques can be suggested. Most of them however are complicated, time consuming and their application in POC settings require fully integrated automated platforms such as Cepheid GeneXpert assay, MAMEF assay, aQcare Chlamydia TRF kit [16–19].

Antimicrobial peptides (AMPs) have proven to be a very potent class of antimicrobial agents in vitro, being active in wide range of pathogens including Gram-positive and Gram-negative bacteria and fungi [20, 21]. Some peptides are able to efficiently lyse pathogen cells, releasing the DNA in the crude sample. The cell surface of the bacteria has a highly negative charge density suggesting that electrostatic interactions are responsible for their selectivity. The initial adhesion of the peptides to the cell membrane takes place with the helical axis parallel to the membrane surface [22–24] followed by insertion into the bilayer and disruption of the cell membrane [25, 26]. Therefore antimicrobial peptides could be potentially applied as fast and efficient sample preparation agents prior to isothermal amplification.

Loop-mediated isothermal amplification (LAMP) stands out to be a novel, highly sensitive and specific diagnostic tool because of the ease of performing and capability to diagnose a negligible amount of pathogen genetic material within an hour [27]. It has been reported that LAMP shows high tolerance to different inhibitors that are naturally present in various biological samples [28]. LAMP is carried out at a constant temperature (60–65 °C) and does not require a sophisticated and expensive thermal cycler. The amount of DNA product at the end of the LAMP reaction is considerably higher that than in PCR and can be simply visualized using metal ion indicators like calcein or such DNA biding dyes as SYBR green, ethidium bromide, picogreen, propidium iodide, hydroxy naphthol blue [29–34].

Here we combined *C. trachomatis* specific LAMP assay with antimicrobial peptide lysis for the rapid and sensitive pathogen detection from human urine which offers a good base for POC diagnostics platform. Application of antimicrobial peptides allows detection of *C. trachomatis* directly from urine sample, providing rapid, sensitive diagnosis with minimal need for training. Initial clinical analysis showed up to 73 % sensitivity and 100 % specificity of the developed *C. trachomatis* specific LAMP assay. The assay requires only 21 min and the product can be detected using lateral flow (LF) strips which is very beneficial for application in the point-of-care (POC) settings.

Methods

Design and selection of the primers

All *C. trachomatis* specific LAMP assay primer sets (Additional file 1: Table S1) were designed to target highly conserved region of the *C. trachomatis* cryptic plasmid within coding sequence 2 - CDS2 [13] using Basic Local Alignment Search Tool-BLAST (http://blast.ncbi.nlm.nih.gov) and LAMP Designer 1.10

software (PREMIER Biosoft USA). Additionally loop primers (LF/LB) were designed to accelerate amplification time and increase sensitivity. Primers were screened for their high sensitivity towards DNA target and for the absence of the non-specific background on LF strips. Oligonucleotides that contain sequence elements that promote secondary structures, hairpins or primer-primer interactions were avoided (using OligoAnalyser tool). Primers FIP and LF were 5′ labelled with biotin and BIP and LB primers with FAM to allow product detection on the LF strips. Primers were obtained from Microsynth AG (Balgach, Switzerland).

LAMP reaction

C. trachomatis specific LAMP reaction was carried out according to the protocol supplied by Eiken Chemical Co. Ltd [35] with reaction total volume 50 µl. Bst polymerase was replaced with Bsm polymerase (Thermo Fisher Scientific Inc. USA) and 1.2 µl of template DNA and 15 µl of ddH20 were used. For untreated samples 5 µl of urine sample and 11.2 µl of ddH20 were used. All LAMP reactions were performed at 63 °C for 21 min and analysed on the LF strips (AMODIA Bioservice GmbH) according to manufacturer's protocol. In order to confirm *C. trachomatis* amplification product specificity the reaction product was cut with PmlI restrictase (Thermo Fisher Scientific Inc. USA). The amplification product was considered specific if the signal on the LF disappeared after treatment with restrictase.

Quantitative LAMP reaction

For quantitative analysis 0.5 µl EvaGreen (Biotium) fluorescent and 0.3 µl ROX (Thermo Fisher Scientific Inc. USA) reference dyes were added into standard LAMP reaction prepared as described above. Primers without Biotin/FAM labelling were used and product was detected using Applied Biosystems 7900HT Real-Time PCR System. A standard curve was constructed using serial dilutions of BglII linearized pGL3-CDS2 plasmid [13] at concentrations from 10^8- 10^4 with a 4 parallels. qLAMP was performed at 63 °C with 40 cycles, each 1 min long, data reading after 30 s.

C. trachomatis strain UW-36/Cx genomic DNA (ATCC® VR-886D™) was obtained from ATCC (American Culture Collection) and CDS2 target copy number was determined by qPCR (Applied Biosystems) using pGL3-CDS2 plasmid and following primers: Fw 5′- CTC CTTGGAGCATTGTCTGG- 3′ and Rw 5′-CGGATGCGATGAACAGTTTG- 3′.

Sample pre-treatment

Lysates used for LAMP reaction were prepared by treating 30 µl of clinical patient's urine sample with 4 µl of 1 × antimicrobial peptide lysis mix (SelfD Technologie GmbH, Leipzig, Germany; commercial component) for 5 min according to the protocol supplied by SelfD Technologie GmbH. Each lysate contained 12 % (from final volume) of peptide lysis mix and subsequently 1.2 % of peptide lysis mix in each LAMP reaction. Heat-treated samples were prepared by pre-heating urine at 90 °C for 5 min and then cooled down on ice. 5 µl of each lysates (heated urine or treated with antimicrobial peptide lysis mix) were then applied for *C. trachomatis* specific LAMP amplification. Pooled urine was only used (*C. trachomatis* negative urine mix from 5 men and 5 women in equal volumes) for assay sensitivity/specificity analysis.

Statistical analysis

Statistical analyses of *C. trachomatis* specific LAMP assay's limit of detection were performed with XLSTAT, 95 % confidence interval (CI) was calculated using logistic regression model. Assay sensitivity and specificity was calculated using online tool from MedCalc (http://www.medcalc.org/calc/diagnostic_test.php) confidence interval for 95 %.

Clinical specimen collection and storage

First-void morning urine samples were collected from 650 patients from 18 to 25 year old (316 females and 334 males) attending Sexual Health Clinique (Tartu, Estonia) from October 2013 to December 2014. Urine samples were self-collected into a clean polypropylene container (average sample volume of 25–35 ml) without preservative and led by patients to the Sexual Health Clinique on the same day. Criteria for patient enrolment in the study were recent change of the sexual partner, multiple sexual partners, unprotected sexual intercourse, STI of the partner, and symptoms of the sexually transmitted disease.

Urine samples were tested by Cobas® 4800 CT/NG Test (Roche) for the presence of *C. trachomatis* according to manufacturer's instruction by the United Laboratories of the Tartu University Hospital regularly on the second day of the sample collection, no longer than 72 h after collection.

The 91 non-frozen urine samples selected randomly out of 650 clinical specimens were tested by *C. trachomatis* specific LAMP assay within 6 h after collection. Approval for the study was obtained from the Research Ethics Committee of the University of Tartu.

Results

Validation of *C. trachomatis* specific LAMP assay and sample pre-treatment procedure

Human urine contains variety of critical components that may inhibit the amplification entirely or only partially and by that prolong the amplification time. For instance, high concentration of urea in the sample (more than 50 mmol l^{-1}) can lead even to the degradation of the polymerase [15, 36, 37]. In order to simplify pathogen detection procedure and make it more applicable for POC device settings, the DNA purification step prior the amplification was excluded. The amplification procedure has to take place directly in urine sample without previous concentration of the pathogen genetic material. Therefore, it is essential that developed amplification method has to tolerate as higher percentage of urine in the reaction mixture as possible allowing to increase the whole assay sensitivity as more targets are available for amplification. Our results demonstrated that reactions containing 15 % of urine did not give any signal when analysed on lateral flow strips, indicating that 21 min of amplification time was insufficient for target amplification. 5–10 % of urine in reaction mixture gave positive signal in all replicates ($n = 5$) (Fig. 1b). This observation was also confirmed by quantitative LAMP analysis where addition of 5–10 % urine did not affect amplification time (Fig. 1a). In the presence of 15–20 % of urine however, the amplification time should be prolonged up to 30 min indicating inhibitory effect of the urine components on LAMP reaction (Fig. 1a). Therefore based on this data, 10 % of urine was used as a sample material in all subsequent experiments. Our results showed that minimum reaction time required for product formation on LF strips was 21 min when as low as 100 copies of template per reaction were used in LAMP reaction containing not more than 10 % of crude urine sample (Additional file 1: Table S2). This enabled to reduce assay amplification procedure from recommended 1 h to 21 min without losing reaction sensitivity.

LAMP urine tolerance was tested in the presence of 0 %, 5 %, 10 %, 15 % and 20 % of pooled patient urine. Results were analyzed quantitatively (A) and using LF strips (B). For quantitative analysis, remaining amplification time was calculated as an average time compared to 0 % urine reaction at standard DNA dilutions 10^8, 10^7, 10^6, 10^5 and 10^4 target copies per reaction. For LF strips detection, reaction was performed in the presence of 100 template copies in five parallels; two bands confirm the successful outcome of DNA amplification and a negative result is indicated by the presence of a single black band on the test strip.

To eliminate the possibility that antimicrobial peptide lysis mix itself could inhibit LAMP reaction and find out the best concentration of lysis mix that could be applied in LAMP reaction, different lysis mix concentrations were tested. As a result addition of up to 1.2 % of antimicrobial peptide mix did not inhibit LAMP reaction as the amplification time was not altered. Based on this data up to 1.2 % of peptide lysis mix was used in LAMP assay without significant inhibition of amplification efficiency (Fig. 2).

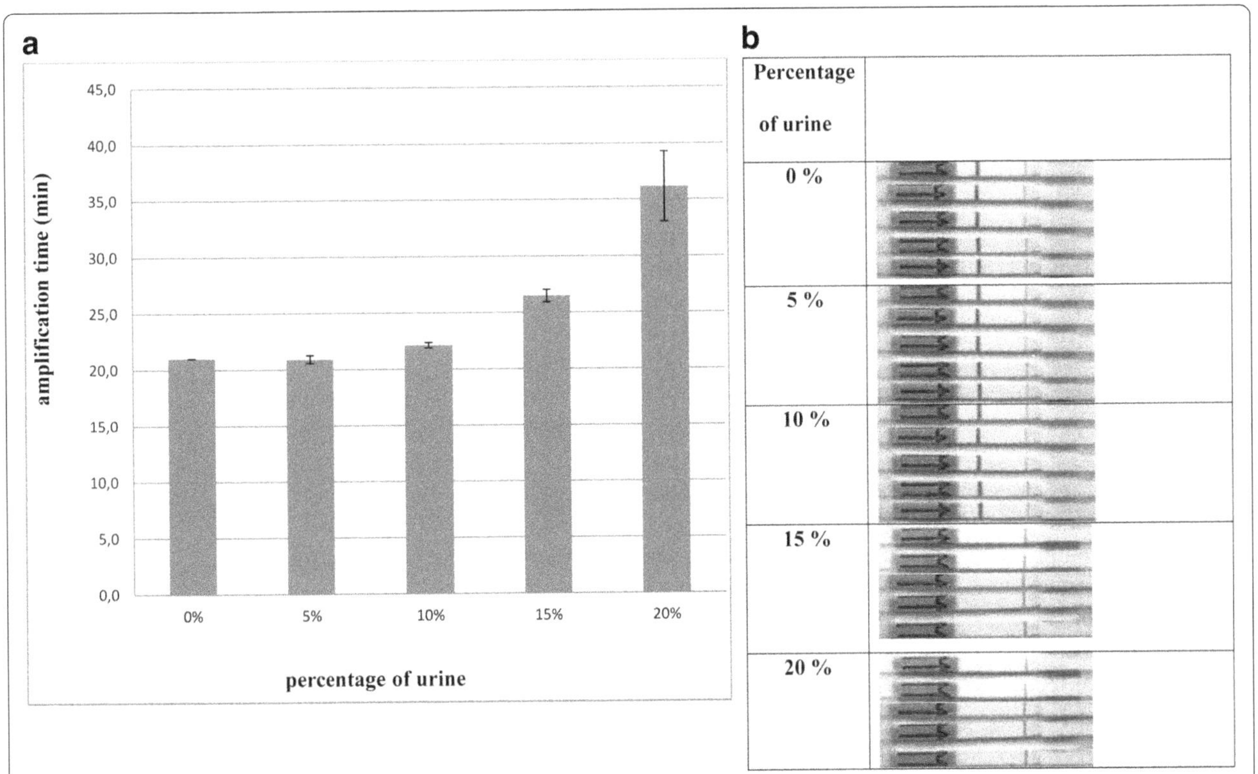

Fig. 1 Urine tolerance of LAMP

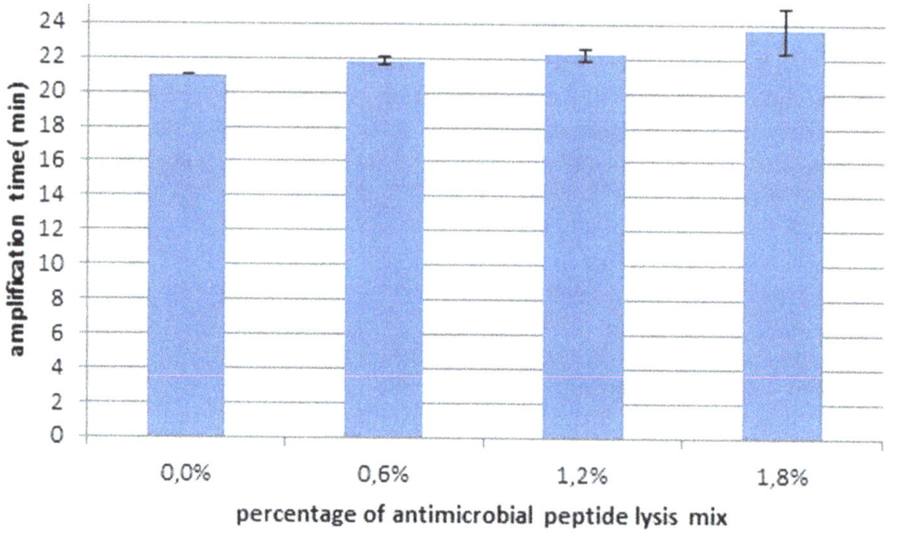

Fig. 2 Tolerance of antimicrobial peptide lysis mix by LAMP

Assay tolerance was tested in the presence of 0 %, 0.6 %, 1.2 %, and 1.8 % of 1 × antimicrobial peptide lysis mix (SelfD Technologie GmbH, Leipzig, Germany; commercial component). Results were analysed quantitatively. For quantitative analysis, remaining amplification time was calculated as an average time compared to 0 % antimicrobial peptide lysis mix reaction at standard DNA dilutions 10^8, 10^7, 10^6, 10^5 and 10^4 target copies per reaction.

Assessment of limit of detection (LOD) for *C. trachomatis* specific LAMP assay

Probit analysis showed that assay was sensitive enough to detect 25 plasmid copies per reaction in water (0.95 value) (Additional file 1: Figure S1). As developed assay does not contain DNA purification step it was important to estimate if 10 % of crude urine can affect the sensitivity. For that pooled urine samples were spiked with different amount of *C. trachomatis* genomic DNA. As a result, in the presence of 10 % urine sensitivity of LAMP assay reduced approximately three times and established LOD was 70 target copies per reaction (0.95 value) (Table 1).

These results are in good correlation with urine inhibition experiment, where addition of 10 % urine prolonged LAMP amplification time (Fig. 1a) and can be the reason why amplification activity was decreased approximately three times (Table 1).

Determination of *C. trachomatis* specific LAMP assay specificity

Although LAMP primers were designed targeting pathogen specific region, their specificity had to be experimentally verified. *C. trachomatis* specific LAMP assay was further analysed for possible non-specific reactivity using excess amount of genomic DNA from human and 30 microorganisms potentially present in human urine (Additional file 1: Table S3). As a result *C. trachomatis* specific LAMP assay did not give cross-reactivity with any examined pathogen's DNA and is highly specific in detection of chlamydia from human urine, fitting well for molecular diagnostic system.

Clinical validation of *C. trachomatis* specific LAMP assay

To determine the prevalence of chlamydia in symptomatic and asymptomatic patients the urine samples subjected to clinical study ($N = 650$) were additionally evaluated. 157 out of 650 patients (24 %), had symptoms of STI and 493 patients (76 %) were asymptomatic. 51 % of the patients were males and 49 % females, with an average age of 22 years (18–25 years old). Chlamydia was diagnosed in 39 male patients and 47 female patients out of which only 12 (31 %) and 13 (28 %) had symptoms, respectively. Clinical data confirmed that *C. trachomatis* infection is mainly asymptomatic, which makes it difficult to diagnose and estimate the real prevalence in human population (Additional file 1: Table S4; Table S5).

Table 1 LOD determination for *C. trachomatis* specific LAMP assay[a]

	Copies per reaction	Lower bound 95 %	Upper bound 95 %
Limit of detection in water (0.95 value)	25	21	33
Limit of detection in pooled urine (0.95 value)	70	61	96

[a]For LOD determination in water 0, 4, 6, 12, 24, 48 and 120 plasmid copies were applied per reaction in 22 parallels each. For LOD determination in urine 0, 40, 50, 75, 100 and 200 plasmid copies were applied. Each reaction was performed in 20 parallels. Numbers of positive and negative signals visualized on LF strips were analysed by XLSTAT

C. trachomatis specific LAMP assay clinical sensitivity and specificity was validated in a study, comprising 91 freshly collected patient urine samples selected randomly from 650 clinical specimens. Although the number of specimens is not enough to provide high statistical power of the clinical study it was calculated to be minimal sample size to perform cost-effective assay validation with peptide lysis mix. First-void morning urine samples were self-collected by 56 male and 34 female patients and the overall prevalence of *C. trachomatis* among tested group was 12 %. Collected urine samples were subjected in parallel for *C. trachomatis* specific LAMP assay and Roche Cobas 4800 CT/NG test, a conventional technique for *C. trachomatis* detection. According to Roche Cobas 4800 CT/NG test 11 out of 91 had chlamydia infection. Two different sample pre-treatment strategies were tested and compared to untreated samples: heating at 90 °C for 5 min and incubation with peptide lysis mix for 5 min. From 80 *C. trachomatis* negative samples all tested negative in all treatments and no false-negatives were detected. Results showed that highest assay sensitivity (73 %) was obtained when using peptide/detergent lysis mix (out of 11 *C. trachomatis* positive urine samples 8 tested positive and 3 tested negative in the LAMP reaction) whereas pre-treatment with heat showed 64 % of assay sensitivity, and sensitivity dropped to 55 % when urine samples were left untreated (Table 2).

These data clearly shows that pre-treatment of urine samples prior to amplification provide a better access of pathogen DNA material. All 80 chlamydia negative samples were detected as negative by developed LAMP assay, thus clinical specificity was estimated to 100 %.

Discussion

Sexually transmitted infections (STIs), including highly prevalent *Chlamydia trachomatis*, remain an important focus area of the global public health [38]. Current *C. trachomatis* POC tests cannot offer the sensitivity comparable to laboratory nucleic acid amplification based techniques. Also concerns over the trueness of results, accuracy and general usefulness in non-emergency settings have slowed the adoption of these POC tests in general practice. Consequently successful detection and fast identification of chlamydia is necessary for early diagnosis and treatment of the disease. For that reason the need for simple and rapid on-site cost- efficient applicable *C. trachomatis* test which enables highly specific and sensitive pathogen detection remains.

This paper demonstrates for the first time, that the introduction of the antimicrobial peptide lysis step in the specific LAMP assay improves the detection of *C. trachomatis* directly in urine samples without prior extraction, purification and concentration of the pathogen genetic material. *C. trachomatis* cryptic plasmid has been chosen as a target for current diagnostic testing because it is present at up to 10 copies per genome [39]. Cryptic plasmid is relatively stable nucleic acid target being more resistant to nuclease damage than the genomic DNA. Selected CDS2 region shares high homology between different *C. trachomatis* serovars and is present in the Swedish mutant strains [13]. The use of six primers in LAMP reaction (F3, B3/FIP, BIP/LF, LB) provides not only a greater specificity than other amplification method but also accelerate the amplification time. Our data showed that novel *C. trachomatis* specific LAMP assay can detect at least 25 copies of the cryptic plasmid target in water. In urine, however, the sensitivity was 70 plasmid copies per reaction, probably due to potential inhibitors naturally present in crude sample material. Consequently, the newly developed LAMP assay is 100 % specific in detection of chlamydia. The whole assay takes less than 30 min, does not require additional equipment or trained personnel and the amplification product can be easily visualized by LF dipsticks and can be easily applied in the POC settings.

As simple and easy to apply sample pre-treatment method is one of the major criteria for the true self-diagnostic tests it is very important to find the best strategy for lysis of such challenging pathogen as chlamydia directly in crude urine. The lysis of the pathogen cells enables to liberate genetic material in such a way, that it would be suitable for the subsequent rapid

Table 2 *C. trachomatis* detection in 91 first-void urine samples with the Roche Cobas Amplicor CT assay and *C. trachomatis* specific LAMP assay

Fresh urine samples		*C. trachomatis* LAMP assay					
		Untreated urine[a]		Heat treated urine[b]		Peptide lysis mix pre-treated urine[c]	
		Positive	Negative	Positive	Negative	Positive	Negative
Roche Cobas Amplicor CT assay	Positive	6	5	7	4	8	3
	Negative	0	80	0	80	0	80
Sensitivity % [95 % CI]		55 % [23,38–83,25 %]		64 % [30, 79–89, 07 %]		73 % [39, 03–93, 98 %]	
Specificity % [95 % CI]		100 % [95, 5–100 %]		100 % [95, 5–100 %]		100 % [95, 5–100 %]	

[a]5 μl of fresh urine was added to LAMP reaction
[b]5 μl of urine was incubated at 90 °C for 5 min and after that added to LAMP reaction
[c]30 μl of urine was incubated with 4 μl (peptide lysis mix) for 5 min and after that 5 μl was taken out and added to LAMP reaction

amplification by LAMP method. To our knowledge only few reports related to detection of bacteria directly from biological sample using LAMP method are available [40, 41]. Current study shows for the first time novel and advantageous application of antimicrobial peptide mixture for the development of chlamydia specific LAMP assay directly in crude urine sample. Considering that majority of currently available POC tests have only 10–30 % of pathogen detection sensitivities, novel diagnostic approaches are required [42]. Our novel strategy successfully combined LAMP amplification with fast and simple sample preparation technique applying them directly in clinical samples. As a result the overall sensitivity of the novel *C. trachomatis* specific LAMP assay increased from 55 % (untreated, crude urine samples) up to 73 % when using antimicrobial peptide lysis mix and 64 % when samples were heat pre-treated prior addition into the amplification reaction. Thus by optimizing sample pre-treatment (for example urine sample enrichment) sensitivity of LAMP assay could be further increased to the levels comparable with commercially available nucleic acid amplification assays.

Our data shows that the application of antimicrobial peptide lysis mix provides promising sample pre-treatment strategy that suits all above mentioned requirements. Therefore there is no need to prior DNA extraction and purification, like in nucleic acid amplification -based chlamydia detection assays, which makes the whole detection less laborious and time consuming. Such features as increased sensitivity, controllability, simplicity, rapid response time and high specificity of pathogen detection compared to different POC immunoassays make antimicrobial peptide lysis combined *C. trachomatis* specific LAMP assay appealing for the application as reliable molecular diagnostic tool compatible for POC settings.

Conclusions

We have developed for the first time simple, rapid and sensitive LAMP assay combined with antimicrobial peptide lysis mix for the specific detection of *C. trachomatis* directly from crude urine samples. *C. trachomatis* specific LAMP assay has great potential for the application in numerous POC settings.

Additional file

Additional file 1: Table S1. LAMP primer set selected for *C. trachomatis* specific detection. **Table S2.** *C. trachomatis* specific LAMP assay amplification time. **Figure S1.** Probit curve for *C. trachomatis* -LAMP assay LOD in water (closed circle) and pooled urine (closed triangle) with lower and upper bounds 95 % in water and urine as described in lower panel of the image. **Table S3.** List of organisms used to determine specificity of the *C. trachomatis* LAMP assay. **Table S4.** Clinical characteristics of the studied group ($N = 650$). **Table S5.** Data for the patients with co-infection with NG. Additional information for the manuscript "Efficient and Rapid Loop-Mediated Isothermal Amplification Based Method for *Chlamydia trachomatis* Detection Directly from Urine".

Acknowledgments

We thank the Sexual Health Clinique for collaboration during the clinical study, in particular Pille Veskilt and Bianka Peetson; Raili Randoja (Tartu University Hospital United Laboratories).

Funding

This work was supported by the Sächsische AufbauBank provided under project SAB#100144699 and the Estonian Research Council provided under research grant PUT753.

Authors' contributions

JJ carried out the assay validation and clinical studies, participated in the design of the experiments, analyzed and interpreted raw data, drafted the manuscript. JU participated in the design of the study and performed the statistical analysis, participated in drafting the manuscript. LA and ML participated in collecting clinical samples from the patients. KK carried out quantitative LAMP analysis. TG performed the detection with LF dipsticks. IT participated in the design of the study, revised the manuscript. ÜL conceived of the study, and participated in its design and coordination and helped to draft the manuscript. All authors read and approved the final manuscript.

Competing interests

The authors declare that they have no competing interests. There are no non-financial competing interests (political, personal, religious, ideological, academic, intellectual, commercial or any other) to declare.

Consent for publication

Not applicable.

Author details

[1]University of Tartu, Institute of Technology Laboratory of Molecular Biotechnology, Nooruse 1, Tartu 50411, Estonia. [2]SelfD Technologie GmbH, Leipzig, Germany. [3]The Tartu University Hospital's Women's Clinic and Tartu Sexual Health Clinic, Tartu Estonia. [4]University of Tartu, Institute of Chemistry, Tartu, Estonia. [5]Stockholm University, Stockholm, Sweden.

References

1. McGregor JA, French JI. Chlamydia trachomatis infection during pregnancy. Am J Obstet Gynecol. 1991;164(6 Pt 2):1782–9.
2. Miller KE. Diagnosis and treatment of Chlamydia trachomatis infection. Am Fam Physician. 2006;73(8):1411–6.
3. Peralta L, Durako SJ, Ma Y. Correlation between urine and cervical specimens for the detection of cervical Chlamydia trachomatis and Neisseria gonorrhoeae using ligase chain reaction in a cohort of HIV infected and uninfected adolescents. J Adolesc Health. 2001;29(3 Suppl):87–92.
4. Bandea CI, Koumans EH, Sawyer MK, Dover J, O'Connor A, Papp JR, et al. Evaluation of the rapid BioStar optical immunoassay for detection of Chlamydia trachomatis in adolescent women. J Clin Microbiol. 2009;47(1):215–6.
5. Yin YP, Peeling RW, Chen XS, Gong KL, Zhou H, Gu WM, et al. Clinic-based evaluation of Clearview Chlamydia MF for detection of Chlamydia

trachomatis in vaginal and cervical specimens from women at high risk in China. Sex Transm Infect. 2006;82 Suppl 5:v33–7.
6. Sabido M, Hernandez G, Gonzalez V, Valles X, Montoliu A, Figuerola J, et al. Clinic-based evaluation of a rapid point-of-care test for detection of Chlamydia trachomatis in specimens from sex workers in Escuintla, Guatemala. J Clin Microbiol. 2009;47(2):475–6.
7. De Baetselier I, Mwambarangwe L, Cuylaerts V, Musengamana V, Agaba S, Kestelyn E, et al. Evaluation of an enzymatic Chlamydia trachomatis point-of-care rapid assay in Rwanda: the BioChekSwab Rapid Test. Sex Transm Infect. 2015;052202. doi:10.1136/sextrans-2015-052202.
8. Nunez-Forero L, Moyano-Ariza L, Gaitan-Duarte H, Angel-Muller E, Ruiz-Parra A, Gonzalez P, et al. Diagnostic accuracy of rapid tests for sexually transmitted infections in symptomatic women. Sex Transm Infect. 2016;92(1):24–8.
9. van der Helm JJ, Sabajo LO, Grunberg AW, Morre SA, Speksnijder AG, de Vries HJ. Point-of-care test for detection of urogenital chlamydia in women shows low sensitivity. A performance evaluation study in two clinics in Suriname. PLoS One. 2012;7(2):e32122.
10. Dean D, Turingan RS, Thomann HU, Zolotova A, Rothschild J, Joseph SJ, et al. A multiplexed microfluidic PCR assay for sensitive and specific point-of-care detection of Chlamydia trachomatis. PLoS One. 2012;7(12):e51685.
11. Cheng A, Qian Q, Kirby JE. Evaluation of the xott RealTime CT/NG assay in comparison to the Roche Cobas Amplicor CT/NG assay. J Clin Microbiol. 2011;49(4):1294–300.
12. Nakano R, Nakano A, Ishii Y, Ubagai T, Kikuchi-Ueda T, Kikuchi H, et al. Rapid detection of the Klebsiella pneumoniae carbapenemase (KPC) gene by loop-mediated isothermal amplification (LAMP). J Infect Chemother. 2015;21(3):202–6.
13. Krõlov K, Frolova J, Tudoran O, Suhorutsenko J, Lehto T, Sibul H, et al. Sensitive and rapid detection of Chlamydia trachomatis by recombinase polymerase amplification directly from urine samples. J Mol Diagn. 2014;16(1):127–35.
14. Edwards T, Burke PA, Smalley HB, Gillies L, Hobbs G. Loop-mediated isothermal amplification test for detection of Neisseria gonorrhoeae in urine samples and tolerance of the assay to the presence of urea. J Clin Microbiol. 2014;52(6):2163–5.
15. Khan G, Kangro HO, Coates PJ, Heath RB. Inhibitory effects of urine on the polymerase chain reaction for cytomegalovirus DNA. J Clin Pathol. 1991; 44(5):360–5.
16. Gaydos CA, Van Der Pol B, Jett-Goheen M, Barnes M, Quinn N, Clark C, et al. Performance of the Cepheid CT/NG Xpert Rapid PCR Test for Detection of Chlamydia trachomatis and Neisseria gonorrhoeae. J Clin Microbiol. 2013;51(6):1666–72.
17. Melendez JH, Huppert JS, Jett-Goheen M, Hesse EA, Quinn N, Gaydos CA, et al. Blind evaluation of the microwave-accelerated metal-enhanced fluorescence ultrarapid and sensitive Chlamydia trachomatis test by use of clinical samples. J Clin Microbiol. 2013;51(9):2913–20.
18. Causer LM, Hengel B, Natoli L, Tangey A, Badman SG, Tabrizi SN, et al. A field evaluation of a new molecular-based point-of-care test for chlamydia and gonorrhoea in remote Aboriginal health services in Australia. Sex Health. 2014;12(1):27-33.
19. Ham JY, Jung J, Hwang BG, Kim WJ, Kim YS, Kim EJ, et al. Highly sensitive and novel point-of-care system, aQcare Chlamydia TRF kit for detecting Chlamydia trachomatis by using europium (Eu) (III) chelated nanoparticles. Ann Lab Med. 2015;35(1):50–6.
20. Carriel-Gomes MC, Kratz JM, Barracco MA, Bachere E, Barardi CR, Simoes CM. In vitro antiviral activity of antimicrobial peptides against herpes simplex virus 1, adenovirus, and rotavirus. Mem Inst Oswaldo Cruz. 2007;102(4):469–72.
21. Suttmann H, Retz M, Paulsen F, Harder J, Zwergel U, Kamradt J, et al. Antimicrobial peptides of the Cecropin-family show potent antitumor activity against bladder cancer cells. BMC Urol. 2008;8:5.
22. Silvestro L, Axelsen PH. Membrane-induced folding of cecropin A. Biophys J. 2000;79(3):1465–77.
23. Bechinger B. The structure, dynamics and orientation of antimicrobial peptides in membranes by multidimensional solid-state NMR spectroscopy. Biochim Biophys Acta. 1999;1462(1–2):157–83.
24. Sato H, Feix JB. Peptide-membrane interactions and mechanisms of membrane destruction by amphipathic alpha-helical antimicrobial peptides. Biochim Biophys Acta. 2006;1758(9):1245–56.
25. Huang HW. Action of antimicrobial peptides: two-state model. Biochemistry. 2000;39(29):8347–52.
26. Huang HW. Molecular mechanism of antimicrobial peptides: the origin of cooperativity. Biochim Biophys Acta. 2006;1758(9):1292–302.
27. Dhama K, Karthik K, Chakraborty S, Tiwari R, Kapoor S, Kumar A, et al. Loop-mediated isothermal amplification of DNA (LAMP): a new diagnostic tool lights the world of diagnosis of animal and human pathogens: a review. Pak J Biol Sci. 2014;17(2):151–66.
28. Francois P, Tangomo M, Hibbs J, Bonetti EJ, Boehme CC, Notomi T, et al. Robustness of a loop-mediated isothermal amplification reaction for diagnostic applications. FEMS Immunol Med Microbiol. 2011;62(1):41–8.
29. Parida M, Sannarangaiah S, Dash PK, Rao PV, Morita K. Loop mediated isothermal amplification (LAMP): a new generation of innovative gene amplification technique; perspectives in clinical diagnosis of infectious diseases. Rev Med Virol. 2008;18(6):407–21.
30. Dukes JP, King DP, Alexandersen S. Novel reverse transcription loop-mediated isothermal amplification for rapid detection of foot-and-mouth disease virus. Arch Virol. 2006;151(6):1093–106.
31. Curtis KA, Rudolph DL, Owen SM. Rapid detection of HIV-1 by reverse-transcription, loop-mediated isothermal amplification (RT-LAMP). J Virol Methods. 2008;151(2):264–70.
32. Hill J, Beriwal S, Chandra I, Paul VK, Kapil A, Singh T, et al. Loop-mediated isothermal amplification assay for rapid detection of common strains of Escherichia coli. J Clin Microbiol. 2008;46(8):2800–4.
33. Tomita N, Mori Y, Kanda H, Notomi T. Loop-mediated isothermal amplification (LAMP) of gene sequences and simple visual detection of products. Nat Protoc. 2008;3(5):877–82.
34. Soliman H, El-Matbouli M. Loop mediated isothermal amplification combined with nucleic acid lateral flow strip for diagnosis of cyprinid herpes virus-3. Mol Cell Probes. 2010;24(1):38–43.
35. Notomi T, Okayama H, Masubuchi H, Yonekawa T, Watanabe K, Amino N, et al. Loop-mediated isothermal amplification of DNA. Nucleic Acids Res. 2000; 28(12):E63.
36. Saulnier P, Andremont A. Detection of genes in feces by booster polymerase chain reaction. J Clin Microbiol. 1992;30(8):2080–3.
37. Wilson IG. Inhibition and facilitation of nucleic acid amplification. Appl Environ Microbiol. 1997;63(10):3741–51.
38. Da Ros CT. Schmitt CaS. Global epidemiology of sexually transmitted diseases. Asian J Androl. 2008;10(1):110–4.
39. Pickett MA, Everson JS, Pead PJ, Clarke IN. The plasmids of Chlamydia trachomatis and Chlamydophila pneumoniae (N16): accurate determination of copy number and the paradoxical effect of plasmid-curing agents. Microbiology. 2005;151(Pt 3):893–903.
40. Iwamoto T, Sonobe T, Hayashi K. Loop-mediated isothermal amplification for direct detection of Mycobacterium tuberculosis complex, M. avium, and M. intracellulare in sputum samples. J Clin Microbiol. 2003;41(6):2616–22.
41. Gahlawat SK, Ellis AE, Collet B. A sensitive loop-mediated isothermal amplification (LAMP) method for detection of Renibacterium salmoninarum, causative agent of bacterial kidney disease in salmonids. J Fish Dis. 2009;32(6):491–7.
42. van Dommelen L, van Tiel FH, Ouburg S, Brouwers EE, Terporten PH, Savelkoul PH, et al. Alarmingly poor performance in Chlamydia trachomatis point-of-care testing. Sex Transm Infect. 2010;86(5):355–9.

4

Leucocyte esterase dip-stick test as a point-of-care diagnostic for urogenital chlamydia in male patients: A multi-center evaluation in two STI outpatient clinics in Paramaribo and Amsterdam

Menne Bartelsman[1*], Henry J. C. de Vries[1,2,3], Maarten F. Schim van der Loeff[2,4], Leslie O. A. Sabajo[5] and Jannie J. van der Helm[1,4]

Abstract

Background: Point-of-care (POC) tests are an important strategy to address the epidemic of sexually transmitted infections (STIs). The leucocyte esterase test (LET) can be used as a POC test for chlamydia. The aim of this study was to determine the diagnostic accuracy of the LET to detect urogenital chlamydia among men at STI clinics in Paramaribo, Suriname and Amsterdam, the Netherlands.

Methods: Recruitment of patients took place in 2008–2010 in Suriname and in 2009–2010 in the Netherlands. Urine of patients was examined with the LET. The reference test was a nucleic acid amplification test (NAAT).

Results: We included 412 patients in Suriname and 645 in the Netherlands. Prevalence of chlamydia in Suriname and the Netherlands was respectively 22.8 and 13.6 %. The sensitivity of the LET was 92.6 % (95 % CI = 85.3–97.0) and 77.3 % (95 % CI = 67.1–85.5) respectively, the specificity was 38.1 % (95 % CI = 32.7–43.6 %) and 58.1 % (95 % CI = 53.9–62.3) respectively. The positive predictive value was 30.6 % (95 % CI = 27.3–36.4) and 22.6 % (95 % CI = 18.0–27.7) respectively and the negative predictive value was 94.5 % (95 % CI = 89.1–97.8) and 94.2 % (95 % CI = 91.1–96.4) respectively. The kappa was respectively 0.179 and 0.176.

Conclusions: To diagnose urogenital chlamydia in men the LET performs poorly. It has a high negative but low positive predictive value. If the LET result is negative, chlamydia is accurately excluded, yet a positive result has a low predictive value. Whether the advantages of direct management based on LET outweigh the disadvantages of overtreatment is a subject for further studies.

Keywords: Sensitivity, Specificity, Chlamydia, Point-of-care test, Leucocyte esterase test, *Chlamydia trachomatis*

Background

Chlamydia trachomatis (Ct) is the most common cause of nongonoccal urethritis in men [1]. In resource-limited settings management of male urethritis is generally based on a syndromic approach: when a patient has typical symptoms like urethral discharge, penile itching or dysuria, immediate treatment with antibiotics is given. Yet, with a syndromic approach, a significant proportion of men infected with Ct are missed, as the majority of men does not have symptoms [2]. The proportion of cases that are asymptomatic varies by population and ranges from 40 to 96 % [3–5]. Moreover, a syndromic approach also can lead to overtreatment, antibiotic overconsumption, induction of side effects and antimicrobial resistance of infections like *Neisseria gonorrhoeae* (Ng). Also, effective contact tracing and treatment is challenging based on a presumptive diagnosis only.

* Correspondence: mbartelsman@ggd.amsterdam.nl
[1]Department of Infectious Diseases, STI Outpatient Clinic, Public Health Service of Amsterdam (GGD Amsterdam), Weesperplein 1, 1018, XA, Amsterdam, The Netherlands
Full list of author information is available at the end of the article

Point of care (POC) management can partly overcome the disadvantages of syndromic management. POC testing is defined as medical testing at or near the site of patient care [6]. Ideally a POC test should meet the ASSURED criteria of the World Health Organization; Affordable, Sensitive, Specific, User-friendly, Rapid and Robust, Equipment-free, Deliverable to those who need them [7]. Recently, several companies have developed commercial POC tests based on bacterial antigens that provide rapid results for the detection of Ct, but the sensitivity of these tests is low (17–65 %) and this precludes more widespread use in clinical settings [6, 8–10]. The Cepheid GeneXpert Ct/Ng assay is a rapid (<2 h to results) nucleic acid amplification test (NAAT) assay that can be performed in on-site laboratories, but the high costs are an obstacle for implementation in low-and middle-income countries. Moreover it is questionable if patients are willing to wait 2 h for their test result [11]. As long as no other promising POC test is available, sexually transmitted infections (STI) clinics are dependent on convential techniques like light microscopy and dipstick urinalysis with the leucocyte esterase test (LET).

Light microscopy is used in the POC management of various STIs [1]. However, light microscopy requires a laboratory infrastructure that is often lacking in resource-limited settings. In these settings the LET might be an alternative for light microscopy, because it is cheap, easy to perform and does not require a laboratory [12, 13]. LET is available as dipstick assay and is used to detect a urinary inflammatory reaction through the presence of an esterase enzyme produced by polymorph nuclear leucocytes (PMNL) in the urine, possibly associated with either a urinary tract infection or STI in males [14].

Suriname is a middle-income country in South America with most of the population concentrated in the coastal region, and the remainder in sparsely populated, predominantly remote areas. For these settings, an equipment-free POC test could be of great benefit. The Netherlands is a high-income country in Europe, but also there an equipment-free POC test may be useful in certain primary health care settings like general practitioners clinics.

Previous studies that investigated the performance of the LET to detect urogenital Ct in males have reported sensitivities and specificities ranging from 46 to 100 % and 60 to 96 % respectively [15–19]. The variety of outcomes can be explained by a difference in settings, patient groups, experimental test thresholds and reference tests. In most of the studies obsolete reference tests like ligase chain reaction (LCR) were used and/or investigated the LET in either symptomatic or asymptomatic patients in one setting [16, 20–28].

The aim of our study was to evaluate the diagnostic performance of the LET as a POC test for urogenital Ct compared to NAAT in male patients irrespective of symptoms attending STI outpatient clinics in two different settings; an outpatient clinic in a middle-income country, Suriname, and in a high-income country, the Netherlands.

Methods

Study design, selection of patients

Participants were recruited at:

1. The Dermatological Service in Paramaribo, an integrated outpatient clinic that offers free-of-charge examination and treatment of STIs and infectious skin diseases such as leprosy and leishmaniasis. Recruitment took place between March 2008 and July 2010.
2. The STI Outpatient Clinic of the Public Health Service of Amsterdam, which is a low threshold clinic serving over 40,000 patients annually. Patients were prioritized based on a short questionnaire to estimate the risk of having an STI, as described before [29]. The following categories were regarded as high risk: age <25 years, men who have sex with men, born in an STI and HIV endemic country, receiving money/goods for sex, paying for sex, ≥3 partners in the previous 6 months, reporting a sexual partner with a partner born in an STI and HIV endemic country, being notified by a sex partner or having STI related symptoms. Patients regarded as high-risk were eligible to participate; recruitment took place between November 2009 and May 2010.

In both countries demographic characteristics and data regarding symptoms were obtained using a questionnaire. Patients were regarded as symptomatic when either dysuria, urethral discharge or scrotal pain was reported in the questionnaire.

Leucocyte esterase test (LET)

The LET (Combur^2 Test LN, Roche Diagnostics, GmbH, Mannheim, Germany) is a non-specific rapid dipstick assay used to detect the presence of an esterase enzyme produced by PMNL's in urine. The presence of PMNL's in urine indicates an inflammatory response, possibly caused by an infection. In Suriname and the Netherlands patients provided urine samples that were immediately brought to the on-site laboratory by nurses. A laboratory technician performed the LET within two hours of sample collection and placed the dipstick in a urine sample according to the manufacturer's instructions. The results were read after 2 and 5 min. Using a reference color table, the dipstick differentiated between negative, 1+ (ca. 10–25 PMNL/μl), 2+ (ca. 75 PMNL/μl), 3+ (ca. 500 PMNL/μl). The LET was regarded positive when the dipstick colored ≥ 1+. Patients with a failed or missing LET were excluded from the analyses.

Reference tests

The Aptima Ct assay (Hologic Gen-Probe, USA) was used as the reference NAAT to detect urogenital Ct both in the Netherlands and Suriname. Reference testing was performed on the same urine sample that was used for the LET. In the Netherlands the samples were tested the same week at the Public Health Laboratory in Amsterdam. In Suriname, the samples were collected according to the manufacturer's (Hologic) instructions, stored in a fridge (at temperature between 2° and 7 °C) and packed according to international air transport association (IATA) rules for transport by plane to the Public Health Laboratory in Amsterdam for NAAT testing. According to the manufacturer's instructions the samples had to be analysed within 30 days after collection. In our study 349 of the 412 samples (84.7 %) were analysed within 30 days and 63 samples (15.3 %) were tested between 31 and 48 days (median time: 35 days (IQR 33–36 days)). More details about the data collection were previously described [8, 30].

Diagnostic performance and statistical analysis

The diagnostic performance of the LET was investigated by calculating the sensitivity, specificity, positive predictive value (PPV), negative predictive value (NPV), the percentage agreement and kappa. A kappa value >0.61 was considered as good test agreement, $\kappa = 0.41–0.60$ as fair agreement, $\kappa = 0.21–0.40$ as slight agreement, $\kappa = 0.01–0.20$ as poor agreement, and $\kappa \leq 0.00$ as no agreement) [31].

As prescribed by the manufacturer the LET was read 2 min after it was placed in urine (from here onwards described as "LET 2 m"). We also read the result of the LET 5 min after it was placed in urine (from now on described as "LET 5 m") to evaluate the influence of timing on the diagnostic performance.

We compared the diagnostic performance of the LET 2 m between symptomatic and asymptomatic patients and conducted a subgroup analysis for individuals <25 years.

Characteristics of the study populations were compared using the Pearson's chi-square test. When the expected cell-count was <5 the Fisher's exact test was used. We considered a p-value <0.05 as statistically significant. Analyses were performed with SPSS package version 21 (SPSS Inc., Chicago, Illinois, USA) and STATA software V11.2 (Stata Corp, College Station, Texas, USA).

Results

Study populations

Suriname

In total 415 patients provided samples for the study, of which three patients had an invalid LET result and were excluded. From the remaining 412 patients 279 (67.7 %) of the patients were symptomatic and 133 (32.3 %) were asymptomatic. The median age was 28 years (interquartile range (IQR) 24.0–37.0). Ct prevalence was 22.8 % (95 % CI 19.0–27.1) (Table 1).

The Netherlands

In total 647 patients provided samples for the study of which two patients had an invalid LET result and were excluded. Data regarding symptoms were missing for nine patients. Among the remaining 636 patients 257 (40.4 %) of the patients were symptomatic and 379 (59.6 %) were asymptomatic. The median age was 34 years (IQR 26.5–43.0). Ct prevalence was 13.6 % (95 % CI 11.2–16.5).

Table 1 Characteristics of male patients included at the Dermatological Service Paramaribo, Suriname, 2008–2010 and the STI Outpatient Clinic, Amsterdam, The Netherlands, 2009–2010

	Suriname ($N = 412$)	The Netherlands ($N = 645$)	*P* value
Demographic characteristics	*n* (%)	*n* (%)	
Median age (years) (IQR)	28.0 (24.0–37.0)	34.0 (26.5–43.0)	<0.001
Age (years)			<0.001
< 25	109 (26.5)	110 (17.1)	
25–29	115 (27.9)	123 (19.1)	
30–34	59 (14.3)	108 (16.7)	
≥ 35	129 (31.3)	304 (47.1)	
Symptoms*			<0.001
No	133 (32.3)	379 (59.6)	
Yes	279 (67.7)	257 (40.4)	
HIV status**			<0.001
Negative	392 (95.1)	519 (80.5)	
Positive	2 (0.49)	113 (17.5)	
Unknown	18 (4.4)	13 (2.0)	
Sexual preference*			<0.001
Heterosexual men	402 (98.3)	282 (43.7)	
Men who have sex with men	7 (1.7)	363 (56.3)	
Ct prevalence			
Total population	94 (22.8)	88 (13.6)	<0.001
< 25 years	29 (26.6)	21 (19.1)	0.185
Symptomatic patients*	77 (27.6)	53 (20.6)	0.060
Asymptomatic patients*	17 (12.8)	34 (9.0)	0.207

Abbreviations: *STI* sexual transmitted infections; *IQR* interquartile range; *Ct Chlamydia trachomatis*

*Numbers do not add up to column total due to missing data; data on symptoms were missing for 9 patients in the Netherlands and data on sexual preference were missing for 3 patients in Suriname. Percentages were calculated based on those with non-missing data and thus add up to 100 %

**In the Netherlands a positive HIV status was based on a positive HIV test in the past or on the date of inclusion (noted in the patient records); a negative HIV status was based on a negative HIV test result on the date of inclusion. The HIV status was unknown when a HIV test was lacking on the date of inclusion. In Suriname the HIV status was self-reported at the date of inclusion

Ct prevalence and symptomatology in Suriname and the Netherlands

In Suriname significantly more patients reported symptoms compared with the Netherlands; 67.7 % (279/412) versus 40.4 % (257/636) ($p < 0.001$). Also a significantly higher prevalence of Ct was found in Suriname than in the Netherlands; 22.8 % (94/412) versus 13.6 % (88/645) ($p < 0.001$).

Diagnostic performance

Suriname

With LET 2 m 284/412 had a positive and 128/412 a negative result. The LET 2 m showed a sensitivity of 92.6 % (95 % CI 85.3–97.0), a specificity of 38.1 % (95 % CI 32.7–43.6 %), a PPV of 30.6 % (95 % CI 27.3–36.4), an NPV of 94.5 % (95 % CI 89.1–97.8) and a kappa of 0.179 (Table 2). The LET 5 m had a comparable sensitivity of 96.8 % ($p = 0.1936$) but a significantly lower specificity of 16.7 % ($p < 0.001$). The LET 2 m had a comparable sensitivity among symptomatic and asymptomatic patients, 92.2 % versus 94.1 % ($p = 0.786$), but the specificity was significantly lower among the symptomatic patients compared with the asymptomatic patients; 30.2 % versus 51.7 % ($p < 0.001$).

Among patients <25 years of age the sensitivity was 100 % (95 % CI 90.2–100) for the LET 2 m, although this was not significantly different compared with the sensitivity of the those ≥ 25 years; 89.2 % (95 % CI 79.1–95.6) ($p = 0.066$). Also the specificity was not significantly different; 41.3 % (95 % CI 30.9–52.3) versus 37.0 % (95 % CI 30.8–43.4) ($p = 0.496$).

The Netherlands

With LET 2 m 301/645 had a positive result and 344/645 had a negative result. The LET 2 m had a sensitivity of 77.3 % (95 % CI 67.1–85.5), a specificity of 58.1 % (95 % CI 53.9–62.3), a PPV of 22.6 % (95 % CI 18.0–27.7), an NPV of 94.2 % (95 % CI 91.1–96.4) and a kappa of 0.176 (Table 3). The sensitivity of the LET 5 m was 90.9 %; significantly higher than the sensitivity of the LET 2 m ($p = 0.013$). The specificity of the LET 5 m was 40.8 %; significantly lower than the specificity of the LET 2 m ($p < 0.001$).

The sensitivity of the LET 2 m was not significantly different between symptomatic and asymptomatic patients ($p = 0.096$), but the specificity was significantly lower among symptomatic patients (51.0 %) than among asymptomatic patients (62.6 %) ($p = 0.008$). In the younger age group (<25 years) a high prevalence of Ct was found (19.1 %) but the sensitivity and specificity of the LET 2 m in this group were not significantly different compared with the age group ≥ 25 years ($p = 0.290$ and $p = 0.377$).

Compared with Suriname the sensitivity of the LET 2 m was significantly lower; 77.3 % versus 92.6 % ($p = 0.004$).

Discussion

To our knowledge this is the first multi-center study that evaluated the LET to detect urogenital Ct among men in clinics in both a middle-income country and in a high-income country with high Ct prevalences (22.8 % and 13.6 %, respectively).

Both in Suriname and the Netherlands the LET 2 m had a reasonably high sensitivity (respectively 92.6 and 77.3 %) but a poor specificity (respectively 38.1 and 58.1 %) and a poor agreement (respectively kappa 0.179 and 0.176). The significantly higher sensitivity of the LET 2 m we found in Suriname compared with the Netherlands can be caused by a difference in study populations. In the Netherlands significantly more patients were asymptomatic (59.6 %) compared with Suriname (32.3 %). Wiggins et al. suggested that asymptomatic patients have infections with a lower infection-load and therefore fewer leucocytes which might cause false negative test results [32]. The same group showed that the number of leucocytes (predominantly PMNL's) was strongly correlated with urethritis and proved that men with asymptomatic urethritis have fewer PMNL's than symptomatic men [33]. A Swedish study conducted among 480 male patients of an STI clinic (also with Ct as outcome and ≥1+ as cutoff point) supports this hypothesis: the LET had a significantly higher sensitivity (69.6 % versus 25.9 %) but a lower specificity (76.3 % versus 85.8 %) among symptomatic patients compared with asymptomatic patients [17].

Moreover, in both countries the LET 2 m showed a significantly higher specificity in asymptomatic patients compared with symptomatic patients. A possible explanation can be that symptomatic patients had relatively more often infections like Neisseria gonorrhoeae (Ng), Mycoplasma genitalum (Mg) or Trichomonas Vaginalis (Tv) compared to asymptomatic patients which could have caused a relative higher proportion of 'false positive' results [34–36]. Also in a previous study we showed that light microscopic examination of Gram stained urethral smears is less specific to detect urogenital Ct infections when done in samples of symptomatic males only [37].

In the Netherlands the sensitivity of the LET increased and in both countries the specificity decreased when the incubation time was prolonged from 2 to 5 min. A study of Morré et al. found also a higher sensitivity when the reading time was prolonged from 2 to 5 min [38].

The strength of our study is that we explored the diagnostic accuracy of the LET among both symptomatic and asymptomatic male patients in a high- and in a middle-income country with a different Ct prevalence. A shortcoming is that we only focused on Ct and not on other causative micro-organisms of urethritis like Ng, Mg or Tv. Evaluation of other micro-organisms could have

Table 2 Diagnostic performance* of the Leucocyte Esterase Test (LET) after a reading time of 2 min ("LET 2 m") and 5 min ("LET 5 m") in the detection of urogenital *Chlamydia Trachomatis* (Ct) among male patients, Dermatological Service in Paramaribo, Suriname, 2008–2010

	N	LET + NAAT+	LET-NAAT+	LET + NAAT-	LET- NAAT-	Sens. (95 % CI)	Spec. (95 % CI)	PPV (95 % CI)	NPV (95 % CI)	Agr.	Kappa
LET 2 m											
ALL	412	87	7	197	121	92.6 % (85.3–97.0)	38.1 % (32.7–43.6)	30.6 % (27.3–36.4)	94.5 % (89.1–97.8)	50.5 %	0.179
Sympto-matic patients	279	71	6	141	61	92.2 % (83.8–97.1)	30.2 % (24.0–37.0)	33.5 % (27.2–40.3)	91.0 % (81.5–96.6)	47.3 %	0.145
Asympto-matic patients	133	16	1	56	60	94.1 % (71.3–99.9)	51.7 % (42.3–61.1)	22.2 % (13.8–32.9)	98.4 % (91.2–100)	57.1 %	0.193
<25 years	109	29	0	47	33	100 % (88.1–100)	41.3 % (30.4–52.8)	38.2 % (27.2–50.0)	100 % (89.4–100)	56.9 %	0.272
LET 5 m											
ALL	412	91	3	265	53	96.8 % (91.0–99.3)	16.7 % (12.7–21.2)	25.6 % (21.1–30.4)	94.6 % (85.1–98.9)	35.0	0.068

*Sensitivity (Sens.), Specificity (Spec.), Positive Predictive Value (PPV), Negative Predictive Value (NPV), Agreement (Agr.) and Kappa

Table 3 Diagnostic performance* of the Leucocyte Esterase Test (LET) after a reading time of 2 min ("LET 2 m") and 5 min ("LET 5 m") in the detection of urogenital *Chlamydia Trachomatis* (Ct) among male patients, STI outpatient clinic, Amsterdam, The Netherlands, 2009–2010

	N	LET+ NAAT+	LET- NAAT+	LET+ NAAT-	LET- NAAT-	Sens. (95 % CI)	Spec. (95 % CI)	PPV (95 % CI)	NPV (95 % CI)	Agr.	Kappa
LET 2 m											
ALL	645	68	20	233	324	77.3 % (67.1–85.5)	58.1 % (53.9–62.3)	22.6 % (18.0–27.7)	94.2 % (91.1–96.4)	60.8 %	0.176
Sympto-matic patients	257	44	9	100	104	83.0 % (70.2–91.9)	51.0 % (43.9–58.0)	30.6 % (23.2–38.8)	92.0 % (85.4–96.3)	57.6 %	0.208
Asympto-matic patients	379	23	11	129	216	67.6 % (49.5–82.6)	62.6 % (57.2–67.7)	15.1 % (9.8–21.8)	95.1 % (91.4–97.5)	63.1 %	0.026
<25 years	110	18	3	41	48	85.7 % (63.7–97.0)	53.9 % (43.0–64.6)	30.5 % (19.2–43.9)	94.1 % (84.8–98.8)	60.0 %	0.068
LET 5 m											
ALL	645	80	8	330	227	90.9 % (82.9–96.0)	40.8 % (36.7–45.0)	19.6 % (15.9–23.8)	96.6 % (93.4–98.5)	47.6 %	0.125

*Sensitivity (Sens.), Specificity (Spec.), Positive Predictive Value (PPV), Negative Predictive Value (NPV), Agreement (Agr.) and Kappa

been helped to interpret the difference of false positive results between symptomatic and asymptomatic patients. Another shortcoming is that not all NAAT samples from Suriname were analyzed within 30 days after collection (according to manufacturer's instructions) at the Public Health Laboratory in Amsterdam; 63 samples (15.3 %) were analyzed between 31 and 48 days, although it is unlikely that this small delay has influenced the performance of the NAAT [39]. Recently, several companies have developed commercial POC tests that provide rapid results for the detection of Ct, however, the sensitivity of these tests is low (25–65 %) and precludes more widespread use in clinical settings [8–10, 40, 41]. An exception of a POC test with a high sensitivity is the GeneXpert Ct/Ng (Cepheid), a cartridge-based automated test that can identify Ct and Ng infections by NAAT within 2 h, but the high costs hinder the implementation in low-and middle-income countries [42]. Moreover, not all patients may be willing to wait for the results for 2 h. Earlier we showed that in the Surinamese setting only 26.7 % of the female STI visitors would be willing to wait for their POC test results for more than one hour [8].

Syndromic management based on symptoms falls short and leaves many asymptomatic infections untreated [40, 43]. As long as no accurate and affordable POC tests for Ct are available, the LET could be a cheap and an easy to perform alternative to exclude urogenital Ct infections among men in settings where any Ct diagnostics are lacking. The sensitivity we found for the LET in Suriname (91.6 %) was reasonably high. It is estimated that a POC test of even moderate sensitivity (63 %) combined with immediate treatment on-site may lead to the treatment of more infected individuals than an ultra-sensitive and specific NAAT alone when patient return is low [44].

Settings lacking any STI laboratory diagnostics now mainly rely on syndromic management for STI treatment. Further studies into the diagnostic performance of the LET test as opposed to routine syndromic management are needed; the effect on overtreatment due to low specificity would be an important end point.

Our previous study on the cost-effectiveness of microscopic examination of Gram stained urethral smears compared to NAAT at the STI outpatient clinic in Amsterdam showed a sensitivity of 83.8 % and specificity of 74.1 %, comparable with the sensitivity and specificity of the LET we found in the current study [37]. However, if available, microscopy is preferable above the LET because it can also detect Ng infections by finding Gram negative diplococci in a Gram stained smear.

Conclusion

In conclusion, we showed that the LET has a reasonably high sensitivity but a low specificity to diagnose urogenital Ct in male STI clinic visitors. Future studies that also include the detection of other main causative infections of urethritis are needed to compare the cost-effectiveness of the LET in comparison with syndromic management.

Abbreviations

ASSURED: Affordable, Sensitive, Specific, User-friendly, Rapid and Robust Equipment-free, Deliverable; Ct: Chlamydia trachomatis; IATA: International air transport association; IQR: Interquartile range; LCR: Ligase chain reaction; LET: Leucocyte esterase test; Mg: Mycoplasma genitalum; NAAT: Nucleic acid amplification test; Ng: Neisseria gonorrhoeae; NPV: Negative predictive value; PMNL: Polymorph nuclear leucocytes; POC: Point of care; PPV: Positive predictive value; STI: Sexually transmitted infections; Tv: Trichomonas Vaginalis

Acknowledgements

The authors would like to thank all nurses and laboratory technicians of the Dermatological Service in Paramaribo and the STI outpatient clinic in Amsterdam for data collection.

Funding

This study was financed by the Research and Development department of the Public Health Service of Amsterdam, no 2382.

Authors' contributions

HJCdV, JJvdH and LOAS were responsible for the design of the study. JJvdH and LOAS collected the data in Suriname. JJvdH collected the data in the Netherlands. MB and JJvdH did the statistical analysis of the diagnostic outcomes. MB drafted the paper. MFSvdL advised on statistical analysis and interpretation. HJCdV supervised the overall study. All authors reviewed and approved the final article.

Competing interests

Maarten Schim van der Loeff and Henry de Vries served on an Advisory Board of GSK.

Consent for publication

Not applicable.

Author details

[1]Department of Infectious Diseases, STI Outpatient Clinic, Public Health Service of Amsterdam (GGD Amsterdam), Weesperplein 1, 1018, XA, Amsterdam, The Netherlands. [2]Center for Infection and Immunology Amsterdam (CINIMA), Academic Medical Center (AMC), University of Amsterdam, Amsterdam, The Netherlands. [3]Department of Dermatology, Academic Medical Center (AMC), University of Amsterdam, Amsterdam, The Netherlands. [4]Department of Research, Public Health Service of Amsterdam (GGD Amsterdam), Nieuwe Achtergracht 100, 1018, WT, Amsterdam, The Netherlands. [5]Dermatological Service, Ministry of Health Suriname, Tourtonnelaan 5, Paramaribo, Suriname.

References

1. Brill JR. Diagnosis and treatment of urethritis in men. Am Fam Physician. 2010;81:873–8.
2. Alary M, Lowndes CM, Mukenge-Tshibaka L, et al. Sexually transmitted infections in male clients of female sex workers in Benin: risk factors and reassessment of the leucocyte esterase dipstick for screening of urethral infections. Sex Transm Infect. 2003;79:388–92.

3. Cecil JA, Howell MR, Tawes JJ, et al. Features of Chlamydia trachomatis and Neisseria gonorrhoeae infection in male Army recruits. J Infect Dis. 2001;184:1216–9.
4. Detels R, Green AM, Klausner JD, et al. The incidence and correlates of symptomatic and asymptomatic Chlamydia trachomatis and Neisseria gonorrhoeae infections in selected populations in five countries. Sex Transm Dis. 2011;38:503–9.
5. Kent CK, Chaw JK, Wong W, et al. Prevalence of rectal, urethral, and pharyngeal chlamydia and gonorrhea detected in 2 clinical settings among men who have sex with men: San Francisco, California, 2003. Clin Infect Dis. 2005;41:67–74.
6. Huppert J, Hesse E, Gaydos CA. What's the point? How Point-of-Care STI tests can impact infected patients. Point Care. 2010;9:36–46.
7. Peeling RW, Holmes KK, Mabey D, et al. Rapid tests for sexually transmitted infections (STIs): the way forward. Sex Transm Infect. 2006;82 Suppl 5:v1–6.
8. van der Helm JJ, Sabajo LO, Grunberg AW, et al. Point-of-care test for detection of urogenital chlamydia in women shows low sensitivity. A performance evaluation study in two clinics in Suriname. PLoS One. 2012;7:e32122.
9. van Dommelen L, van Tiel FH, Ouburg S, et al. Alarmingly poor performance in Chlamydia trachomatis point-of-care testing. Sex Transm Infect. 2010;86:355–9.
10. de Herbst CS, Bristow CC, Joseph DD, et al. A systematic review of point of care testing for Chlamydia trachomatis, Neisseria gonorrhoeae, and Trichomonas vaginalis. Infect Dis Obstet Gynecol. 2016;2016:4386127.
11. Gaydos CA, Van Der Pol B, Jett-Goheen M, et al. Performance of the Cepheid CT/NG Xpert Rapid PCR Test for Detection of Chlamydia trachomatis and Neisseria gonorrhoeae. J Clin Microbiol. 2013;51:1666–72.
12. Centers for Disease Control and Prevention. STD Treatment Guidelines 2015. Available at: https://www.cdc.gov/std/tg2015/.
13. Horner PJ, Blee K, Falk L, et al. 2016 European guideline on the management of non-gonococcal urethritis. Int J STD AIDS. 2016;27:928-37.
14. Rahman MS, Beever W, Skov S, et al. Using urinary leucocyte esterase tests as an indicator of infection with gonorrhoea or chlamydia in asymptomatic males in a primary health care setting. Int J STD AIDS. 2014;25:138–44.
15. Blake DR, Lemay CA, Gaydos CA, et al. Performance of urine leukocyte esterase in asymptomatic male youth: another look with nucleic acid amplification testing as the gold standard for Chlamydia detection. J Adolesc Health. 2005;36:337–41.
16. Sellors JW, Mahony JB, Pickard L, et al. Screening urine with a leukocyte esterase strip and subsequent chlamydial testing of asymptomatic men attending primary care practitioners. Sex Transm Dis. 1993;20:152–7.
17. Hedin G, Abrahamsson G, Dahlberg E. Urethritis associated with Chlamydia trachomatis: comparison of leukocyte esterase dipstick test of first-voided urine and methylene blue-stained urethral smear as predictors of chlamydial infection. APMIS. 2001;109:595–600.
18. Marrazzo JM, Whittington WL, Celum CL, et al. Urine-based screening for Chlamydia trachomatis in men attending sexually transmitted disease clinics. Sex Transm Dis. 2001;28:219–25.
19. Wood BJ, Gaydos JC, McKee Jr KT, et al. Comparison of the urine Leukocyte Esterase Test to a Nucleic Acid Amplification Test for screening non-health care-seeking male soldiers for Chlamydia trachomatis and Neisseria gonorrhoeae infections. Mil Med. 2007;172:770–2.
20. Bowden FJ. Reappraising the value of urine leukocyte esterase testing in the age of nucleic acid amplification. Sex Transm Dis. 1998;25:322–6.
21. Grosskurth H, Mayaud P, Mosha F, et al. Asymptomatic gonorrhoea and chlamydial infection in rural Tanzanian men. BMJ. 1996;312:277–80.
22. Jackson DJ, Rakwar JP, Chohan B, et al. Urethral infection in a workplace population of East African men: evaluation of strategies for screening and management. J Infect Dis. 1997;175:833–8.
23. Mayaud P, Changalucha J, Grosskurth H, et al. The value of urine specimens in screening for male urethritis and its microbial aetiologies in Tanzania. Genitourin Med. 1992;68:361–5.
24. O'Brien SF, Bell TA, Farrow JA. Use of a leukocyte esterase dipstick to detect Chlamydia trachomatis and Neisseria gonorrhoeae urethritis in asymptomatic adolescent male detainees. Am J Public Health. 1988;78:1583–4.
25. Patrick DM, Rekart ML, Knowles L. Unsatisfactory performance of the leukocyte esterase test of first voided urine for rapid diagnosis of urethritis. Genitourin Med. 1994;70:187–90.
26. Shafer MA, Schachter J, Moscicki AB, et al. Urinary leukocyte esterase screening test for asymptomatic chlamydial and gonococcal infections in males. JAMA. 1989;262:2562–6.
27. Tyndall MW, Nasio J, Maitha G, et al. Leukocyte esterase urine strips for the screening of men with urethritis–use in developing countries. Genitourin Med. 1994;70:3–6.
28. Watson-Jones D, Mugeye K, Mayaud P, et al. High prevalence of trichomoniasis in rural men in Mwanza, Tanzania: results from a population based study. Sex Transm Infect. 2000;76:355–62.
29. Heijman TL, Van der Bij AK, de Vries HJ, et al. Effectiveness of a risk-based visitor-prioritizing system at a sexually transmitted infection outpatient clinic. Sex Transm Dis. 2007;34:508–12.
30. Bom RJ, van der Helm JJ, Bruisten SM, et al. The role of Surinamese migrants in the transmission of Chlamydia trachomatis between Paramaribo, Suriname and Amsterdam, The Netherlands. PLoS One. 2013;8:e77977.
31. Zweig MH, Campbell G. Receiver-operating characteristic (ROC) plots: a fundamental evaluation tool in clinical medicine. Clin Chem. 1993;39:561–77.
32. Wiggins R, Graf S, Low N, et al. Real-time quantitative PCR to determine chlamydial load in men and women in a community setting. J Clin Microbiol. 2009;47:1824–9.
33. Wiggins RC, Holmes CH, Andersson M, et al. Quantifying leukocytes in first catch urine provides new insights into our understanding of symptomatic and asymptomatic urethritis. Int J STD AIDS. 2006;17:289–95.
34. Shahmanesh M, Radcliffe KW. Is the urethral smear necessary in asymptomatic men attending a genitourinary medicine clinic? Sex Transm Infect. 2007;83:79–81.
35. Ross JD, Jensen JS. Mycoplasma genitalium as a sexually transmitted infection: implications for screening, testing, and treatment. Sex Transm Infect. 2006;82:269–71.
36. Falk L, Fredlund H, Jensen JS. Symptomatic urethritis is more prevalent in men infected with Mycoplasma genitalium than with Chlamydia trachomatis. Sex Transm Infect. 2004;80:289–93.
37. Bartelsman M, van Rooijen MS, Alba S, et al. Point-of-care management of urogenital Chlamydia trachomatis via Gram-stained smear analysis in male high-risk patients. Diagnostic accuracy and cost-effectiveness before and after changing the screening indication at the STI Clinic in Amsterdam. Sex Transm Infect. 2015;91:479–84.
38. Morre SA, Spaargaren J, Veldhuijzen IK, et al. Evaluation of the leukocyte esterase test (LET) as pre-screening test to reduce costs for national population-based Chlamydia trachomatis screening programs. J Adolesc Health. 2006;38:332–3.
39. Boyadzhyan B, Yashina T, Yatabe JH, et al. Comparison of the APTIMA CT and GC assays with the APTIMA combo 2 assay, the Abbott LCx assay, and direct fluorescent-antibody and culture assays for detection of Chlamydia trachomatis and Neisseria gonorrhoeae. J Clin Microbiol. 2004;42:3089–93.
40. Natoli L, Maher L, Shephard M, et al. Point-of-care testing for chlamydia and gonorrhoea: implications for clinical practice. PLoS One. 2014;9:e100518.
41. Causer LM, Hengel B, Natoli L et al. A field evaluation of a new molecular-based point-of-care test for chlamydia and gonorrhoea in remote Aboriginal health services in Australia. Sex Health. 2015;12:27-33.
42. Cepheid. Product information Xpert Ct/Ng. Available at: http://www.cepheid.com/us/cepheid-solutions/clinicalivd-tests/sexual-health/xpert-ct-ng.
43. Watchirs Smith LA, Hillman R, Ward J, et al. Point-of-care tests for the diagnosis of Neisseria gonorrhoeae infection: a systematic review of operational and performance characteristics. Sex Transm Infect. 2013;89:320–6.
44. Gift TL, Pate MS, Hook III EW, et al. The rapid test paradox: when fewer cases detected lead to more cases treated: a decision analysis of tests for Chlamydia trachomatis. Sex Transm Dis. 1999;26:232–40.

5

Antimicrobial susceptibility of *Neisseria gonorrhoeae* isolates from Hefei (2014–2015): genetic characteristics of antimicrobial resistance

Fa-Xing Jiang[1†], Qian Lan[1†], Wen-Jing Le[2] and Xiao-Hong Su[2*]

Abstract

Background: Antimicrobial resistance (AMR) and genetic determinants of resistance of *N. gonorrhoeae* isolates from Hefei, China, were characterized adding a breadth of information to the molecular epidemiology of gonococcal resistance in China.

Methods: 126 *N. gonorrhoeae* isolates from a hospital clinic in Hefei, were collected between January, 2014, and November, 2015. The minimum inhibitory concentration (MIC) of *N. gonorrhoeae* isolates for seven antimicrobials were determined by the agar dilution method. Isolates were tested for mutations in *penA* and *mtrR* genes and 23S rRNA, and also genotyped using *N. gonorrhoeae* multi-antigen sequence typing (NG-MAST).

Results: All *N. gonorrhoeae* isolates were resistant to ciprofloxacin; 81.7% (103/126) to tetracycline and 73.8% (93/126) to penicillin. 39.7% (50/126) of isolates were penicillinase producing *N. gonorrhoeae* (PPNG), 31.7% (40/126) were tetracycline resistant *N. gonorrhoeae* (TRNG) and 28.6% (36/126) were resistant to azithromycin. While not fully resistant to extended spectrum cephalosporins (ESCs), a total of 14 isolates (11.1%) displayed decreased susceptibility to ceftriaxone (MIC $\geq$ 0.125 mg/L, n = 10), cefixime (MIC $\geq$ 0. 25 mg/L, n = 1) or to both ESCs (n = 3). *penA* mosaic alleles XXXV were found in all isolates that harbored decreased susceptibility to cefixime, except for one. Four mutations were found in *mtrR* genes and mutations A2143G and C2599T were identified in 23S rRNA. No isolates were resistant to spectinomycin. Gonococcal isolates were distributed into diverse NG-MAST sequence types (STs); 86 separate STs were identified.

Conclusions: *N. gonorrhoeae* isolates from Hefei during 2014–2015, displayed high levels of resistance to antimicrobials that had been recommended previously for treatment of gonorrhea, e.g., penicillin, tetracycline and ciprofloxacin. The prevalence of resistance to azithromycin was also high (28.6%). No isolates were found to be fully resistant to spectinomycin, ceftriaxone or cefixime; however, 11.1% isolates, overall, had decreased susceptibility to ESCs.

Keywords: *Neisseria gonorrhoeae*, Antimicrobial resistance, Azithromycin, Cephalosporins, Resistance determinants

* Correspondence: suxh@ncstdlc.org
†Equal contributors
[2]STD clinic, Institute of Dermatology, Chinese Academy of Medical Sciences & Peking Union Medical College, Nanjing 210042, China
Full list of author information is available at the end of the article

Background

Neisseria gonorrhoeae is the etiologic agent of gonorrhea, one of the most common bacterial sexually transmitted infections (STIs) worldwide. WHO estimated that 78.3 million of new cases of gonorrhea occurred among adults globally in 2012 [1].100, 245 cases of gonorrhea were reported nationally by the China Centers for Disease Control and Prevention in 2015, making it the fifth most commonly reported communicable disease in China [2]. At this time there are no effective vaccines for gonococcal infections and antimicrobial treatment continues to be the mainstay of control. However, *N. gonorrhoeae* has developed resistance to antimicrobials that had been used previously for treatment of this infection including sulfonamides, penicillins, tetracyclines and quinolones. Presently, extended spectrum cephalosporins (ESCs) that include ceftriaxone and cefixime are recommended as the first-line treatment of gonorrhea in most parts of the world. In many countries azithromycin has been added not just to treat chlamydia infection that often co-infects, but also to supplement treatment for *N. gonorrhoeae* itself [3]. Diminished susceptibility of *N. gonorrhoeae* and emergence of full resistance and treatment failures with ESCs (mainly pharyngeal gonorrhea) have been documented in several countries [4]. Furthermore, *N. gonorrheae* strains with high-level azithromycin resistance have been reported in France [5], the United States [6], Australia [7] and China [8]. Resistance to azithromycin threatens efficacy of dual antimicrobial therapy (ESCs plus azithrothmycin) that may result in decreased treatment options and enhance the possibility of untreatable infection.

A key component of a successful response plan to gonococcal antimicrobial resistance (AMR) is to conduct timely surveillance of resistance and treatment failures across geographic regions (e.g. GISP [U.S] and GASP (WHO/Europe) [9, 10]) and to characterize the genetic elements of resistant strains. Antimicrobial susceptibility patterns vary by geographic region. AMR surveillance programs have been conducted in several cities in China [11, 12]. The aims of the present study were to describe the prevalence of gonococcal AMR and the molecular epidemiological characteristics of *N. gonorrhoeae* strains from 2014 to 2015 in Hefei, a city in eastern China.

Methods

Clinical isolates

Clinical isolates of *N. gonorrhoeae* (n = 126) investigated in this study were collected consecutively from men with urethritis (urethral discharge and/or dysuria) and women with cervical infection in the STD clinic at Anhui Provincial Hospital, China, between January, 2014 and November 2015. Cotton swabs, used to obtain cervical and urethral specimens, were immediately streaked onto Thayer-Martin (T-M) selective medium to isolate *N. gonorrhoeae*. Inoculated plates were incubated at 36 °C in 5% carbon dioxide for 24–48 h. and *N. gonorrhoeae* was identified by colonial morphology, Gram's stain, and oxidase testing. Gonococcal strains were subcultured onto chocolate agar plates, preserved in tryptone-based soy broth and then stored at −70 °C until used.

Antimicrobial susceptibility testing

Minimum inhibitory concentrations (MICs; mg/L) of *N. gonorrhoeae* isolates to penicillin, tetracycline, ciprofloxacin, spectinomycin, azithromycin, ceftriaxone and cefixime were determined on Difco GC medium base agar supplemented with 1% BBL™, IsoVitaleX™ enrichment (Becton, Dickinson and Company) using the agar dilution method recommended by the Clinical and Laboratory Standards Institute (CLSI) [13]. Gonococcal isolates were subcultured from frozen stocks onto chocolate agar and the resulting colonies were re-subcultured at 36 °C in 5% CO_2 for 18–20 h before antimicrobial susceptibility testing was performed. Concentrations of antibiotics used were: penicillin, 0.06–8 mg/L; tetracycline, 0.125–16 mg/L; ciprofloxacin, 0.06–8 mg/L; spectinomycin, 4–128 mg/L; azithromycin,0.015–2048 mg/L; ceftriaxone, 0.002–0.5 mg/L and cefixime,0.002–0.5 mg/L. All antibiotics were purchased from Sigma Aldrich (USA), except for azithromycin, which was purchased from Shanghai yuanye Bio-Technology Co., Ltd. 95% ethanol was used to dissolve azithromycin powder to obtain a stock solution of 4096 mg/L; azithromycin stock was further diluted with distilled water to prepare twofold working dilutions. ATCC49226 and WHO reference strains G, K, M, O, P were used as quality controls for MIC determinations. Results were interpreted according to the CLSI standard, except for azithromycin that used breakpoints recommended by the European Committee on Antimicrobial Susceptibility Testing (EUCAST); www.eucast.org [14].Criteria for decreased susceptibility to ceftriaxone (MIC ≥ 0.125 mg/L) and cefixime (MIC ≥ 0.25 mg/L) were defined by WHO [9].

Identification and typing of β-lactamase and *tetM* encoding plasmids

β-lactamase production was determined by the paper acidometric method [15]. Isolates were classified as high level resistant to tetracycline (TRNG) if MICs were ≥16 mg/L and resistant (plasmid-mediated) to penicillin (PPNG) if they were β-lactamase positive [16]. The type of β-lactamase and *tetM* encoding plasmids were determined by PCR [17].

Genetic determinants associated with decreased susceptibility to ESCs and resistance of *N. gonorrhoeae*to azithromycin

Amplification of *penA* and *mtrR* genes and 23S rRNA were performed using published primers and conditions [18–20]. 14 gonococcal isolates with decreased susceptibility to ceftriaxone or cefixime were tested for *penA* mutations, including 3 isolates that had decreased susceptibility to both cefixime and ceftriaxone; all isolates were tested for mutations in *mtrR* and 41strains (including all 36 azithromycin-resistant and 5 randomly selected azithromycin sensitive strains) were tested for 23S rRNA mutations. PCR products were sequenced twice in both directions using an Applied Biosystems 3730XL DNA automatic sequencer. The nucleotide and deduced amino acid sequences were analyzed using the EditSeq program (LaserGene software [version 7.1; DNAStar Corp.]) and aligned against their respective prototypes using the Megalign program (LaserGene software). Standard sequences used for alignment in the study were: PBP2; wild strain LM306 (GenBank accession no. M32091 [18]); 4 alleles of 23S rRNA (GenBank accession no. AF450074 to AF450081 [20]) and mtrR (GenBank accession no. Z25796 [19]).

Molecular epidemiologic typing

N. gonorrhoeae multiantigen sequence typing (NG-MAST) was performed on all isolates (n = 126) as described [21]. The allele numbers of *por* and *tbpB*, and the sequence types (STs) were assigned using the NG-MAST website (www.ng-mast.net).

Statistical analysis

Statistical analysis was performed using statistical software IBM SPSS Statistics version 19.0 for comparisons of proportions. The level of significance was set at $P < 0.05$.

Results

Antimicrobial susceptibility testing

Antimicrobial susceptibility testing of 126 gonococcal isolates obtained from Hefei, China, between January, 2014 and November, 2015, is indicated in Table 1. Resistance to penicillin and tetracycline was 73.8% (93/126) and 81.7% (103/126), respectively; all isolates were resistant to ciprofloxacin. 28.6% (36/126) of isolates were resistant to azithromycin; among them,36.1% (13/36) displayed high-level azithromycin resistance (MIC ≥ 256 mg/L). No isolates were found to be fully resistant to spectinomycin, ceftriaxone or cefixime. However,14 isolates (11.1%) displayed decreased susceptibility to ceftriaxone (MIC ≥ 0.125 mg/L, n = 10), cefixime (MIC ≥ 0. 25 mg/L, n = 1) or to both ESCs (n = 3).Two azithromycin-resistant isolates also exhibited reduced susceptibility to ceftriaxone. Overall, plasmid mediated resistance to either penicillin or tetracycline was exhibited by 60.3% (76/126) of isolates: 39.7% (50/126) were PPNG; 31.7% (40/126) were TRNG and 11.1% (14/126) were PPNG/TRNG. 80% (40/50) PPNG isolates carried the Asia type β-lactamase encoding plasmid and 20% (10/50) harbored the African type plasmid. No Toronto plasmid was detected. 97.5% (39/40) of TRNG isolates carried the Dutch type *tetM* containing plasmid and the remainder carried the American-type.

Characterization of resistance in *penA* and *mtrR* genes and 23S rRNA

Mutations in the penA gene

We sequenced the *penA* gene from 14 isolates that displayed decreased susceptibility to ceftriaxone (n = 10), cefixime (n = 1) or to both ESCs (n = 3) (Table 2). Six PBP2 amino acid sequence patterns were identified, including a mosaic allele (XXXV) [18]. PBP2 allele XIII [19] was the predominant type (n = 5), followed by mosaic allele XXXV (n = 3) and alleles XVIII (n = 3), V (n = 1), XVII (n = 1) and XXI (n = 1) [19, 22, 23]. The three isolates that harbored mosaic allele XXXV had decreased susceptibility to cefixime; one (of the 3) displayed decreased susceptibility to both ceftriaxone and cefixime. Among 11 non-mosaic isolates that included 10 with decreased susceptibility to ceftriaxone and 1 to both ESCs, seven harbored alleles XIII, XVII and XXI and displayed an A501V mutation in PBP2. Three isolates with allele XVIII possessed an A501T mutation and one had a G542S mutation.

Mutations in the mtrR gene

All 126 isolates had mutations in the *mtrR* gene. Adenine (A) was deleted in the promoter region of *mtrR* in 107(87.3%) strains; there was no difference (p = 0.181) in isolates with MICs ≥1 mg/L to azithromycin (33/36 [91.7%]) compared to isolates with an MIC ≤0.5 mg/L (74/90 [82.2%]). However, the G45D mutation in the *mtrR* gene was identified more often in azithromycin-resistant isolates (25/36 [69.4%]) than in susceptible isolates (9/90 [10%]) ($p < 0.01$). The A40D mutation was present in three isolates with (lower) azithromycin MICs of 0.125 mg/L; these isolates also exhibited reduced cefixime and/or ceftriaxone susceptibility. The A39T mutation was found in 16 more sensitive isolates, having MICs to azithromycin >0.125 mg/L but <0.5 mg/L.

Mutations in domains of 23S rRNA

All 36 azithromycin-resistant isolates and five –susceptible isolates were tested for mutations in 23S rRNA. The A2143G (*N. gonorrhoeae* numbering) mutation was identified in four alleles in the13 isolates with high-level

Table 1 Antimicrobial susceptibility of *Neisseria gonorrhoeae* isolates (n = 126) from Hefei, China (2014–2015)

Antimicrobial breakpoints (susceptible/resistant [mg/L])	Number			MIC (mg/L)		
	Susceptible	Intermediate	Resistant	Range	MIC_{50}	MIC_{90}
Penicillin G (S ≤ 0.06/*R* ≥ 2)	0	33	93	0.125 to >8	2	>8
Tetracycline (S ≤ 0.25/*R* ≥ 2)	2	21	103	0.25 to >16	4	>16
Ciprofloxacin (S ≤ 0.06/*R* ≥ 1)	0	0	126	0.25 to >8	>8	>8
Azithromycin(S ≤ 0.25/*R* ≥ 1)	48	42	36	≤0.015 to >2048	0.5	> 2048
Spectinomycin (S ≤ 32/*R* ≥ 128)	126	0	0	8 to 32	16	32
Cefixime (S ≤ 0.25)	126	0	0	0.004 to 0.25	0.03	0.06
Ceftriaxone(S ≤ 0.25)	126	0	0	0.004 to 0.25	0.06	0.125

MIC minimum inhibitory concentration

azithromycin resistance (MICs ≥ 256 mg/L). AC259 9 T mutation in four alleles was found in four isolates (MICs, 8 to 32 mg/L).No mutations were found in the five azithromycin-susceptible isolates.

Sequence-based molecular epidemiologic typing

The 126 *N. gonorrhoeae* isolates were assigned to 86 different NG-MASTs (abbreviated henceforth as STs); 53 (61.6%) STs were novel. 19 STs were shared by ≥ 2 isolates and 67 STs were represented only in single isolate. The most common ST was7469, represented by 6 isolates (4.8%), followed by ST1866 (5 isolates; 4.0%). All ST7469 isolates were comprised exclusively of the Dutch-type TRNG; all ST1866 isolates were resistant to azithromycin (MIC ≥ 1 mg/L).Three isolates, which possessed the *penA* mosaic allele XXXV and had decreased susceptibility to cefixime (MIC = 0.25 mg/L), belonged to different STs (ST12200, ST12647, ST13044) but shared identical *tbpB*10.

Discussion

A high prevalence of resistance to antimicrobials previously used for the treatment of gonorrhea was documented in Hefei (2014–15) in this study: penicillin (68.9%); tetracycline (80.6%) and ciprofloxacin (100%). Similar levels of resistance to ciprofloxacin, tetracycline and penicillin have been reported in *N. gonorrhoeae* isolates from other cities in China: Nanjing (penicillin 67.7%, tetracycline 97.9% and ciprofloxacin 98.8%, in 2011–2012) [17]; Shanghai (penicillin 90%, tetracycline 82.56% and ciprofloxacin 100%, in 1988–2013) [11] and Guangzhou (penicillin 90.1% and ciprofloxacin 98%, in 2008–2013) [12]. A high percentage of PPNG and TRNG isolates was also identified in Hefei. Because penicillin and tetracycline are no longer used for the treatment of gonorrhea in China, continued high resistance may have been the result of having used these antimicrobials to treat other infections, particularly in patients who self-medicate, which is common in China [24].

Resistance to azithromycin was 28.6%, higher than had been reported from certain other countries, such as Japan [25] and Spain [26] during this period. We found that 10.3% (13/126) of isolates were highly resistant to azithromycin (MIC > 2048 mg/L). *N. gonorrhoeae* isolates with high-level azithromycin resistance have also been reported from other Chinese cities; Hanghzou [27] and Guangzhou [28]. Similar to other reports [29, 30], our isolates with high-level azithromycin resistance all contained the mutation A2143G in 4 alleles in the peptidyltransferase loop of domain V of 23S rRNA. The C2599T mutation was found in 23S rRNA alleles in four moderately azithromycin-resistant *N. gonorrhoeae* isolates (representing MICs of 8, 16, and 32 mg/L).

There are no reports of ceftriaxone treatment failures in China. The percentage of isolates with decreased susceptibility to ceftriaxone (MIC ≥ 0.125 mg/L) was 10.3%

Table 2 Characteristics of *N gonorrhoeae* isolates (n = 14) with increased MICs to ceftriaxone (MIC, 0.125 mg/L) or cefixime (MIC, 0.25 mg/L)

Strain number	MIC(mg/L)		PBP2 allele	NG-MAST
	Ceftriaxone	Cefixime		
HF17	0.125	0.06	XVIII	ST12197[b]
HF20	0.125	0.25	XIII	ST1577
HF37	0.125	0.25	XXXV[a]	ST12200[b]
HF 42	0.125	0.125	XIII	ST12192[b]
HF 109	0.06	0.25	XXXV[a]	ST12647[b]
HF 141	0.125	0.125	XIII	ST12662[b]
HF 149	0.125	0.125	XIII	ST12192[b]
HF 152	0.125	0.06	V	ST12198[b]
HF 154	0.125	0.06	XIII	ST 2318
HF 156	0.125	0.25	XXXV[a]	ST13044[b]
HF 163	0.125	0.06	XVIII	ST3356
HF 169	0.125	0.06	XVII	ST13133[b]
HF 170	0.125	0.125	XXI	ST13134[b]
HF 175	0.125	0.06	XVIII	ST12479[b]

[a]Mosaic penA alleles
[b]Novel STs

(13/126) in Hefei in 2014–2015, which is higher than the corresponding 4.5% reported from another eastern Chinese city, Nanjing, between 2011 and 2012 [17]. The proportions of ceftriaxone non-susceptible isolates (MIC ≥ 0.125 mg/L) in Shanghai, the largest city in eastern China, were 7%–13% from 2011 to 2013 [11]. This suggests the possibility that resistance to extended spectrum cephalosporins (ESCs) may be increasing in eastern China. PBP2 is targeted by cephalosporins and mutations in PBP2 may lead to a decline in susceptibility to ESCs [31]. Four (3.2%) of our isolates had reduced susceptibility to cefixime (MIC = 0.25 mg/L); three (ST12200, ST12647, ST13044) had the mosaic allele XXXV. The majority (7/11 [63.6%]) of non-mosaic isolates with decreased susceptibility to ceftriaxone harbored mutations in PBP2 at position 501 (A501V or A501T). Other studies have also found that A501 mutations in non-mosaic *penA* alleles play an important role in decreased sensitivity to ESCs [32]. A G542S mutation in PBP2 has been tentatively linked epidemiologically to higher ceftriaxone MICs [33] but an absolute correlation with a *penA* fixed-point mutation has not been shown. ST1407 *N. gonorrhoeae* strains, which display decreased susceptibility to ESCs or full resistance [34], and have spread worldwide, were not identified in Hefei. Five different STs (ST10367, ST12649, ST12650, ST12657, ST13132) that shared the same *tbpB*110 with ST1407 were identified but their *por* alleles were different (by 13 to 37 nucleotides) than *por*908 of ST1407; all isolates with these STs were susceptible to both ceftriaxone and cefixime. ST1407, however, has been isolated in Shanghai [35].

Significant diversity of isolates was identified among 126 isolates that were divided into 86 NG-MAST STs. Notably, ST1866 has been reported only from China and identified to be associated with high level azithromycin resistance [28]. The 5 ST1866 isolates in this study were azithromycin-resistant strains; three had high level resistance to azithromycin.

Conclusions

This is the first study that describes antimicrobial resistance profiles and molecular determinants of *N. gonorrhoeae* strains isolated from Hefei, China. *N. gonorrhoeae* isolates from Hefei, during 2014–2015, possessed high level resistance to antimicrobials previously recommended for the treatment of gonorrhea, e.g., penicillin, tetracycline and ciprofloxacin. Azithromycin-resistance was documented in 28.6% of isolates, higher than that reported from other areas of the world. No isolates were found to be resistant to ceftriaxone, cefixime or spectinomycin. However, 11.1% isolates had decreased susceptibility to ESCs, which was often associated with mutations in the *penA* gene. Gonococcal isolates were distributed into diverse NG-MAST sequence types.

Abbreviations

AMR: Antimicrobial resistance; CLSI: Clinical and Laboratory Standards Institute; ESCs: Extended-spectrum cephalosporins; GASP: Gonococcal antimicrobial surveillance programme; GISP: Gonococcal Isolate Surveillance Project; MIC: Minimum inhibitory concentration; NG-MAST: *Neisseria gonorrhoeae* multi-antigen sequence typing; PBP: Penicillin-binding protein; PPNG: Penicillinase-producing *N. gonorrhoeae*; ST: Sequence type; STD: Sexually transmitted disease; STI: Sexually transmitted infection; TRNG: Tetracycline-resistant *N. gonorrhoeae*; WHO: World Health Organization

Acknowledgements

We thank Dr. Na Wang for assistance in collection of gonococcal isolates, Dr. Magnus Unemo for providing WHO reference strains and Dr. Peter A. Rice for assistance in writing the manuscript.

Funding

This study was supported by Nature Science foundation of Anhui Province (No. 090413143).

Authors' contributions

FXJ co-directed the project and supervised the collection of bacterial isolates. QL assisted with antimicrobial susceptibility testing, performed sequencing, assigned NG-MAST designations and prepared the first draft of the manuscript. XHS also co-directed the project and was involved in preparation of the manuscript. WJL carried out antimicrobial susceptibility testing and identified *tetM* and β-lactamase. All authors read and approved the final manuscript.

Competing interests

The authors declare no competing interests.

Consent for publication

Not applicable.

Author details

[1]Department of Dermatology, Anhui Provincial Hospital, Hefei 230001, China. [2]STD clinic, Institute of Dermatology, Chinese Academy of Medical Sciences & Peking Union Medical College, Nanjing 210042, China.

References

1. Newman L, Rowley J, Vander Hoorn S, Wijesooriya NS, Unemo M, Low N, et al. Global estimates of the prevalence and incidence of four curable sexually transmitted infections in 2012 based on systematic review and Global reporting. PLoS One. 2015;10:e0143304.
2. National health and Family Planning Commision of China. General situation of national legal infectious diseases in 2015. Available at: http://www.nhfpc.gov.cn/jkj/s3578/201602/b9217ba14e17452aad9e45a5bcce6b65. Accessed February 18, 2016.
3. Bignell C, Unemo M. European STI Guidelines Editorial Board. 2012 European guideline on the diagnosis and treatment of gonorrhoea in adults. Int J STD AIDS. 2013;24:85–92.
4. Unemo M. Current and future antimicrobial treatment of gonorrhoea - the rapidly evolving *Neisseria gonorrhoeae* continues to challenge. BMC Infect Dis. 2015;15:364.
5. Bercot B, Belkacem A, Goubard A, Mougari F, Sednaoui P, La Ruche G, Cambau E. High-level azithromycin-resistant *Neisseria gonorrhoeae* clinical isolate in France, March 2014. Euro Surveill. 2014;19(44): pii= 20951. Available online: http://www.eurosurveillance.org/ViewArticle.aspx?ArticleId=20951.
6. Katz AR, Komeya AY, Soge OO, Kiaha MI, Lee MV, Wasserman GM, et al. *Neisseria gonorrhoeae* with high-level resistance to azithromycin: case report of the first isolate identified in the United States. Clin Infect Dis. 2012;54:841–3.

7. Stevens K, Zaia A, Tawil S, Bates J, Hicks V, Whiley D, et al. *Neisseria gonorrhoeae* isolates with high-level resistance to azithromycin in Australia. J Antimicrob Chemother. 2015;70:1267–8.
8. Ni C, Xue J, Zhang C, Zhou H, van der Veen S. High prevalence of *Neisseria gonorrhoeae* with high-level resistance to azithromycin in Hangzhou. China J Antimicrob Chemother. 2016;71:2355–7.
9. World Health Organization (WHO). Global action plan to control the spread and impact of anti-microbial resistance in *Neisseria gonorrhoeae*. Geneva: WHO. Available from: http://apps.who.int/iris/bitstream/10665/44863/1/9789241503501_eng.pdf.
10. Kirkcaldy RD, Harvey A, Papp JR, Del Rio C, Soge OO, Holmes KK, Hook EW 3rd, Kubin G, Riedel S, Zenilman J, Pettus K, Sanders T, Sharpe S, Torrone E. *Neisseria gonorrhoeae* Antimicrobial Susceptibility Surveillance - The Gonococcal Isolate Surveillance Project, 27 Sites, United States, 2014. MMWR Surveill Summ. 2016;65:1–19.
11. Gu WM, Chen Y, Yang Y, Wu L, Hu WZ, YL J. Twenty-five-year changing pattern of gonococcal antimicrobial susceptibility in Shanghai: surveillance and its impact on treatment guidelines. BMC Infect Dis. 2014;14:731.
12. Cao W, Liang JY, Li XD, Bi C, Yang RD, Liang YH, et al. Trends in antimicrobial resistance in *Neisseria gonorrhoeae* isolated from Guangzhou, China, 2000 to 2005 and 2008 to 2013. Sex Transm Dis. 2015;42:27–9.
13. CLSI: *Neisseria gonorrhoeae*. In Performance Standards for Antimicrobial Susceptibility Testing; Twenty-Second Informational Supplement. CLSI document M100-S25. Wayne, PA: Clinical and Laboratory Standards Institute. 2015:80–82.
14. Breakpoint tables for interpretation of MICs and zone diameters: version 1.3. European Committee on Antimicrobial Susceptibility Testing. Available from: http://www.eucast.org/clinical_breakpoints/. Accessed January 15, 2012.
15. Sng EH, Yeo KL, Rajan VS. Simple method for detecting penicillinase-producing *Neisseria gonorrhoeae* and *Staphylococcus aureus*. Br J Vener Dis. 1981;57:141–2.
16. Barry PM, Klausner JD. The use of cephalosporins for gonorrhea: the impending problem of resistance. Expert Opin Pharmacother. 2009;10:555–7.
17. Li S, Su XH, Le WJ, Jiang FX, Wang BX, Rice PA. Antimicrobial susceptibility of *Neisseria gonorrhoeae* isolates from symptomatic men attending the Nanjing sexually transmitted diseases clinic (2011–2012): genetic characteristics of isolates with reduced sensitivity to ceftriaxone. BMC Infect Dis. 2014;14:622.
18. Allen VG, Farrell DJ, Rebbapragadą A, Tan J, Tijet N, Perusini SJ, et al. Molecular analysis of antimicrobial resistance mechanisms in *Neisseria gonorrhoeae* isolates from Ontario, Canada. Antimicrob Agents Chemother. 2011;55:703–12.
19. Liao M, Gu WM, Yang Y, Dillon JA. Analysis of mutations in multiple loci of *Neisseria gonorrhoeae* isolates reveals effects of PIB, PBP2 and MtrR on reduced susceptibility to ceftriaxone. J Antimicrob Chemother. 2011;66:1016–23.
20. Ng LK, Martin I, Liu G, Bryden L. Mutation in 23S rRNA associated with macrolide resistance in *Neisseria gonorrhoeae*. Antimicrob Agents Chemother. 2002; 46:3020–5.
21. Martin IM, Ison CA, Aanensen DM, Fenton KA, Spratt BG. Rapid sequence-based identification of gonococcal transmission clusters in a large metropolitan area. J Infect Dis. 2004;189:1497–505.
22. Whiley DM, Limnios EA, Ray S, Sloots TP, Tapsall JW. Diversity of penA alterations and subtypes in *Neisseria gonorrhoeae* strains from Sydney, Australia, that are less susceptible to ceftriaxone. Antimicrob Agents Chemother. 2007;51:3111–6.
23. Martin I, Sawatzky P, Allen V, Hoang L, Lefebvre B, Mina N, et al. Emergence of *Neisseria gonorrhoeae* isolates with decreased susceptibilities to ceftriaxone and cefixime in Canada : 2001-2010. Sex Transm Dis. 2012;39:316–23.
24. Bi P, Tong S, Parton KA. Family self-medication and antibiotics abuse for children and juveniles in a Chinese city. Soc Sci Med. 2000;50:1445–50.
25. Shigemura K, Osawa K, Miura M, Tanaka K, Arakawa S, Shirakawa T, et al. Azithromycin resistance and its mechanism in *Neisseria gonorrhoeae* strains in Hyogo Japan. Antimicrob Agents Chemother. 2015;59:2695–9.
26. Cobo F, Cabezas-Fernández MT, Cabeza-Barrera MI. Antimicrobial susceptibility and typing of *Neisseria gonorrhoeae* strains from southern Spain, 2012–2014. Enferm Infecc Microbiol Clín. 2016;34:3–7.
27. Xue J, Ni C, Zhou H, Zhang C, van der Veen S. Occurrence of high-level azithromycin-resistant *Neisseria gonorrhoeae* isolates in China. J Antimicrob Chemother. 2015;70:3404–5.
28. Liang JY, Cao WL, Li XD, Bi C, Yang RD, Liang YH, et al. Azithromycin-resistant *Neisseria gonorrhoeae* isolates in Guangzhou, China (2009–2013): coevolution with decreased susceptibilities to ceftriaxone and genetic characteristics. BMC Infect Dis. 2016;16:152.
29. Lynagh Y, Mac Aogáin M, Walsh A, Rogers TR, Unemo M, Crowley B. Detailed characterization of the first high-level azithromycin-resistant *Neisseria gonorrhoeae* cases in Ireland. J Antimicrob Chemother. 2015;70:2411–3.
30. Chisholm SA, Wilson J, Alexander S, Tripodo F, Al-Shahib A, Schaefer U, et al. An outbreak of high-level azithromycin resistant *Neisseria gonorrhoeae* in England. Sex Transm Infect. 2015;92:365–7.
31. Bharat A, Demczuk W, Martin I, Mulvey MR. The effect of variants of penicillin-binding protein 2 (PBP2) on cephalosporin and carbapenem susceptibilities in *Neisseria gonorrhoeae*. Antimicrob Agents Chemother. 2015;59:5003–6.
32. Olsen B, Lan PT, Golparian D, Johansson E, Tran HK, Unemo M. Antimicrobial susceptibility and genetic characteristics of *Neisseria gonorrhoeae* isolates from Vietnam, 2011. BMC Infect Dis. 2013;13:40.
33. Whiley DM, Goire N, Lambert SB, Ray S, Limnios EA, Nissen MD, et al. Reduced susceptibility to ceftriaxone in *Neisseria gonorrhoeae* is associated with mutations G542S, P551S and P551L in the gonococcal penicillin-binding protein 2. J Antimicrobial Chemother. 2010;65:1615–8.
34. Unemo M, Golparian D, Nicholas R, Ohnishi M, Gallay A, Sednaoui P. High-level cefixime- and ceftriaxone-resistant *N. gonorrhoeae* in Europe (France): novel penA mosaic allele in a successful international clone causes treatment failure. Antimicrob. Agents Chemother. 2012;56:1273–80.
35. Chen SC, Yin YP, Dai XQ, Unemo M, Chen XS. First nationwide study regarding ceftriaxone resistance and molecular epidemiology of *Neisseria gonorrhoeae* in China. J Antimicrob Chemother. 2016;71:92–9.

6

Sero-epidemiological assessment of *Chlamydia trachomatis* infection and sub-fertility in Samoan women

S. Menon[1†], S. H. Stansfield[1†], M. Walsh[2†], E. Hope[3†], L. Isaia[4], A. A. Righarts[2], T. Niupulusu[5], S. V. A. Temese[6], L. Iosefa-Siitia[7], L. Auvaa[3], S. A. Tapelu[8], M. F. Motu[7], T. Suaalii-Sauni[9], P. Timms[10], P. C. Hill[2] and W. M. Huston[1,11,12*]

Abstract

Background: In our recent village-based cross-sectional study, the prevalence of nucleic acid amplification technique (NAAT) diagnosed *Chlamydia trachomatis* (CT) in sexually active Samoan women was very high (36 %), and test positivity was associated with sub-fertility. We conducted a serological and epidemiological analysis in these participants to identify if serological data can provide further insight into the potential contribution of CT to sub-fertility in this population.

Methods: Serological prediction of CT associated sub-fertility was conducted using a series of commercial tests. The correlation between fertility or sub-fertility, behavioral factors, and serologically predicted CT associated sub-fertility was determined.

Results: A positive antibody reaction against the *Chlamydia* Major Outer Membrane Protein (MOMP) was significantly associated with sub-fertility, with 50 % of infertile women being positive. Serum IgG and IgA antibodies against MOMP correlated with current infection measured by urine NAAT, suggesting longer term infections are common in this population. *Chlamydia pneumoniae* antibodies were frequently detected in this population (84 %), and unexpectedly, were significantly associated with sub-fertility.

Conclusions: The high prevalence of chlamydial infection and of positive chlamydial sub-fertility results suggests that CT is an important and frequent contributory factor to sub-fertility in this population.

Keywords: Chlamydia, Pacific islands, samoa, female sub-fertility, diagnosis, serology

Background

Chlamydia trachomatis (CT) is the most common bacterial sexually transmitted infection (STI) in the world. The infection can result in the development of serious sequelae such as pelvic inflammatory disease (PID), ectopic pregnancy and tubal factor infertility (TFI) in women. The reported prevalence of CT infection is in the range 1.4–8.7 % when the general population in high income countries is screened [1–3]. The prevalence of CT infection in Samoa was previously estimated by Sullivan et al. [4] to be 30.9 % based on antenatal screening. Similarly, in women who attended antenatal clinics between 2004 and 2005 in the Pacific Islands (Fiji, Kiribati, Samoa, Solomon Islands, Tonga, and Vanuatu), CT prevalence was 26.1 % in women under 25 years old, and 11.9 % in women over 25 [5].

The proportion of infertility attributable to CT in the Samoan population is not known. Such infertility results from tissue damage to the fallopian tubes (tubal factor infertility, TFI) that remains after the active infection is cleared, meaning that diagnosis using nucleic acid amplification tests (NAAT) is not necessarily suitable. There are numerous serological or chlamydia antibody tests (CAT) that have been developed to diagnose CT infertility, that have been validated on cohorts of women with evidence of tubal damage detected by hysterosalpingography or

* Correspondence: Wilhelmina.Huston@uts.edu.au
†Equal contributors
[1]Institute of Health and Biomedical Innovation, Queensland University of Technology, Brisbane, Australia
[11]School of Life Sciences, Faculty of Science, University of Technology Sydney, Broadway, Sydney, NSW, Australia
Full list of author information is available at the end of the article

laparoscopy [6–11]. In a meta-analysis of published evaluations of various assays, Broeze and co-workers identified that micro immune-fluorescence (MIF) was the most sensitive, but relatively low in specificity [6]. In the same study the MEDAC and ANIlabsystems enzyme linked immunosorbant assays (ELISA) appeared to most specific, although less sensitive than MIF, to diagnose women with uni or bi-lateral tubal damage detected by surgical or sonographic technologies [6]. However, a proportion of women with infertility and who are serologically positive by CAT have no detectable tubal blockage but still require IVF (*in vitro* fertilization) to conceive, and this could be at least partially due to tubal damage not detectable by the current surgical or sonographic methods [7, 12–14]. In lower and middle income countries (LMIC) studies generally report higher prevalence of CT in infertile or sub-fertile women (39-55 %), although the prevalence of CT infection in fertile women is also generally high [15–17].

We recently reported a high prevalence (36.0 % by NAAT) of CT in Samoan women using community-based screening and survey of sexually active women aged 18–29 years having unprotected sex, and current infection was associated with women who were defined as being sub-fertile [14, 18]. Here, we conducted a serological study to evaluate the prevalence of CT associated sub-fertility in these same women.

Methods

The study design and sampling protocol has been previously reported [15, 18]. Women (n = 239) were recruited into a cross-sectional study on CT and sub-fertility from the Pacific nation of Samoa during 2011. Participant inclusion criteria were age between 18 and 29 years, living in the village for at least a year and being sexually active without using any forms of contraception (including condoms, birth control pills, or other forms of contraception) for at least a year. Women were excluded if they had a medical condition, or had undergone a procedure that made it impossible to become pregnant. Participants provided informed written consent, completed an interviewer-led questionnaire and provided biological samples. The nurse who conducted the interview asked the sexual behavioral questions using socially acceptable language and used a two step approach to gauge sexual behavior (as previously described) [18]. The questionnaire responses were used to assign women to 'sub-fertile' (or otherwise 'fertile'). Sub-fertility was defined as at least 12 months of unprotected intercourse without conceiving a pregnancy [18]. The NAAT results have been previously analysed and presented [18], all participants provided a urine specimen that was analysed for CT infection status using the BD ProbeTec ET assay in accordance with the manufacturer's instructions and using positive and negative controls (BD Biosciences, USA) [18].

The participant sera were tested for CT antibodies using the following commercial ELISAs: CT-IgG ELISA-plus MEDAC (peptides from the MOMP protein, referred to as MEDAC MOMP, used to diagnose past or current infection), cHSP60-IgG ELISA MEDAC (cSHP60 protein), ANIlabsystems CT IgG (peptides from MOMP, marketed to diagnose CT infertility), CT IgA ELISA MEDAC (used to diagnose current CT infection), *Chlamydia pneumoniae* (CP)-IgG-ELISA MEDAC (used to diagnose current CP infection) (summarized in Table 1). The assay positive or negative results in accordance with the manufacturer's instructions were used for this study (positive, negative, unequivocal (excluded), invalid (excluded)). Titres were not included in this study as they are not part of these commercial tests. All sera were tested with all assays, however, any that were unequivocal or invalid more than once were excluded from the data for that assay and any participants that did not have a complete dataset and valid test result in every assay were completely excluded from the analysis in Table 2 and Fig. 2. The serological testing of CT associated sub-fertility is difficult because the gold standard (MIF) has low specificity leading to high false positives (although it had the highest accuracy using area under the curve), but is reported to be highly subjective and labor intensive [6]. Therefore we chose to test the population using ELISA as we prioritised highest specificity in order to

Table 1 Commercial serological assays and previously reported sensitivity and specificity

Assay name	Antigen	Study reference name	Sensitivity	Specificity	Detected group	Ref
MEDACCT-IgG ELISA-plus MEDAC	MOMP	MEDAC MOMP	55 %	87 %	Women with infertility (n = 315)	[7]
cHSP60-IgG ELISA MEDAC	cHSP60	MEDAC cHSP60	69 %	93 %	Women with TFI (n = 70)	[22]
MEDAC IgG CT pELISA and cHSP60 IgG ELISA	Combination of both assays	MEDAC Infertile				[22]
ANIlabsystems CT IgG	MOMP peptides	ANIlab	91 %	84 %	CT NAAT diagnosed infection and infertility (*n* = 303)	[16]
CT IgA ELISA MEDAC	MOMP peptides	MEDAC IgA			NAAT diagnosed current infection	[23]
C. pneumoniae-IgG-ELISA MEDAC	MOMP peptides	MEDAC Cpn	91.3 %	93.3 %	Current pneumonia and MIF positive status for *C. pneumoniae*	[24]

Table 2 Participant data included/excluded in the Table 3 analysis

Variable	Included, n	Excluded, n	OR (95 % C.I.)	*P* value for OR
Age				
18–24	97	48	1	
25–29	64	29	1.11 (0.63–1.94)	0.720
Smoking				
Never	129	59	1	
Ex-smoker/ current	33	18	0.84 (0.44–1.61)	0.600
Fertility status				
Sub-fertile	59	28	1	
Fertile	103	49	1.00 (0.57–1.75)	0.990

Comparison of Age, smoking and fertility status for participants included or excluded in the study. Participants excluded had no statistical difference in age, smoking or fertility status ($P > 0.05$)

indicate the amount of CT associated sub-fertility in Samoa, and a format that could enable us to compare several tests in a timely manner. We selected multiple ELISAs to compare the different IgG responses and we also included IgA to indicate how many of the infections were recent. Finally, we included a *Chlamydia pneumoniae* ELISA to enable comparison of the sero-prevalence of a related and very common pathogen.

All statistical analyses were conducted in R statistical environment (3.0.3) using the 'EpiR (0.9-57) and 'metafor' package (1.9-2) for calculation and presentation (forest plots) of odds ratios (OR). All analyses were conducted to measure the association of assay results with sub-fertility. OR and 95 % confidence intervals (CI) were calculated with restricted maximum likelihood estimates of error.

Results

Antibody test results for CT associated sub-fertility

Two hundred thirty-nine women meeting the inclusion and exclusion criteria participated in the study; 90 were defined as being sub-fertile and 149 were defined as fertile with a history of having had a pregnancy. The association of CT with sub-fertility was analysed using each of the commercial serological assays. As shown in Fig. 1a, women who were sub-fertile were significantly more likely to have a positive serological reaction in the MEDAC MOMP assay ($p = 0.045$). 42 out of 82 sub-fertile women were positive in the MEDAC MOMP assay, whereas 52 out of a total of 139 fertile women were positive. It is important to note that 34 sub-fertile women have been excluded for this assay from Fig. 1a because they had unequivocal results. One of the most common immunological reactions that was associated with infertility in previous studies [9, 12], an antibody response to cHSP60, was not significantly associated with sub-fertility: the sero-prevalence of antibodies to cHSP60 did not differ based on fertility with 57 % of both infertile and fertile women being positive (44 out of 76 sub-fertile women were positive and 73 out of 129 fertile women were positive). The

a

Assay (+ / -)	Equivocal/ Invalid	Sub-fertile Assay +	Sub-fertile Assay -	Fertile Assay +	Fertile Assay -	Total	Odds Ratio [95% CI]	P
MEDAC Infertile (+ / -)	38	29	45	36	91	239	1.63 [0.89 , 2.98]	0.113
MEDAC MOMP (+ / -)	18	42	40	52	87	239	1.76 [1.01 , 3.05]	0.045
MEDAC cHSP60 (+ / -)	34	44	32	73	56	239	1.05 [0.59 , 1.87]	0.855
MEDAC IgA (+ / -)	10	13	69	15	132	239	1.66 [0.75 , 3.68]	0.211
ANIlab (+ / -)	26	43	35	59	76	239	1.58 [0.90 , 2.77]	0.108
MEDAC C.pneumoniae (+ / -)	6	82	3	119	29	239	6.66 [1.96 , 22.60]	<0.001

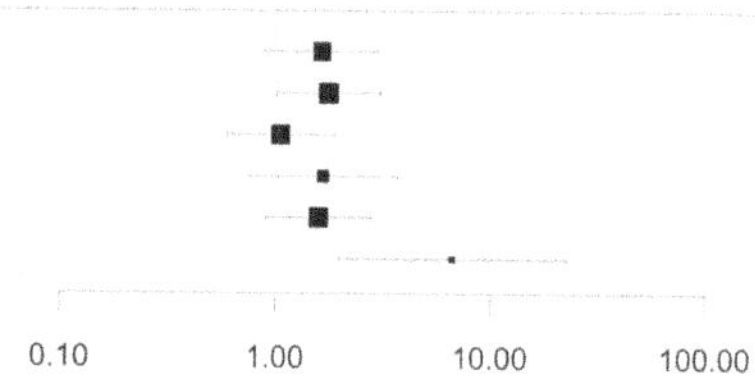

b

Assay (+ / -)	Equivocal/ Invalid	Chlamydia + Assay +	Chlamydia + Assay -	Chlamydia - Assay +	Chlamydia - Assay -	Total	Odds Ratio [95% CI]	P
MEDAC Infertile (+ / -)	38	41	36	24	100	239	4.75 [2.52 , 8.92]	<0.001
MEDAC MOMP (+ / -)	18	53	28	41	99	239	4.57 [2.55 , 8.20]	<0.001
MEDAC cHSP60 (+ / -)	34	56	20	61	68	239	3.12 [1.68 , 5.78]	<0.001
MEDAC IgA (+ / -)	10	17	66	11	135	239	3.16 [1.40 , 7.13]	0.004
ANIlab (+ / -)	26	57	21	45	90	239	5.43 [2.93 , 10.04]	<0.001
MEDAC C.pneumoniae (+ / -)	6	74	9	127	23	239	1.49 [0.65 , 3.39]	0.340

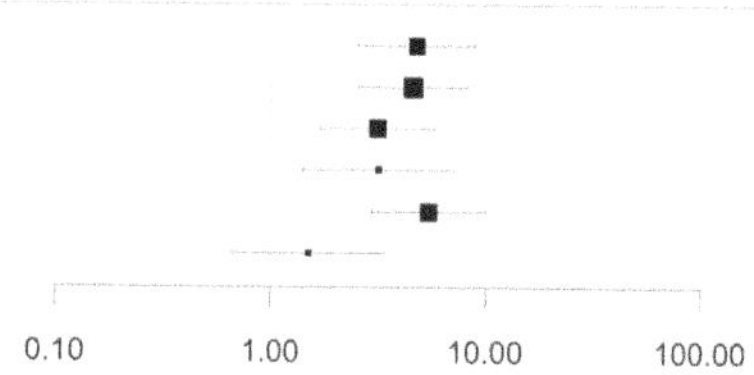

Fig. 1 Analysis of the association of serological responses to *Chlamydia* with fertility and CT infection status. **a**. The figure shows Forest plots and Odds Ratio of the association of a positive reaction in the serological assay listed to the right with being infertile. The assay is indicated in the left column. The number of participants that were positive or negative in the serum assay(s) according to their fertile or infertile status are shown on the figure. All 239 participant specimens were tested in each assay. Samples that were unequivocal or not reproducible upon multiple testing were excluded for each assay and these are indicated in the column titled invalid/unequivocal on the table. **b.** The number of participants positive or negative in each serological assay, grouped according to also being positive or negative for current CT infection by urine NAAT (Chlamydia +/–) are shown on the figure. OR with 95 % CI and P values are indicated at the right of the figures

MEDAC Infertile assay, which is recommended by the manufacturer to be a positive reaction in both the MEDAC MOMP and MEDAC cHSP60 assays, was not significantly associated with sub-fertility in this study (in the infertile group 29 women were positive out of 74 total who had results in the assay, and 36 were positive out of a total of 127 women with reportable results in the fertile group).

The overall IgG sero-positivity to CT in this population was 43 % according to the MEDAC MOMP results, and 50 % according to the ANIlab assay. The numbers reported in Fig. 1 vary depending on the number of women that had consistent reportable results in the assay (i.e. we did not include unequivocal or invalid results, these are indicated to the left of the figure).

We included testing for a common respiratory pathogen (*Chlamydia pneumoniae*) to provide an indication of serological responses in our population tested. Women who were sub-fertile were significantly more likely to have a positive reaction in MEDAC CP assay ($p < 0.001$) (Fig. 1a). The overall presence of sero-positivity to this pathogen (CP) was 86 %. A positive urine NAAT result did not correlate with a positive CP serological result, supporting that this assay is not likely to be detecting CT cross reactivity. Although, pairwise analysis did show that MEDAC MOMP positivity significantly correlated with MEDAC CP (chisel $p = 0.042$), meaning that women positive in MEDAC MOMP were more likely to be positive in MEDAC CP (OR 3.63 [95 % CI: 0.92–21.11]).

We previously reported that the current infection by urine NAAT was 36 % in this cohort [18], therefore, we evaluated if the serological results correlate with current infection status. Women who were NAAT positive were significantly more likely to be positive in the serological assays for CT by all of assays tested (Fig. 1b). The high association of IgG against MOMP and cHSP60 and current infection by urine NAAT in this cohort could imply these are longer term infections, consistent with the lack of STI screening and treatment programs in this country. A positive result in the MEDAC IgA significantly correlated with NAAT positive status (Fig. 1b) ($p = 0.004$). This higher frequency of IgG (compared to IgA) correlating with NAAT diagnosed current infection further supports the possibility that in this population there are frequent repeat or longer term infections, given that IgA tends to be produced early and in primary infections.

In the evaluation of demographic factors in relation to subfertility and serological results, we only included data for participants that had a recordable result in every test and answered every demographic question ($n = 162$). The details of the participants excluded from this analysis are provided in Table 2, and there were no significant differences in the sub-fertility status or other factors in those excluded compared to those included. Age (older women were more likely to be fertile, $p < 0.010$), MEDAC MOMP ($p = 0.040$), NAAT positive for CT ($p = 0.003$) and MEDAC CP ($p = 0.007$) were all significant factors that associated with sub-fertility in this subset of participants (Table 3).

We used the same subset of specimens to assess test concordance. As shown in the Venn diagram (Fig. 2) there was often concordance between the serological

Table 3 Analysis of demographic factors and serological results that associate with sub-fertility

Variable	Sub-fertile, n	Fertile, n2[a]	OR (95 % C.I.)	*P* value for OR
Age				
18–24	47	50	1	
25–29	12	53	0.24 (0.11–0.51)	<0.01
BMI				
Normal Weight	12	21	1	
Overweight	27	35	0.74 (0.31–1.80)	0.498
Obese	20	47	0.74 (0.31–1.80)	0.512
Smoking				
Never	46	83	1	
Ex-smoker/current	13	20	1.17 (0.53–2.57)	0.691
MEDAC Infertile				
Negative	34	72	1	
Positive	25	31	1.71 (0.88–3.33)	0.115
MEDAC MOMP				
Negative	28	66	1	
Positive	31	37	1.97 (1.03–3.78)	0.040
MEDAC cHSP60				
Negative	25	41	1	
Positive	34	62	0.9 (0.47-1.72)	0.749
MEDAC IgA				
Negative	49	89	1	
Positive	10	14	1.3 (0.55-3.14)	0.563
ANIlab				
Negative	29	59	1	
Positive	30	44	1.39 (0.73–2.64)	0.318
MEDAC CP				
Negative	2	22	1	
Positive	57	81	7.74 (1.75–34.21	0.007
CT Infection (NAAT)				
Negative	28	73	1	
Positive	31	30	2.69 (1.39–5.24)	0.003

[a]This table only includes women who had consistent results in all assays ($n = 162$), 59 sub-fertile and 103 fertile women

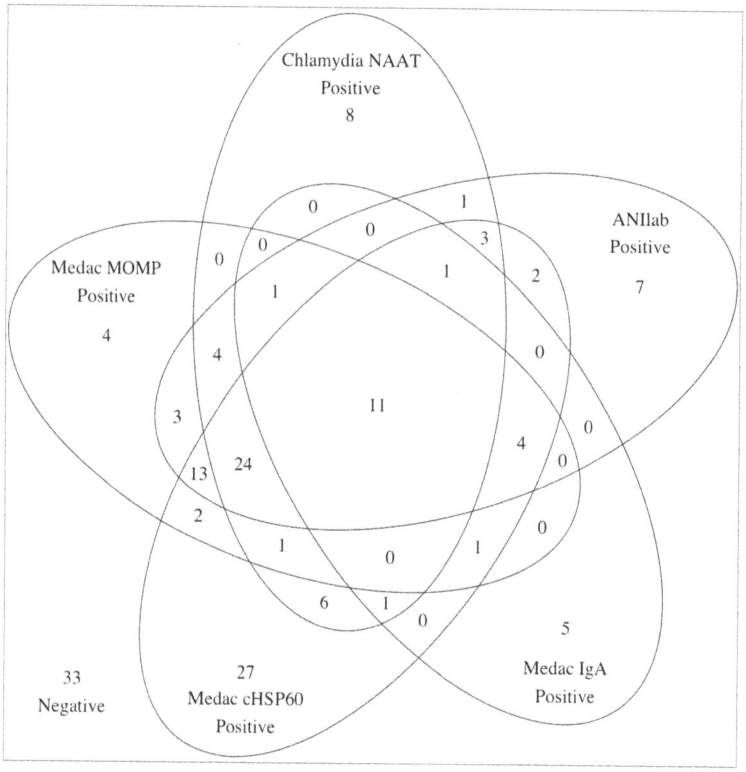

Fig. 2 Venn diagram to demonstrate concordance between serological assays and CT NAAT results. The diagram shows the number of participants positive in each of the assays and those who were positive in more than one assay. The two MOMP assays (MEDAC IgG and ANIlab) and NAAT results showed considerable concordance. The samples that were negative in all assays are also indicated on the figure, only the 162 samples that had a valid result in all of these assays are included in the Venn diagram

assays and NAAT results, particularly between NAAT, MEDAC MOMP, and ANIlab. This supports the notion that these assays are reporting serological responses to CT and are not likely to be a consequence of non-specific reactivity.

Discussion

The results of this study imply that up to half (51 % infertile women positive for MEDAC MOMP) of women who are sub-fertile in this population could have CT as a cause or contributing factor. To our knowledge this is one of the highest burdens of CT associated sub-fertility reported to date. This is higher than most studies report, even those conducted in fertility clinics, but is consistent with a fertility clinic study in India that found a similar prevalence [15]. This may be a reflection of the absence of routine screening and treatment for CT infections in this population.

A possible limitation of our study is that the serological results may be influenced by a higher number of repeat infections given the high prevalence of infection in this population. These repeat infections may lead to higher positives in these assays which use absorbance thresholds that have been designed on clinically defined infertile cohorts, often in settings with a much lower background prevalence. The MEDAC Infertile assay was not significantly associated with sub-fertility in this study. Nevertheless, the high prevalence of cHSP60 antibodies (one of the components of the MEDAC test) could suggest that chronic infections or sequelae are high in this population. Most studies that found a significant association had TFI as the specified measure for infertility [9]. In this population we have limited knowledge of the other fertility factors as this was a village-based survey in the absence of any gynecological investigations that would normally be conducted in a fertility clinic. In addition it is of course possible, considering the sensitivities of obtaining sexual behavior information that some women were mis-classified with respect to sub-fertility. The amount of sexual activity was of course not the same for each woman, affecting their individual probabilities of becoming pregnant.

The study findings indicated a higher fertility rate in the older ages (although the inclusion criteria were limited to the most reproductive years). The higher fertility in the older women is not that unexpected and is likely because this study is based on sexually active women who were all within the ideal reproductive age, so the longer the period of sexual activity the more likely the women are to have conceived. Alternatively, this could be explained by an increased desire of these women (25–29 year olds) to achieve pregnancy leading to increased sexual activity.

It was unexpected to find a significant correlation of sero-positivity to *C. pneumoniae* with sub-fertility in this population. It is difficult to determine if this is actually serological cross reactivity (or a genuine association). Serology to *C. pneumoniae,* or the presence of the organism, has been previously found to significantly correlate with various diseases [19–21], but not with sub-fertility. One possible explanation for this finding could be that the infertile women in this population have tissue lesions or adhesions in the fallopian tube that may form a reservoir for the pathogen and perhaps the immune response to this reserve of CP may exacerbate the CT pathology that results in development of tubal sub-fertility. This persistence in the scarring site could explain the high prevalence of CP serology that, whilst significant, is not causal for sub-fertility. Alternatively, this could be a chance result. Firstly, as the prevalence of *Chlamydia pneumoniae* antibodies is very high (in both fertile and infertile women), statistical analysis tends to lead to an overestimation of the odds ratio. Secondly, the number of participants included in the analysis is relatively low (n = 233).

MEDAC MOMP and MEDAC CP were the only assays that significantly correlated with sub-fertility, suggesting that whilst serology is a much more feasible manner to measure possible chlamydial infertility in the developing world setting the current assays may be confounded by the high prevalence, and only MEDAC MOMP may be suitable.

Conclusions

The high prevalence of *C. trachomatis* infections in Samoa is likely to be leading to high rates of preventable sub-fertility in this population. The results reported here using serological and epidemiological data collection indicate that CT-associated sub-fertility could be a factor for as much as half of the burden of sub-fertility in sexually active women in this reproductive age range in Samoa.

Ethics approval and consent to participate

Participants provided informed written consent, completed an interviewer-led questionnaire and provided biological samples. The initial ethical approval was from National University of Samoa, Samoa National Health Service Board approval for the use of the Laboratory and staff, and the Samoa Ministry of Women approved the village based survey, and the Samoan Ministry of Health. Ethical approval was previously reported [19] and Queensland University of Technology Human Research Ethics Committee approval was also obtained (approval number 1100000276).

Consent for publication

Not applicable.

Abbreviations

CI: confidence interval; CT: *Chlamydia trachomatis*; MEDAC Cpn: MEDAC *Chlamydia pneumoniae* pELISA; MEDAC MOMP: MEDAC *Chlamydia trachomatis* pELISA; MEDAC cHSP60: MEDAC *C. trachomatis* cHSP60 ELISA; MEDAC Infertile: combined results from MEDAC MOMP and MEDAC cHSP60 to predict infertile/chronic sequelae outcomes from *C. trachomatis* infections as per the manufacturer's recommendations; OR: odds ratio; NAAT: nucleic acid amplification test.

Competing interests

The authors declare that they have no competing interests.

Authors' contributions

SM conducted laboratory serology assays. EH, IL, TN, SVAT, ISL, LA, SAT, MMF, and TSS all contributed to recruitment, questionnaire implementation and field work. SM, SSH, MW, EH, AAR, PT, PH, WMH analysed data and contributed to design. All authors had input into manuscript preparation. All authors read and approved the final manuscript.

Acknowledgements

We would like to thank the participants, village leaders, and various stakeholders in Samoa.

Funding

The field study was funded by the New Zealand Aid Programme. The serological assay component was funded by a Queensland Government Smart State National and International Research Alliance for research into *Chlamydia* awarded to P Timms, sub-project leader W Huston.

Author details

[1]Institute of Health and Biomedical Innovation, Queensland University of Technology, Brisbane, Australia. [2]Centre for International Health, University of Otago, Dunedin, New Zealand. [3]National University of Samoa, Apia, Samoa. [4]National Health Service Laboratory Division, Apia, Samoa. [5]Samoa Family Health Association, Apia, Samoa. [6]Centre for Samoan Studies, National University of Samoa, Apia, Samoa. [7]Samoa National Council of Churches, Apia, Samoa. [8]Samoa AIDS Foundation, Apia, Samoa. [9]Victoria University of Wellington, Wellington, New Zealand. [10]Faculty of Science, Health, Education and Engineering, University of the Sunshine Coast, Maroochydore, Australia. [11]School of Life Sciences, Faculty of Science, University of Technology Sydney, Broadway, Sydney, NSW, Australia. [12]School of Life Sciences, University of Technology Sydney, PO BOX 123, Broadway, Sydney, NSW 2007, Australia.

References

1. Adams EJ, Charlett A, Edmunds WJ, Hughes G. Chlamydia trachomatis in the United Kingdom: a systematic review and analysis of prevalence studies. Sex Transm Infect. 2004;80(5):354–62.
2. Kohli R, Konya WP, Obura T, Stones W, Revathi G. Prevalence of genital *Chlamydia* infection in urban women of reproductive age, Nairobi, Kenya. BMC Res Notes. 2013;6:44.

3. Lewis D, Newton DC, Guy RJ, Ali H, Chen MY, Fairley CK, Hocking JS. The prevalence of *Chlamydia trachomatis* infection in Australia: a systematic review and meta-analysis. Bmc Infect Dis. 2012;12:113.
4. Sullivan EA, Koro S, Tabrizi S, Kaldor J, Poumerol G, Chen S, O'Leary M, Garland SM. Prevalence of sexually transmitted diseases and human immunodeficiency virus among women attending prenatal services in Apia, Samoa. Int J Std Aids. 2004;15(2):116–9.
5. Cliffe SJ, Tabrizi S, Sullivan EA, Pacific Islands Second Generation HIVSG. *Chlamydia* in the Pacific region, the silent epidemic. Sex Transm Dis. 2008; 35(9):801–6.
6. Broeze KA, Opmeer BC, Coppus SF, Van Geloven N, Alves MF, Anestad G, Bhattacharya S, Allan J, Guerra-Infante MF, Den Hartog JE, et al. *Chlamydia* antibody testing and diagnosing tubal pathology in subfertile women: an individual patient data meta-analysis. Hum Reprod Update. 2011;17(3):301–10.
7. Land JA, Gijsen AP, Kessels AGH, Slobbe MEP, Bruggeman CA. Performance of five serological chlamydia antibody tests in subfertile women. Hum Reprod. 2003;18(12):2621–7.
8. Tiitinen A, Surcel HM, Halttunen M, Birkelund S, Bloigu A, Christiansen G, Koskela P, Morrison SG, Morrison RP, Paavonen J. *Chlamydia trachomatis* and chlamydial heat shock protein 60-specific antibody and cell-mediated responses predict tubal factor infertility. Hum Reprod. 2006;21(6):1533–8.
9. Witkin SS, Askienazy-Elbhar M, Henry-Suchet J, Belaisch-Allart J, Tort-Grumbach J, Sarjdine K. Circulating antibodies to a conserved epitope of the Chlamydia trachomatis 60 kDa heat shock protein (hsp60) in infertile couples and its relationship to antibodies to *C. trachomatis* surface antigens and the Escherichia coli and human HSP60. Hum Reprod. 1998;13(5):1175–9.
10. Witkin SS, Linhares IM. *Chlamydia trachomatis* in subfertile women undergoing uterine instrumentation - An alternative to direct microbial testing or prophylactic antibiotic treatment. Hum Reprod. 2002;17(8):1938–41.
11. Spandorfer SD, Neuer A, LaVerda D, Byrne G, Liu HC, Rosenwaks Z, Witkin SS. Previously undetected *Chlamydia trachomatis* infection, immunity to heat shock proteins and tubal occlusion in women undergoing *in-vitro* fertilization. Hum Reprod. 1999;14(1):60–4.
12. Coppus SF, Land JA, Opmeer BC, Steures P, Eijkemans MJ, Hompes PG, Bossuyt PM, van der Veen F, Mol BW, van der Steeg JW. *Chlamydia trachomatis* IgG seropositivity is associated with lower natural conception rates in ovulatory subfertile women without visible tubal pathology. Hum Reprod. 2011;26(11):3061–7.
13. Coppus SF, Opmeer BC, Logan S, van der Veen F, Bhattacharya S, Mol BW. The predictive value of medical history taking and *Chlamydia* IgG ELISA antibody testing (CAT) in the selection of subfertile women for diagnostic laparoscopy: a clinical prediction model approach. Hum Reprod. 2007;22(5):1353–8.
14. Keltz MD, Sauerbrun-Cutler MT, Durante MS, Moshier E, Stein DE, Gonzales E. Positive *Chlamydia trachomatis* serology result in women seeking care for infertility is a negative prognosticator for intrauterine pregnancy. Sex Transm Dis. 2013;40(11):842–5.
15. Malik A, Jain S, Rizvi M, Shukla I, Hakim S. *Chlamydia trachomatis* infection in women with secondary infertility. Fertil Steril. 2009;91(1):91–5.
16. Muvunyi CM, Dhont N, Verhelst R, Temmerman M, Claeys G, Padalko E. *Chlamydia trachomatis* infection in fertile and subfertile women in Rwanda: prevalence and diagnostic significance of IgG and IgA antibodies testing. Hum Reprod. 2011;26(12):3319–26.
17. Siemer J, Theile O, Larbi Y, Fasching PA, Danso KA, Kreienberg R, Essig A. *Chlamydia trachomatis* infection as a risk factor for infertility among women in Ghana, West Africa. Am J Trop Med Hyg. 2008;78(2):323–7.
18. Walsh MS, Hope E, Isaia L, Righarts A, Niupulusu T, Temese SV, Iosefa-Siitia L, Auvaa L, Tapelu SA, Motu MF, et al. Prevalence of *Chlamydia trachomatis* infection in Samoan women aged 18 to 29 and assessment of possible risk factors: a community-based study. Trans Royal Soc Trop Med Hyg. 2015; 109(4):245–51.
19. Ramirez JA. Isolation of Chlamydia pneumoniae from the coronary artery of a pateient with coronary atherosclerosis. The Chlamydia pneumoniae/ atherosclerosis Study group. Ann Intern Med. 1996;125(12):979–82.
20. Balin BJ, Gerard HC, Arking EJ, Appelt DM, Branigan PJ, Abrams JT, Whittum-Hudson JA, Hudson AP. Identification and localization of *Chlamydia pneumoniae* in the Alzheimer's brain. Med Microbiol Immunol. 1998;187(1):23–42.
21. Gerard HC, Dreses-Werringloer U, Wildt KS, Deka S, Oszust C, Balin BJ, Frey WH, 2nd, Bordayo EZ, Whittum-Hudson JA, Hudson AP. *Chlamydophila (Chlamydia) pneumoniae* in the Alzheimer's brain. FEMS Immunol Med Microbiol. 2006;48(3):355–66.
22. Hjelholt A, Christiansen G, Johannesson TG, Ingerslev HJ, Birkelund S. Tubal factor infertility is associated with antibodies against *Chlamydia trachomatis* heat shock protein 60 but not human HSP60. Hum Reprod. 2011;26:2069–76.
23. van den Broek IVF, Land JA, van Bergen JEAM, Morr'e SA, van der Sande MAB: *Chlamydia trachomatis* antibody testing in vaginal mucosal material versus blood samples of women attending a fertility clinic and an STI clinic. Obstet Gynecol International 2014, 2014(601932).
24. De Ory F, Guisasola ME, Eiros JM. Detection of *Chlamydophila pneumoniae* IgG in paired serum samples: comparison of serological techniques in pneumonia cases. APMIS. 2006;114(4):279–84.

7

Antimicrobial resistance of *Neisseria gonorrhoeae* in Germany: low levels of cephalosporin resistance, but high azithromycin resistance

Susanne Buder[1*†], Sandra Dudareva[2,3*†], Klaus Jansen[2], Anna Loenenbach[2], Sergejs Nikisins[2,4,5], Andrea Sailer[2], Eva Guhl[1], Peter K. Kohl[1], Viviane Bremer[2] and GORENET study group

Abstract

Background: The widespread antimicrobial resistance of *Neisseria gonorrhoeae* is a serious problem for the treatment and control of gonorrhoea. Many of the previously effective therapeutic agents are no longer viable. Because *N. gonorrhoeae* infections are not reportable in Germany, only limited data on disease epidemiology and antimicrobial susceptibility patterns are available. The Gonococcal Resistance Network (GORENET) is a surveillance project to monitor trends in the antimicrobial susceptibility of *N. gonorrhoeae* in Germany in order to guide treatment algorithms and target future prevention strategies.

Methods: Between April 2014 and December 2015, data on patient-related information were collected from laboratories nationwide, and susceptibility testing was performed on 537 *N. gonorrhoeae* isolates forwarded from the network laboratories to the Conciliar Laboratory for gonococci. Susceptibility results for cefixime, ceftriaxone, azithromycin, ciprofloxacin and penicillin were defined according to EUCAST 4.0 standards. Percentages, medians and interquartile ranges (IQR) were calculated.

Results: Altogether, 90% of isolates were from men. The median age was 32 (IQR 25–44) years for men and 25 (IQR 22–40) years for women (p-value < 0.001). The most frequently tested materials among men were urethral (96.1%) and rectal swabs (1.7%), and among women, it was mainly endocervical and vaginal swabs (84.3%). None of the isolates were resistant to ceftriaxone. Furthermore, 1.9% (in 2014) and 1.4% (in 2015) of the isolates were resistant to cefixime, 11.9% and 9.8% showed resistance against azithromycin, 72.0% and 58.3% were resistant to ciprofloxacin, and 29.1% and 18.8% were resistant to penicillin.

Conclusions: Resistance to ceftriaxone was not detected, and the percentage of isolates with resistance to cefixime was low, whereas azithromycin resistance showed high levels during the observation period. The rates of ciprofloxacin resistance and penicillin resistance were very high across Germany. Continued surveillance of antimicrobial drug susceptibilities for *N. gonorrhoeae* remains highly important to ensure efficient disease management.

Keywords: *Neisseria gonorrhoeae*, Gonorrhoea, Antimicrobial resistance, Resistance surveillance

* Correspondence: dr.susanne.buder@web.de; DudarevaS@rki.de
†Equal contributors
[1]German Consiliary Laboratory for Gonococci, Department of Dermatology and Venerology, Vivantes Hospital Berlin, Berlin, Germany
[2]Department for Infectious Disease Epidemiology, Robert Koch Institute, Berlin, Germany
Full list of author information is available at the end of the article

Background

The worldwide development of antimicrobial resistance in *Neisseria gonorrhoeae* is a serious problem for the treatment and control of gonorrhoea. Treatment opportunities are dramatically limited because many of the previously recommended therapeutic agents are no longer effective.

The World Health Organization (WHO) [1], the Centers for Disease Control and Prevention (CDC) [2], and the European Centre for Disease Prevention and Control (ECDC) [3] have called for action to confine the spread of multidrug-resistant *N. gonorrhoeae* by enhancing the surveillance system of *N. gonorrhoeae* susceptibility testing and by strengthening laboratory capacities to perform culture and antimicrobial resistance testing. Representative coverage of collected data, unified *N. gonorrhoeae* susceptibility testing methods and interpretation standards are of great importance [4–6].

Extended spectrum cephalosporins (ESCs) are the last agents effective against *N. gonorrhoeae*. However, resistance to ESCs is increasingly common [7–13], causing concern that the efficacy of this substance group could expire in the near future [5–10]. Due to the worldwide rising resistance of *N. gonorrhoeae* against cefixime in recent years, the treatment guidelines needed to be changed accordingly. Thus, cefixime is no longer recommended as first-line therapy in many countries [14–16] and new therapy guidelines and action plans have been developed to keep gonorrhoea a treatable disease. In 2014 the German STI Society implemented new therapy guidelines for Germany. These guidelines recommend the use of the ESC ceftriaxone (1000 mg single dose i.m. or i.v.), now in combination with azithromycin as dual therapy (1.5 g single dose p.o.), as the first-line treatment [17]. The use of cefixime (800 mg single dose p.o.) should be reserved for cases where parenteral treatment is not possible and ideally after susceptibility testing.

Because gonorrhoea is not a notifiable disease in Germany, only very limited data about epidemiology and antimicrobial resistance against *N. gonorrhoeae* are available. Furthermore, no standard operating procedures or unified protocols for *N. gonorrhoeae* susceptibility testing have been established in Germany. To date, information about *N. gonorrhoeae* susceptibility can be derived from several cross-sectional, regionally limited studies [18–21] through the German antibiotic resistance surveillance programme (ARS) and 100–120 isolates submitted to Euro-GASP yearly through the Consiliary Laboratory (CL) for gonococci [22]. Within this Euro-GASP collection, isolates resistant against ceftriaxone (MIC >0.125 mg/L) have been observed in Germany. Resistance against ceftriaxone was shown by 6.5% (n = 7) of all German Euro-GASP isolates in 2011, while in the following years 2012–2014, one isolate per year (1%) could be identified with ceftriaxone resistance. Cefixime resistance (MIC >0.125 mg/L) in German Euro-GASP isolates ranged between 5.7% and 12.9% (n = 13, 11.9% in 2010; n = 11, 10.2% in 2011; n = 6, 5.7% in 2012; n = 13, 12.9% in 2013) [22]. In 2014, there was no detection of cefixime-resistant isolates in Euro-GASP.

To implement continuous routine data collection on epidemiology and antimicrobial susceptibility testing for *N. gonorrhoeae* in German laboratories (aim 1) and to collect isolates for testing in the German CL for gonococci with unified methodology (aim 2), we set up a *N. gonorrhoeae* resistance network (GORENET).

We analysed the data and isolates collected through GORENET in 2014 and 2015 to guide treatment algorithms and targeted prevention strategies in Germany.

Methods

To characterise laboratories testing for *N. gonorrhoeae* in Germany and indicate laboratories for recruitment, we performed a cross-sectional survey between June and August 2013, as described previously [23]. From the laboratories that expressed an interest in participating, we recruited private and hospital laboratories for GORENET, prioritizing those with a wider catchment area and a higher number of *N. gonorrhoeae* tests per quarter. The laboratories in Germany have no predefined catchment areas, and practitioners are free to choose laboratories for cooperation. For a better geographical coverage of the data, we strove to recruit laboratories from all regions in Germany and laboratories that use any gradient Etest for *N. gonorrhoeae* susceptibility testing, at least for azithromycin, ceftriaxone and cefixime. Participation was voluntary, and there was no financial compensation for laboratories to participate in the study. The data collection protocol was confirmed by the data protection officer at the Robert Koch Institute (RKI), Berlin. Additional approval from an ethics committee was deemed to be unnecessary.

Continuous routine data collection

From GORENET network laboratories, continuous routine data on all samples tested for *N. gonorrhoeae* antimicrobial susceptibility were collected between April 2014 and December 2015. The network laboratories submitted data to the RKI (further labelled as samples). The collected data included sample identification number, information on test results, sampled material (urethral swab, urine, vaginal swab, cervical swab, rectal swab, pharyngeal swab, and other material), date of sampling, date of testing, district code, gender and year of birth. If the district code of the patient was not available, we used the code of the laboratory instead. Based on the year of birth, we calculated the person's age at the time of sampling. If the date of testing was not available, we used the date when the isolate was received in the CL.

Data were transmitted electronically to the RKI. Laboratories entered the data either in an online questionnaire (VOXCO Command Center 3) or in a preformatted Excel spreadsheet (.xls). Data on *N. gonorrhoeae* susceptibility from laboratories willing to participate in GORENET but already submitting their susceptibility data (including data on a wide range of other agents) to the German Antibiotic Resistance Surveillance Programme (ARS) were extracted from the ARS database. We performed plausibility checks on all reported data.

Based on the district codes, we described the geographical distribution of the samples tested for *N. gonorrhoeae* antimicrobial susceptibility. Each district code or respective 3-digit postal code corresponded to one district in Germany. We used samples tested for susceptibility from participating laboratories to describe tested persons by gender, age, sampled material and treating specialist. Susceptibility results from participating laboratories are used for national surveillance, but not presented in this paper.

An overview of the analysis of samples tested for *N. gonorrhoeae* susceptibility in network laboratories is given in Table 1.

Isolate collection and susceptibility testing

The network laboratories were asked to send *N. gonorrhoeae* isolates from the samples tested for antimicrobial susceptibility between April 2014 and December 2015 to the CL for extended and comparative susceptibility testing (further labelled as isolates). There were no criteria used to preselect isolates that should be sent to CL. The sample identification number was used to link isolates to samples. For all received isolates, we confirmed *N. gonorrhoeae* by using a combination of culture on non-selective agar medium, rapid oxidase production assays and determining the presence of Gram-negative diplococci using microscopy and the Phadebact Monoclonal GC OMNI Test (Pharmacia Diagnostics, Piscataway, NJ, USA). Susceptibility testing was performed and MIC were detected by using Etest (bioMérieux SA, Marcy-l'Étoile, France) according to the manufacturer's instructions for ceftriaxone, cefixime, azithromycin, penicillin and ciprofloxacin. To define resistance, we used the criteria of the European Committee on Antimicrobial Susceptibility Testing EUCAST 4.0 (2014) [24]. The presence of beta-lactamase enzyme production, which provides high-level resistance to penicillins, was detected by using the nitrocefin test (BBL DrySlide™, Becton, Dickinson, NJ, USA). Isolates testing positive for beta-lactamase were defined as penicillinase-producing *N. gonorrhoeae* (PPNG).

The working stock of *N. gonorrhoeae* isolates was stored at −80 °C. *N. gonorrhoeae* strains ATCC 49226 and WHO-reference strains G, K, M, O and P were used with each batch of Etest as quality controls [25]. Ceftriaxone and cefixime were tested twice when the MIC was ≥0.125 mg/L. Isolates tested in the CL were characterized by their resistance patterns.

An overview of the analysis of isolates tested in CL is given in Table 1. Note that a direct comparison of historical German data with current GORENET data was not possible because different methods for isolate collection were in place before GORENET was rolled out and the geographical coverage was different.

For categorical variables we calculated percentages and, for continuous variables, medians together with interquartile ranges (IQR) were determined. Percentages were compared by Chi-squared or Fisher's exact tests, and medians were compared with the Wilcoxon-Mann-Whitney test, where applicable. The Kruskal-Wallis test was used to compare continuous variables between more than two categories. Significance level was set at a p-value < 0.05.

Results

Of the 100 laboratories that were interested in participating in GORENET, 31 were selected for recruitment, and 23 agreed and reported data to GORENET. The reasons for declining participation in GORENET were not using the Etest for *N. gonorrhoeae* susceptibility

Table 1 Isolates tested for susceptibility in network laboratories and in CL, number of laboratories and isolates included in analysis and description of performed analysis for each data source

	Number of laboratories	Number of samples or isolates			In manuscript referred as	Performed analysis
		Total	2014	2015		
Samples tested for *N. gonorrhoeae* susceptibility in network laboratories	23	1654	727	927	Samples	Geographical, age and gender distribution. Sampled material and treating specialist
Isolates tested in CL	16	537	261	276	Isolates	Susceptibility for ceftriaxone, cefixime, azithromycin, penicillin and ciprofloxacin. Presence of beta-lactamases

testing ($n = 5$) and too much time and effort needed for participation ($n = 3$).

Continuous routine data collection

Twenty-three participating laboratories reported to the RKI in total 1654 *N. gonorrhoeae* samples tested for susceptibility. Of them, 727 were collected from April to December 2014, and 927 were collected from January to December 2015. Overview of the reported samples is given in Table 1.

The number of reported samples varied between 2 and 305 per laboratory, with a median of 43 samples (IQR 24–86). In total 47.1% of the samples were reported by three laboratories, which provided information on 209 (in Hamburg), 265 (in Berlin) and 305 (in North Rhine-Westphalia) samples, respectively.

The number of reported *N. gonorrhoeae* samples varied by administrative district between 1 and 209 (Fig. 1). The three laboratories submitting the majority of the data were located in the areas with >50 samples.

Central and northern Germany were represented equally. Data from southern Germany mostly originated from the larger cities.

Overall, 90.0% of samples tested for susceptibility in network laboratories were from men; 9.5% were from women and in nine samples, information on gender was not available. The median age of tested men and women was 33 (IQR 25–44) and 27 (IQR 22–40) years respectively (p-value < 0.001). The distribution of

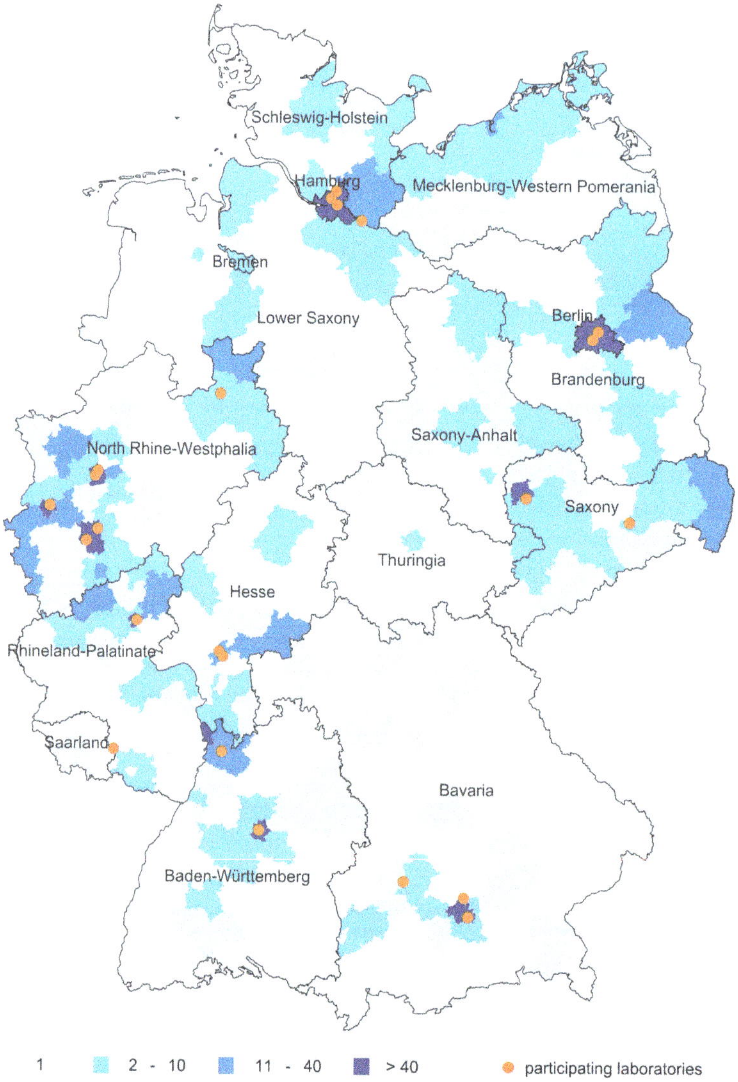

Fig. 1 Distribution of *N. gonorrhoeae* samples by district in Germany. One thousand, six hundred and fifty-four samples from April 2014 to December 2015 (1366 defined by district code of the patient, 288 defined by district code of the laboratory). Map developed with RegioGraph Software

N. gonorrhoeae susceptibility testing by age group and gender is displayed in Fig. 2.

Most tested samples from men were from urethral (96.1%) and rectal swabs (1.7%), while among women samples came from predominately endocervical or vaginal swabs (84.3%). Most of the samples tested from men were ordered by urologists (74.4%) and from women by gynaecologists (79.7%). Distribution by gender (*p*-value = 0.25), age (*p*-value = 0.28 for men and *p*-value = 0.87 for women), tested material (*p*-value = 0.15 for men and p-value = 0.07 for women) and ordering specialist (*p*-value = 0.63 for men and *p*-value = 0.73 for women) did not differ between the years 2014 and 2015.

Isolate collection and susceptibility testing

From the recruited 23 laboratories submitting information on samples tested for *N. gonorrhoeae* susceptibility, 16 sent isolates to the CL. We received 261 viable isolates collected between April and December 2014 and 276 viable isolates collected between January and December 2015. It was determined that 91.4% of isolates were from men, 8.4% were from women, and for one of the samples the gender was unspecified. The median age was 33 (IQR 26–43) for isolates from men and 28 (IQR 23–41) for isolates from women. These 537 isolates were tested for susceptibility in the CL. An Overview of the isolates tested in CL is given in Table 1. The results of the AMR testing of all isolates are summarized in Table 2. The percentage of resistant, intermediate and susceptible isolates did not significantly differ by age or gender.

No resistance to ceftriaxone (MIC >0.125 mg/L) was detected in 2014 or 2015 (Fig. 3). In 2014, two isolates showed MICs at the estimated breakpoint of 0.125 mg/L. One of these isolates displayed further resistance to cefixime, azithromycin and ciprofloxacin and showed an intermediate test result to penicillin (isolate 1, Table 3). Another isolate displayed resistance to ciprofloxacin and penicillin, while it was intermediate to azithromycin and had a MIC value at the breakpoint for cefixime (isolate 10, Table 3).

Altogether, 1.9% (*n* = 5) in 2014 and 1.4% (*n* = 4) in 2015 of the isolates displayed resistance (MIC >0.125 mg/L) to cefixime. The majority of isolates (62.5% in 2014 and 77.9% in 2015) showed low MICs of ≤0.016 mg/L to cefixime (Fig. 4). In 2014, 3.8% (*n* = 10) and in 2015, 1.4% (*n* = 4) of the isolates had a MIC of 0.125 mg/L at the estimated breakpoint.

All isolates with resistance to cefixime displayed resistance to ciprofloxacin. Three of the nine cefixime-resistant strains also showed resistance to azithromycin. No cefixime-resistant strain was susceptible to penicillin (3 resistant, 6 intermediate).

One cefixime-resistant isolate (MIC 0.25 mg/L) displayed additional resistance against azithromycin and ciprofloxacin, intermediate susceptibility against penicillin and showed reduced susceptibility to ceftriaxone at the breakpoint of MIC 0.125 mg/L (isolate 1, Table 3).

All isolates displaying resistance to cefixime were from men.

A total of 11.9% (2014) and 9.8% (2015) of the isolates showed resistance against azithromycin (MIC >0.5 mg/L). In addition, there was a high percentage of *N. gonorrhoeae* strains with intermediate susceptibility (33.7% in 2014 and 28.3% in 2015) and the MIC distribution of the susceptible strains appeared closer to intermediate breakpoint (MIC >0.38 mg/L) (Fig. 5). The MICs of resistant strains were mostly low and showed a distribution concentrating around the breakpoint (MIC >0.5 mg/L).

In 2015, one isolate displayed high-level resistance to azithromycin (MIC >256 mg/L). This isolate also showed high-level resistance to penicillin and resistance to ciprofloxacin, but was susceptible to ceftriaxone and cefixime.

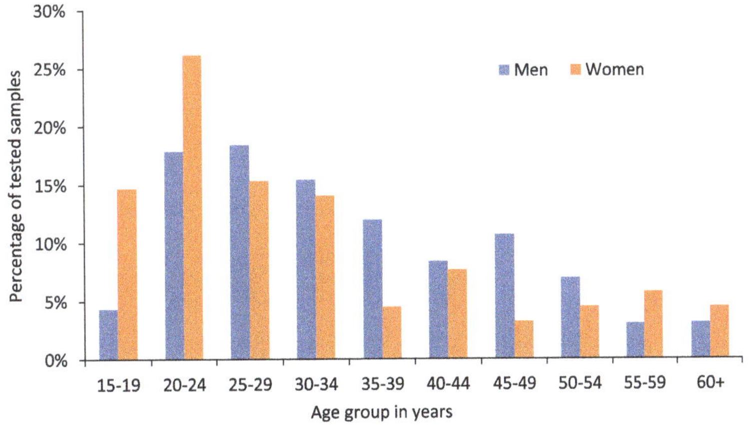

Fig. 2 *N. gonorrhoeae* samples tested in participating laboratories, by age group and gender, *n* = 1642

Table 2 Number and percentage of *N. gonorrhoeae* isolates testing susceptible, intermediate and resistant against cefixime, ceftriaxone, azithromycin, penicillin and ciprofloxacin, $n = 261$ for year 2014 and $n = 276$ for year 2015, *p-value < 0.05

	Susceptible		Intermediate		Resistant	
	Number (percentage, %)		Number (percentage, %)		Number (percentage, %)	
	2014	2015	2014	2015	2014	2015
Cefixime	256 (98.1)	272 (98.6)	/	/	5 (1.9)	4 (1.4)
Ceftriaxone	261 (100)	276 (100)	/	/	0 (0)	0 (0)
Azithromycin	142 (54.4)	171 (62.0)	88 (33.7)	78 (28.3)	31 (11.9)	27 (9.8)
Ciprofloxacin*	73 (28.0)	114 (41.3)	0 (0)	1 (0.4)	188 (72.0)	161 (58.3)
Penicillin*	27 (10.3)	40 (14.5)	158 (60.5)	184 (66.7)	76 (29.1)	52 (18.8)

The percentage of strains with resistance to ciprofloxacin (MIC >0.06 mg/L) was 72.0% in 2014 and 58.3% in 2015 (Table 2).

Overall, 29.1% of the isolates in 2014 and 18.8% in 2015 displayed resistance to penicillin. In addition, there was a very high rate of intermediate *N. gonorrhoeae* strains (Table 2).

Nitrocefin testing for the detection of beta-lactamase activity in *N. gonorrhoeae* was performed in 83.5% ($n = 218$) of isolates in 2014. All 276 isolates (100%) were tested for beta-lactamase activity in 2015. High-level plasmid-mediated resistance against penicillin (penicillinase producing *N. gonorrhoeae*, PPNG) was found in 25% of all tested strains in 2014 and in 14% of the strains in 2015.

Discussion

Using GORENET we aimed at two targets concerning gonococcal infections: data collection on disease epidemiology and monitoring of resistance patterns with unified methodology.

We were able to implement a nationwide data collection of all performed *N. gonorrhoeae* susceptibility testing in the participating laboratories. Routine data collection on all performed *N. gonorrhoeae* susceptibility tests together with epidemiological information, like age and gender, was not in place until GORENET surveillance.

Before starting GORENET, the CL collected isolates from a range of laboratories. This pre-existing network was expanded within GORENET, and the number of collected isolates increased substantially.

We were able to set up electronic data collection for all samples tested for *N. gonorrhoeae* susceptibility in the participating laboratories. Timely transmitted data are a good tool for monitoring *N. gonorrhoeae* susceptibility dynamics. Due to data protection issues, the collected epidemiological information was limited and important information, such as data regarding the transmission route, therapeutic regimen and therapeutic success, could not be gathered.

We reached a relatively even geographical representation of all regions, but the coverage in central and southern Germany should be increased further.

In routine data collection from the network laboratories, we found that over 90% of all samples tested for *N. gonorrhoeae* susceptibility were from men, similar to several other European countries [22]. This percentage

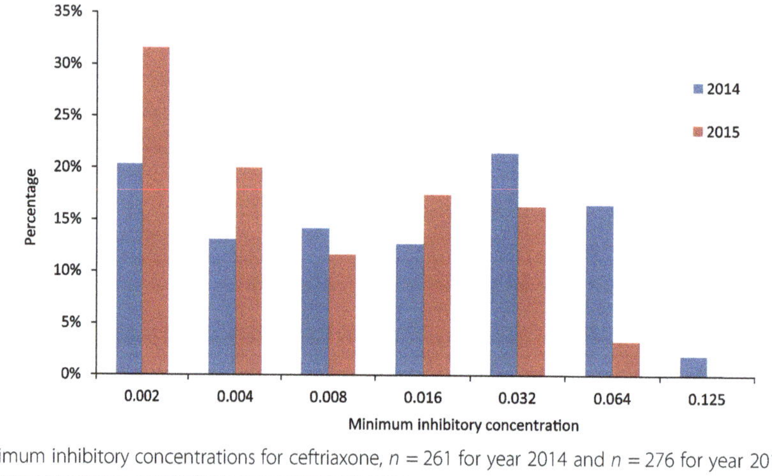

Fig. 3 Distribution of minimum inhibitory concentrations for ceftriaxone, $n = 261$ for year 2014 and $n = 276$ for year 2015

Table 3 Minimum inhibitory concentrations (MIC) of cefixime, ceftriaxone, azithromycin, ciprofloxacin and penicillin for isolates with resistance to cefixime or with MICs at the breakpoint for resistance to cefixime ($n = 24$)

	Minimum inhibitory concentration (MIC)				
Isolate	Cefixime	Ceftriaxone	Azithromycin	Ciprofloxacin	Penicillin
1	0.25	0.125	0.75	32	1
2	0.19	0.047	1	0.25	32
3	0.19	0.094	0.75	32	3
4	0.19	0.023	0.19	32	0.75
5	0.19	0.047	0.125	32	0.75
6	0.19	0.032	0.19	32	1.5
7	0.19	0.032	0.094	12	0.75
8	0.19	0.032	0.19	16	1
9	0.19	0.023	0.125	16	0.75
10	0.125	0.125	0.5	32	2
11	0.125	0.064	1	32	1
12	0.125	0.064	1	32	2
13	0.125	0.032	0.19	32	0.75
14	0.125	0.032	0.19	32	0.75
15	0.125	0.032	0.19	32	0.5
16	0.125	0.032	0.125	32	1.5
17	0.125	0.023	0.125	32	0.38
18	0.125	0.023	0.19	32	0.75
19	0.125	0.023	0.19	32	0.5
20	0.125	0.023	0.125	16	0.75
21	0.125	0.023	0.094	12	0.75
22	0.125	0.016	0.25	32	0.75
23	0.125	0.012	0.125	12	0.38
24	0.016	0.006	256	12	32

was 84% in previous studies in Germany [15], and we can assume that at least half of all isolates from men are attributable to men having sex with men (MSM), comparable to other European countries [22]. Nevertheless, women might still be underrepresented in our sample. This seems possible because men are more often symptomatic and might therefore be tested more often than women [14]. We aim to collect data on transmission routes from physicians to better interpret the collected data.

We also found that the median age of tested men was slightly higher than that of tested women. Again, Euro-GASP data and other previous data from Germany have reported findings [18, 21, 22] similar to our results. In countries that reported the risk of transmission, the proportion of men aged >25 years was higher among MSM than among heterosexual men. This might explain the higher median age of the tested men in our sample. As *N. gonorrhoeae* is not reportable in Germany, we were not able to compare whether the *N. gonorrhoeae* AMR test distribution by age corresponded to the age groups most affected by gonorrhoea.

We exclusively analysed susceptibility data from the CL testing because presently Germany lacks a standard operation protocol and regular quality assurance for *N. gonorrhoeae* testing for all laboratories. From a cross-sectional survey among laboratories performing *N. gonorrhoeae* diagnostics we know that 55% of all laboratories (76% of private laboratories) are accredited and 19% are certified [23]. However, due to the use of different methods, standards and test panels it is unknown if there are substantial differences in quality of testing, and GORENET will be a useful tool for quality assurance in the future.

Susceptibility testing in the CL enabled the monitoring of *N. gonorrhoeae* antimicrobial resistance detected by a unified methodology. Age and gender distribution of the

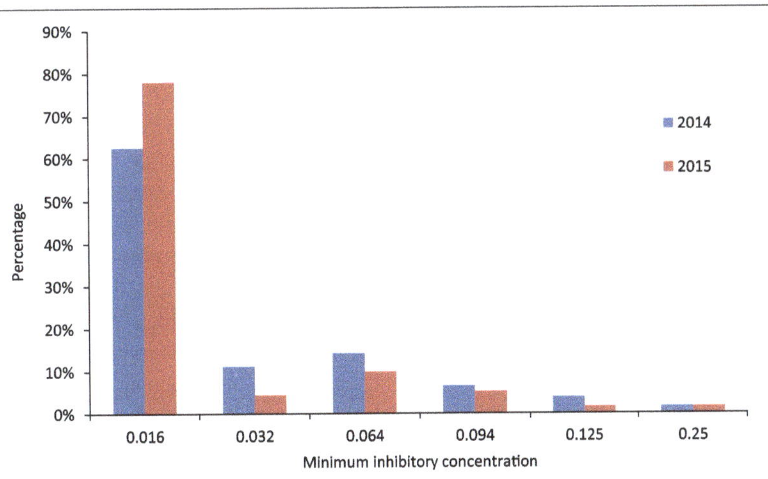

Fig. 4 Distribution of minimum inhibitory concentration for cefixime, $n = 261$ for year 2014 and $n = 276$ for year 2015

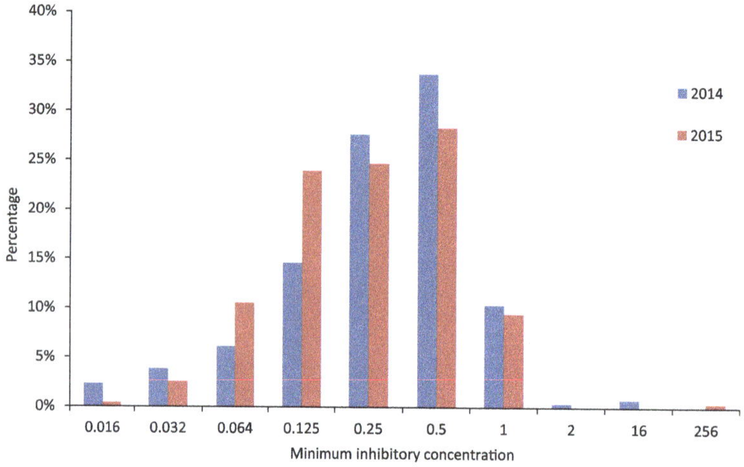

Fig. 5 Distribution of minimum inhibitory concentration for azithromycin, $n = 261$ for year 2014 and $n = 276$ for year 2015

tested isolates did not differ from all samples tested for susceptibility in the participating laboratories.

No resistance to ceftriaxone was detected in 2014 and 2015 in isolates collected with GORENET, and only two isolates showed MICs at the estimated breakpoint of 0.125 mg/L.

Previous German publications also did not show notable levels of ceftriaxone resistance or ESC resistance [18–21] in Germany. However, within the Euro-GASP collection, there was one exception in 2011, when 6.5% of German strains were resistant against ceftriaxone. In the following years 2012–2014, there were no notable levels of ceftriaxone resistance observed [18, 21, 22] in Germany by the Euro-GASP surveillance.

Currently, parenterally administered ceftriaxone remains an effective treatment option for gonorrhoea in Germany. Similar data have been published from surveillance systems in other countries [13, 26].

The percentage of strains with resistance to cefixime remained moderate within the GORENET (<2%), and low MIC values were predominant. German Euro-GASP data from 2014 correspond to this GORENET observation. In 2014 no cefixime-resistant isolate from Germany was detected within the Euro-GASP surveillance [22]. Compared with previous German data from Euro-GASP, this is a decrease from the years 2009–2013, when resistance rates from 5.7% to 12.9% were detected [22]. The decreasing number of strains resistant to cefixime could be observed not only in GORENET: European Euro-GASP data from 2014 and surveillance reports from the United Kingdom, the United States and Canada showed the same trend to less ESC-resistant isolates [26–29]. The decrease in gonococcal resistance to cefixime in 2014/15 suggests that clinicians in Germany may have avoided prescribing this antibiotic as a first-line treatment after the new therapy guidelines were published. However, changes in resistance patterns develop incrementally and are usually not detected so fast.

A presumptive explanation for this observation is the eradication of previously undetected reservoirs [27, 30]. Especially extragenital infections, which are oftentimes asymptomatic, difficult to culture and difficult to treat, are a constant reservoir for the spread of gonorrhoea [9, 30, 31]. Due to regular use of highly sensitive molecular diagnostic tests, like nucleic acid amplification tests (NAAT), in the routine diagnostic, detection of gonococcal infections was improved. Extragenital infections and subclinical urogenital infections are therefore more often confirmed and can be successfully treated [31]. The adjustment of treatment guidelines for ceftriaxone as first-line therapy seems to provide here an additional benefit. Sufficient treatment of these infections prevents a selection of resistant clones and might be a reason for the decrease of cefixime-resistant gonococci [27, 28, 30].

Molecular typing studies, performed with *N. gonorrhoeae* multiantigen sequence typing (NG-MAST, http://www.ng-mast.net) [32], showed one sequence type (ST1407), which was the most frequently observed sequence type associated with ESC- and multi-resistance [33–35]. Therefore, a further reason for the decrease of cefixime resistance could be a replacement of this multidrug-resistant *N. gonorrhoeae* clone ST1407 by clones with different resistance patterns within the infected population [27]. This could be an effect of the sufficient treatment or, as the Euro-GASP authors pointed out, be caused by impaired reinfection with the same clone due to a partial immunity and needs to be evaluated by future typing studies [27]. Additional monitoring and a molecular typing study within GORENET in the next years are therefore intended.

Multidrug resistance was not detected regularly in GORENET. Only one cefixime-resistant isolate displayed further resistance to azithromycin and ciprofloxacin, intermediate susceptibility to penicillin and a reduced susceptibility to ceftriaxone at the breakpoint MIC of 0.125 mg/L. Nevertheless, the combination of resistances is particularly alarming and should be monitored further.

A high prevalence of resistance was detected for azithromycin. Although we observed mostly resistance near the breakpoint (MIC >0.5 mg/L), this trend is concerning. In addition, there was a high rate of intermediate *N. gonorrhoeae* strains: 40–45% of the strains were not fully susceptible to azithromycin. Germany's data from previous years [22] shows that the level of azithromycin resistance was mostly under 5%. The first-line use of azithromycin is very common in STI treatment regimes, especially as a syndromic treatment before or without confirmation of the pathogenic agent. This might explain the increase in azithromycin resistance in the last several years, but data on prescriptions in Germany are not published.

In 2015, we detected the first case of a high-level azithromycin resistant *N. gonorrhoeae* strain in Germany, with a MIC >256 mg/L. This isolate was susceptible to ceftriaxone and cefixime but showed high-level resistance to penicillin and resistance to ciprofloxacin. As rising resistance rates to azithromycin are increasingly observed globally [22, 26] and high-level azithromycin resistance is reported worldwide [35–43], azithromycin is not suitable for first-line treatment. If azithromycin is used as a single-drug treatment in cases of severe penicillin/cephalosporin anaphylaxis, susceptibility testing prior to treatment should be performed.

According to current treatment guidelines, dual therapy with ceftriaxone and azithromycin is recommended, using two antimicrobial agents with different mechanisms of action [5, 44]. Currently, there is no alternative to this dual treatment regime. Ultimately, we will need to discuss whether we have to abandon dual therapy with azithromycin if the trend of increasing azithromycin resistance remains in the years to come [9, 45].

The resistance rates to ciprofloxacin were constantly high in Germany, although a drop was detectable in the surveillance period. A high prevalence of resistance to ciprofloxacin has also been found in Europe and worldwide since the late 1990s [22]. The drug is therefore not recommended for therapeutic use in Germany.

Resistance to penicillin has been prevalent for many decades worldwide. Nearly 25% of all isolates displayed resistance to penicillin and an additional 64% showed intermediate susceptibility in the GORENET surveillance data. Accordingly, approximately 90% of the strains were not fully susceptible to penicillin in Germany. High-level plasmid-mediated resistance to penicillin was also regularly observed but decreased within the surveillance period from 25.9% to 14%, an observation that requires further monitoring.

We have several limitations in our data. First, within the GORENET data collection scheme, we were unable to collect more detailed epidemiological information, such as the risk of transmission, special symptoms, therapy strategies and treatment success rates. Usually, laboratories in Germany have very limited epidemiological information available, provided by the physicians in charge, and need to treat these data confidentially due to strict data-protection regulations.

Second, our data analysis was limited by the small number of isolates collected compared to the overall population of Germany.

Third, we cannot exclude selection bias in our data, because we recruited laboratories based on their catchment area, number of tested *N. gonorrhoeae* samples and use of the Etest from a pool of laboratories that expressed an interest to participate. However, with selected and established network laboratories, which forwarded all of their received isolates, we diminished a collection bias from laboratories being more prone to submit isolates with interesting resistance patterns.

Conclusions

Using GORENET, we were able to implement a nationwide collection of all performed *N. gonorrhoeae* susceptibility data in the participating laboratories and increase the number of collected isolates retested at the CL for confirmation and quality assurance. The majority of susceptibility tests are performed among young men. More detailed epidemiological information would be beneficial.

The resistance rate to ceftriaxone remains low in Germany. Therefore, ceftriaxone is still an appropriate treatment for gonorrhoea at present. In 2014 and 2015, we found low resistance rates for cefixime in Germany. However, this needs further monitoring. Resistance to azithromycin is common and should continue to be monitored in the future. Except for a small decrease in AMR towards ciprofloxacin and penicillin, no substantial changes in the susceptibility patterns between 2014 and 2015 could be detected.

In conclusion, GORENET as a gonococcal antimicrobial surveillance in Germany is highly needed. Current data and ongoing collection of data will be used to update national treatment guidelines and, if necessary, implementation of future prevention measures.

To continue to monitor *N. gonorrhoeae* susceptibility, particularly against ESC and azithromycin, the yearly number of isolates tested in the CL should be substantially increased. Molecular surveillance of the circulating strains is important for monitoring the current situation, the evolving resistances and the transmission networks.

Surveillance of susceptibility is essential to ensure efficient patient management and keep gonorrhoea a treatable disease.

Abbreviations

AMR: Antimicrobial resistance; ARS: Antibiotic resistance surveillance programme; ATCC: American Type Culture Collection; CDC: Centers for Disease Control and Prevention; CL: Consiliary Laboratory for gonococci; ECDC: European Centre for Disease Prevention and Control; ESC: Extended spectrum cephalosporin; EUCAST: European Committee on Antimicrobial Susceptibility Testing; Euro-GASP: European Gonococcal Antimicrobial Surveillance Programme; GORENET: Gonococcal Resistance Network; i.m.: Intramuscular; i.v.: Intravenous; IQR: Interquartile ranges; MSM: Men having sex with men; *N. gonorrhoeae*: *Neisseria gonorrhoeae*; NAAT: nucleic acid amplification test; NG MAST: *Neisseria gonorrhoeae* multiantigen sequence typing; PPNG: Penicillinase producing *N. gonorrhoeae*; RKI: Robert Koch Institute; ST: Sequence type; STI: Sexually transmitted infection; WHO: World Health Organization

Acknowledgements

***GORENET study group.**

Thomas Back (Labor Schottdorf MVZ GmbH, Augsburg).
Anja Berger (Bayerisches Landesamt für Gesundheit und Lebensmittelsicherheit, Oberschleißheim, Sachgebiet GE 2.2 Infektiologie, Humanbakteriologie, Mykologie und Konsiliarlabor Diphtherie).
Valerie Chapot, Jörg Steinmann (Institut für Medizinische Mikrobiologie, Universitätsklinikum Essen).
Stephan Eicke (Labor Dr. Eicke, Berlin).
Claudia Friedrichs (Medizinisches Labor Ostsachsen MVZ GbR, Görlitz).
Andreas Groß, Hans-Jochen Hagedorn (Labor Krone, Bad Salzuflen).
Alexander Halfmann (Institut für Medizinische Mikrobiologie und Hygiene, Universitätsklinikum des Saarlandes, Homburg).
Britt Hornei (MVZ Synlab Leverkusen GmbH, Leverkusen).
Ralf Ignatius (Labor Enders und Kollegen MVZ, Stuttgart).
Simone Korten, Hany Sahly (Labor Lademannbogen MVZ GmbH, Hamburg).
Elzbieta Kozub-Witkowski (LADR GmbH Medizinisches Versorgungszentrum Dr. Kramer & Kollegen, Geesthacht).
Sabine Krämer (MVZ Labor Eveld & Kollegen, Essen).
Margit Kühn (Labor Becker, Olgemöller und Kollegen, München).
Anke Liebetrau (MVZ Labor Dr. Reising-Ackermann und Kollegen, Leipzig).
Thomas Meyer (Institut für Medizinische Mikrobiologie, Virologie und Hygiene, Universitätsklinikum Hamburg-Eppendorf).
Klaus Oberdorfer (Labor Dr. Limbach und Kollegen, Heidelberg).
Roland Pfüller (MDI Laboratorien GmbH, Berlin).
Caroline Ruckert (MVZ für Laboratoriumsmedizin und Mikrobiologie Koblenz-Mittelrhein, Koblenz).
Roman Schwarz (Labor Mönchengladbach, Medizinisches Versorgungszentrum Dr. Stein + Kollegen, Limbach Gruppe).
Daniela Walch, Madeleine Mai (Institut für Labormedizin, Mikrobiologie und Krankenhaushygiene, Krankenhaus Nordwest, Frankfurt am Main).
Thomas A. Wichelhaus (Institut für Medizinische Mikrobiologie und Krankenhaushygiene, Universitätsklinikum Frankfurt, Goethe-Universität).
Hilmar Wisplinghoff (Labor Dr. Wisplinghoff, Köln).
Nicole Wüppenhorst (Institut für Hygiene und Umwelt, Abteilung Medizinische Mikrobiologie, Hamburg).

We acknowledge further persons for their work and involvement:

Lorenz Jäger, Elzbieta Nowakowski, Elisabeth Schlosser, Tanja Sinninger und Doris Streit-Schmid from Labor Schottdorf MVZ GmbH, Augsburg.
Annegret Mahl from Bayerisches Landesamt für Gesundheit und Lebensmittelsicherheit, Oberschleißheim.
Doris Kahle from Medizinisches Labor Ostsachsen MVZ GbR, Görlitz.
Michael Zimmer, Olga Zimmer and Vanessa Dreyer from Labor Krone, Bad Salzuflen.
Thomas Regnath from Labor Enders und Kollegen MVZ, Stuttgart.
Bettina Hebold from MVZ Labor Dr. Reising-Ackermann und Kollegen, Leipzig.
Beatrice Weber from Institut für Medizinische Mikrobiologie, Virologie und Hygiene, Universitätsklinikum Hamburg-Eppendorf.
Mirijam Schlicht, Antje Mewes and Michael Friedrich from MDI Laboratorien GmbH, Berlin.
Denia Frank from Institut für Medizinische Mikrobiologie und Krankenhaushygiene, Universitätsklinikum Frankfurt, Goethe-Universität.
Kerstin Dehmel from Robert Koch Institute.

Funding

The project was designed by Robert Koch Institute and Consiliary Laboratory for Gonococci. The project was funded by German Federal Ministry of Health. German Federal Ministry of Health was not involved in data collection, analysis and writing of the manuscript.

Authors' contributions

SB, SD, PKK and VB developed the concept and methods of the Gonococcal Resistance Network (GORENET). SB, SD, KJ, AL, AS, SN, PKK and VB were responsible for implementation of the GORENET. SB, EG and PKK were responsible for laboratory testing. SD, AS, KJ, SN and VB were in charge of the data collection and analysis. SB and SD drafted the paper and share the first authorship in equal parts. All authors revised the paper. All authors read and approved the final manuscript.

Consent for publication

Not applicable

Competing interests

Klaus Jansen is a member of the editorial board (Associate Editor) of this journal. All other authors declare that they have no competing interests.

Author details

[1]German Consiliary Laboratory for Gonococci, Department of Dermatology and Venerology, Vivantes Hospital Berlin, Berlin, Germany. [2]Department for Infectious Disease Epidemiology, Robert Koch Institute, Berlin, Germany. [3]Charité University Medicine Berlin, Berlin, Germany. [4]Department of Infectious Diseases, Robert Koch Institute, Berlin, Germany. [5]European Public Health Microbiology Training (EUPHEM) programme, European Centre for Disease Prevention and Control (ECDC), Stockholm, Sweden.

References

1. WHO. Global action plan to control the spread and impact of antimicrobial resistance in Neisseria gonorrhoeae. World Health Organization, Department of Reproductive Health and Research; 2012. http://apps.who.int/iris/bitstream/10665/44863/1/9789241503501_eng.pdf.
2. Centers for Disease C, Prevention. CDC grand rounds: the growing threat of multidrug-resistant gonorrhea. MMWR Morb Mortal Wkly Rep. 2013;62(6):103–6.
3. European Centre for Disease Prevention and Control. Response plan to control and manage the threat of multidrug-resistant gonorrhoea in Europe. Stockholm: European Centre for Disease Prevention and Control, 2012; 2012. Report No
4. Bignell CJ. European guideline for the management of gonorrhoea. Int J STD AIDS. 2001;12(Suppl 3):27–9.
5. Unemo M, Shafer WM. Antimicrobial resistance in Neisseria gonorrhoeae in the 21st century: past, evolution, and future. Clin Microbiol Rev. 2014;27(3):587–613.
6. Unemo M, Shafer WM. Antibiotic resistance in Neisseria gonorrhoeae: origin, evolution, and lessons learned for the future. Ann N Y Acad Sci. 2011;1230:E19–28.
7. Bolan GA, Sparling PF, Wasserheit JN. The emerging threat of untreatable gonococcal infection. N Engl J Med. 2012;366(6):485–7.
8. Unemo M, Nicholas RA. Emergence of multidrug-resistant, extensively drug-resistant and untreatable gonorrhea. Future Microbiol. 2012;7(12):1401–22.
9. Unemo M. Current and future antimicrobial treatment of gonorrhoea - the rapidly evolving Neisseria gonorrhoeae continues to challenge. BMC Infect Dis. 2015;15:364.
10. Whiley DM, Goire N, Lahra MM, Donovan B, Limnios AE, Nissen MD, et al. The ticking time bomb: escalating antibiotic resistance in Neisseria gonorrhoeae is a public health disaster in waiting. J Antimicrob Chemother. 2012;67(9):2059–61.
11. Brockmeyer N, Spornraft-Ragaller P, Bremer V, et al. S2k-Leitlinie: Gonorrhoe bei Erwachsenen und Adoleszenten; 2013. http://www.awmf.org/uploads/tx_szleitlinien/059-004l_S25_Gonorrhoe_bei_Erwachsenen_Adoleszenten_2014-verlaengert_01.pdf.
12. Mlynarczyk-Bonikowska B, Serwin AB, Golparian D. Walter de Walthoffen S, Majewski S, Koper M, et al. antimicrobial susceptibility/resistance and genetic characteristics of Neisseria gonorrhoeae isolates from Poland, 2010-2012. BMC Infect Dis. 2014;14:65.

13. La Ruche G, Goubard A, Berçot B, Cambau E, Semaille C, Sednaoui P. Gonococcal infections and emergence of gonococcal decreased susceptibility tocephalosporins in France, 2001 to 2012. Euro Surveill. 2014; 19(34). https://doi.org/10.2807/1560-7917.ES2014.19.34.20885.
14. Bignell C, Unemo M, European STIGEB. 2012 European guideline on the diagnosis and treatment of gonorrhoea in adults. Int J STD AIDS. 2013;24(2):85–92.
15. Bignell C, FitzGerald M. UK national guideline for the management of gonorrhoea in adults, 2011. Int J STD AIDS. 2011;22(10):541–7.
16. Workowski KA. Centers for disease control and prevention sexually transmitted diseases treatment guidelines. Clin Infect Dis. 2015;61(Suppl 8):S759–62.
17. DSTIG. Gonorrhoe bei Erwachsenen und Adoleszenten. Deutsche STI-Gesellschaft e. V., 2013.
18. Horn NN, Kresken M, Korber-Irrgang B, Gottig S, Wichelhaus C, Wichelhaus TA, et al. Antimicrobial susceptibility and molecular epidemiology of Neisseria gonorrhoeae in Germany. Int J Med Microbiol. 2014;304(5–6):586–91.
19. Enders M, Turnwald-Maschler A, Regnath T. Antimicrobial resistance of Neisseria gonorrhoeae isolates from the Stuttgart and Heidelberg areas of southern Germany. Eur J Clin Microbiol Infect Dis. 2006;25(5):318–22.
20. Wagner J, Tebbe B, Hornle R, Chahin M, Arvand M, Wendt C, et al. Antibiotic susceptibility of Neisseria gonorrhoeae isolates in Berlin. Hautarzt. 2000;51(9):666–9.
21. Regnath Thomas, Mertes Thomas, Ignatius Ralf. Antimicrobial resistance of Neisseria gonorrhoeae isolates in south-west Germany, 2004 to 2015: increasing minimal inhibitory concentrations of tetracycline but no resistance to third-generation cephalosporins. Euro Surveill. 2016;21(36). https://doi.org/10.2807/1560-7917.ES.2016.21.36.30335.
22. European Centre for Disease Prevention and Control. Gonococcal antimicrobial susceptibility surveillance in Europe 2015. Stockholm: ECDC; 2017. https://ecdc.europa.eu/sites/portal/files/documents/gonococcal-antimicrobial-susceptibility-surveillance-Europe-2015.pdf.
23. Loenenbach A, Dudareva-Vizule S, Buder S, Sailer A, Kohl PK, Bremer V. Laboratory practices: diagnostics and antibiotics resistance testing of Neisseria gonorrhoeae in Germany. Bundesgesundheitsblatt Gesundheitsforschung Gesundheitsschutz. 2015;58(8):866–74.
24. European Committee on Antimicrobial Susceptibility Testing. Breakpoint tables for interpretation of MICs and zone diameters. Version 4.0. EUCAST 2014. Available from: http://www.eucast.org/clinical_breakpoints/.
25. Unemo M, Fasth O, Fredlund H, Limnios A, Tapsall J. Phenotypic and genetic characterization of the 2008 WHO Neisseria gonorrhoeae reference strain panel intended for global quality assurance and quality control of gonococcal antimicrobial resistance surveillance for public health purposes. J Antimicrob Chemother. 2009;63(6):1142–51.
26. Martin I, Sawatzky P, Liu G, Allen V, Lefebvre B, Hoang L, et al. Decline in decreased cephalosporin susceptibility and increase in Azithromycin resistance in Neisseria gonorrhoeae. Canada Emerg Infect Dis. 2016;22(1):65–7.
27. Cole MJ, Spiteri G, Jacobsson S, Pitt R, Grigorjev V, Unemo M, et al. Is the tide turning again for cephalosporin resistance in Neisseria gonorrhoeae in Europe? Results from the 2013 European surveillance. BMC Infect Dis. 2015;15:321.
28. Public Health England. GRASP 2013 report: the Gonococcal Resistance to Antimicrobial Surveillance Programme (England and Wales). Public Health England; 2014. https://www.gov.uk/government/uploads/system/uploads/attachment_data/file/368477/GRASP_Report_2013.pdf.
29. Centers for Disease Control and Prevention. Sexually transmitted diseases surveillance 2014. Centers for Disease Control and Prevention; 2015. https://www.cdc.gov/std/stats14/surv-2014-print.pdf.
30. Lewis DA. Will targeting oropharyngeal gonorrhoea delay the further emergence of drug-resistant Neisseria gonorrhoeae strains? Sex Transm Infect. 2015;91(4):234–7.
31. Dudareva-Vizule S, Haar K, Sailer A, Wisplinghoff H, Wisplinghoff F, Marcus U, et al. Prevalence of pharyngeal and rectal Chlamydia trachomatis and Neisseria gonorrhoeae infections among men who have sex with men in Germany. Sex Transm Infect. 2014;90(1):46–51.
32. Unemo M, Dillon JA. Review and international recommendation of methods for typing neisseria gonorrhoeae isolates and their implications for improved knowledge of gonococcal epidemiology, treatment, and biology. Clin Microbiol Rev. 2011;24(3):447–58.
33. Chisholm SA, Unemo M, Quaye N, Johansson E, Cole MJ, Ison CA, Van de Laar MJ. Molecular epidemiological typing within the European Gonococcal Antimicrobial Resistance Surveillance Programme reveals predominance of a multidrug-resistant clone. Euro Surveill. 2013;18(3). Available online: http://www.eurosurveillance.org/ViewArticle.aspx?ArticleId=20358.
34. Jeverica S, Golparian D, Maticic M, Potocnik M, Mlakar B, Unemo M. Phenotypic and molecular characterization of Neisseria gonorrhoeae isolates from Slovenia, 2006-12: rise and fall of the multidrug-resistant NG-MAST genogroup 1407 clone? J Antimicrob Chemother. 2014;69(6):1517–25.
35. Morita-Ishihara T, Unemo M, Furubayashi K, Kawahata T, Shimuta K, Nakayama S, et al. Treatment failure with 2 g of azithromycin (extended-release formulation) in gonorrhoea in Japan caused by the international multidrug-resistant ST1407 strain of Neisseria gonorrhoeae. J Antimicrob Chemother. 2014;69(8):2086–90.
36. Galarza PG, Alcala B, Salcedo C, Canigia LF, Buscemi L, Pagano I, et al. Emergence of high level azithromycin-resistant Neisseria gonorrhoeae strain isolated in Argentina. Sex Transm Dis. 2009;36(12):787–8.
37. Palmer HM, Young H, Winter A, Dave J. Emergence and spread of azithromycin-resistant Neisseria gonorrhoeae in Scotland. J Antimicrob Chemother. 2008;62(3):490–4.
38. Chisholm SA, Dave J, Ison CA. High-level azithromycin resistance occurs in Neisseria gonorrhoeae as a result of a single point mutation in the 23S rRNA genes. Antimicrob Agents Chemother. 2010;54(9):3812–6.
39. Starnino S, Stefanelli P. Neisseria gonorrhoeae Italian study G. Azithromycin-resistant Neisseria gonorrhoeae strains recently isolated in Italy. J Antimicrob Chemother. 2009;63(6):1200–4.
40. Katz AR, Komeya AY, Soge OO, Kiaha MI, Lee MV, Wasserman GM, et al. Neisseria gonorrhoeae with high-level resistance to azithromycin: case report of the first isolate identified in the United States. Clin Infect Dis. 2012;54(6):841–3.
41. Unemo M, Golparian D, Hellmark B. First three Neisseria gonorrhoeae isolates with high-level resistance to azithromycin in Sweden: a threat to currently available dual-antimicrobial regimens for treatment of gonorrhea? Antimicrob Agents Chemother. 2014;58(1):624–5.
42. Berçot B, Belkacem A, Goubard A, Mougari F, Sednaoui P, La Ruche G, Cambau E. High-level azithromycin-resistant Neisseria gonorrhoeae clinical isolate in France, March 2014. Euro Surveill. 2014;19(44). https://doi.org/10.2807/1560-7917.ES2014.19.44.20951.
43. Chisholm SA, Wilson J, Alexander S, Tripodo F, Al-Shahib A, Schaefer U, et al. An outbreak of high-level azithromycin resistant Neisseria gonorrhoeae in England. Sex Transm Infect. 2016;92:365–367.
44. Tapsall J. Antimicrobial resistance in Neisseria gonorrhoeae, WHO collaborating Centre for STD and HIV. Sydney: World Health; 2001.
45. Buono SA, Watson TD, Borenstein LA, Klausner JD, Pandori MW, Godwin HA. Stemming the tide of drug-resistant Neisseria gonorrhoeae: the need for an individualized approach to treatment. J Antimicrob Chemother. 2015;70(2): 374–81.

8

Concordance of chlamydia infections of the rectum and urethra in same-sex male partnerships

Vincent J. Cornelisse[1,2*], Christopher J. Sherman[3], Jane S Hocking[1,3], Henrietta Williams[1,3], Lei Zhang[1,4], Marcus Y. Chen[1,2], Catriona S. Bradshaw[1,2], Clare Bellhouse[1,2], Christopher K Fairley[1,2†] and Eric P. F. Chow[1,2†]

Abstract

Background: Our study aimed to describe the concordance of chlamydia infections of the rectum and urethra in men who have sex with men (MSM) and their male partners.

Methods: This was a cross-sectional study of chlamydia in MSM and their male sexual partners both attending Melbourne Sexual Health Centre (MSHC), Australia, between February 2011 and March 2015. We excluded partnerships where testing for chlamydia at both the rectum and urethra were not undertaken.

Results: Our study included 473 partnerships (946 men). 30 men had urethral chlamydia, of whom 14 (47%, 95% CI 28 to 66) had a partner with rectal chlamydia. 46 men had rectal chlamydia, of whom 14 (30%, 95% CI 18 to 46) had a partner with urethral chlamydia. The proportion of men with rectal chlamydia when their partner had urethral chlamydia was significantly higher than the proportion of men with urethral chlamydia when their partner had rectal chlamydia (McNemar's $p = 0.02$).

Conclusions: This is the first study of chlamydia concordance in male sexual partnerships and suggests that transmission of chlamydia between the urethra and rectum may be less efficient than has been reported for transmission between the urethra and cervix in heterosexual couples. It also suggests that transmission from the urethra to the rectum may be more efficient than in the opposite direction.

Keywords: Chlamydia trachomatis [B03.440.190.190.190.750], Homosexuality [F01.145.802.975.500], Sexual Partners [M01.778], Disease Transmission, Infectious [N06.850.310], Chlamydia, Men who have sex with men, Transmission, Partnership, Couple, Dyad

Background

Chlamydia trachomatis remains one of the most common bacterial sexually transmissible infections (STI) worldwide [1, 2]. Chlamydia notifications have been increasing in Australia since the 1990s, and have doubled over the decade from 2004 to 2013, [3] due to both increased testing and a true increase in the prevalence of infection both in heterosexuals and men who have sex with men (MSM) [4–7]. New biomedical HIV prevention strategies such as pre-exposure prophylaxis and treatment as prevention will hopefully result in a significant reduction in new HIV transmissions, but there are concerns that the effective prevention of HIV will result in behavioural changes that will further increase the rates of bacterial STIs among MSM.

To address the rising rates of chlamydia, health departments have sought strategies to control this infection. These strategies include screening programmes, and such programmes have been evaluated in heterosexuals, but the most recent and largest clinical trial did not show a significant effect of screening on the prevalence of infection, even when annual screening rates reached 30% [8].

Screening programmes and other public health interventions can be evaluated using mathematical models. But to date no model of chlamydia transmission in MSM has

* Correspondence: vcornelisse@mshc.org.au
†Equal contributors
[1]Melbourne Sexual Health Centre, Alfred Health, 580 Swanston St, Carlton, Melbourne, VIC 3052, Australia
[2]Central Clinical School, Faculty of Medicine, Nursing and Health Sciences, Monash University, Melbourne, Australia
Full list of author information is available at the end of the article

been published, and there is a paucity of data on key information needed to develop such models. In MSM this information would include the natural duration of infection of the urethra and rectum, the transmission probability between these sites, and the potential role of chlamydia of the pharynx.

The aim of this study was to analyse the concordance of chlamydia infections at the rectum and urethra in male-male partnerships, and to use this data to infer the likelihood of transmission of chlamydia between the urethra and rectum within partnerships. Such information can be used to build mathematical models of chlamydia transmission, and may be useful for clinicians when counselling patients about their chlamydia infections.

Methods

This was a cross-sectional study of chlamydia diagnoses of the urethra and rectum in MSM and their male sexual partners when both attended Melbourne Sexual Health Centre (MSHC) on the same day. MSHC is the major public sexual health clinic in Melbourne, Australia. It provides a free walk-in service and no referrals are required. Over the study period it provided approximately 35,000 consultations annually, and about 37% of consultations were for MSM [9]. All patients complete a computer-assisted self-interview (CASI) that collects their demographic details (e.g., age) and sexual behaviours (e.g., number of casual partners in the last three months, condom use with regular and casual partners during insertive and/or receptive anal sex in the last three months) [10]. From March 2011 onwards, CASI included the additional question "Is your partner also being seen today at this clinic?". Patients who answered "yes" to this question were asked for their partner's name. We initially included all MSM who answered yes to this question and whose partner we could identify, and who had testing for chlamydia between March 2011 and February 2015. Partners were paired and assigned a unique "partnership number". MSHC uses an electronic medical record system in which clinicians enter a diagnosis code when a patient attends for a consultation.

We offered screening for chlamydia on rectal swabs and first void urine samples in all MSM, in line with Australian STI screening guidelines for MSM [11]. During the study period, the screening protocol at MSHC did not include testing for pharyngeal chlamydia. Chlamydia was tested using a strand displacement assay (Becton Dickinson, New Jersey, USA). Urethral and rectal chlamydia positivity was calculated as the number of positive tests divided by the number of tests performed.

All statistical analyses were performed using Stata (version 13.1, StataCorp LP). The 95% confidence interval (CI) for chlamydia positivity was calculated using the 'exact' binomial distribution [12]. The positivity of chlamydia results obtained at the urethra and rectum for each person in each partnership was paired and compared using the McNemar's test of significance. Our primary analysis examined the concordance of chlamydia at the urethra and rectum, and was based on 473 partnerships in which both men were screened for urethral and rectal chlamydia on the same day. A secondary analysis was limited restricted to 406 partnerships where both men did not have symptoms of urethritis or proctitis, to remove possible selection bias as a result of the presence of symptoms as the primary reason of attending the clinic. Another secondary analysis was restricted to 352 partnerships who reported anal sex without condoms to exclude the protective effect of condom use.

Results

During the study period, 1464 MSM attended MSHC with their partner on the same day, consisting of 732 partnerships, their demographics are described in Table 1. In 473 partnerships (946 men, 65% of total), both men were screened for urethral and rectal chlamydia on the same day. In 57 partnerships (114 men) at least one man had symptomatic urethritis, including 6 partnerships where both men had symptomatic urethritis. In 22 partnerships (44 men) at least one man had symptomatic proctitis, including two partnerships in which both men had symptomatic proctitis. There were 406 partnerships (812 men) in which both partners had complete testing for chlamydia and neither partner had symptomatic proctitis or urethritis (Additional file 1: Figure S1). Table 2 describes the frequency and proportion of chlamydia infections amongst these 946 men and 812 men respectively.

Of the 946 men, 30 had urethral chlamydia, of whom 14 (47%, 95% CI 28 to 66) had a partner with rectal chlamydia. Of the 946 men, 46 men had rectal chlamydia, of whom 14 (30%, 95% CI 18 to 46) had a partner with urethral

Table 1 Demographic and behavioural characteristics of the 1464 men attended the Melbourne Sexual Health Centre with their male partner on the same day

	Median (IQR)	Yes/total; % yes
Age (years)	28 (24 to 35)	
Age difference (years) between partners	4 (2 to 9)	
HIV positive		54/1464 (4%)
CSP in last 3 months (yes vs no)		702/963 (73%)
Condoms for RAI with RSP[a]		530/1330 (40%)
Condoms for RAI with CSP[a]		1078/1311 (82%)
Condoms for IAI with RSP[a]		508/1321 (38%)
Condoms for IAI with CSP[a]		1060/1309 (81%)
Number of CSP in last 3 months for those with CSP.	3 (1 to 5)	

IQR interquartile range, *RAI* receptive anal intercourse, *IAI* insertive anal intercourse, *RSP* regular sexual partner, *CSP* casual sexual partner
[a]Consistent condoms use at all times or no anal sex

Table 2 Chlamydia positivity in MSM, by anatomic site (individual MSM data, not grouped into partnerships), including only MSM from partnerships in which both men were tested for chlamydia at both rectum and urethra

	Positivity (all men) n/N; % (95%CI)	Positivity (excluding symptomatic cases) n/N; % (95%CI)
Chlamydia at any site	70/946; 7.4 (5.8 to 9.3)	48/812; 5.9 (4.4 to 7.8)
Urethral chlamydia	30/946; 3.2 (2.1 to 4.5)	18/812; 2.2 (1.3 to 3.5)
Rectal chlamydia	46/946; 4.9 (3.6 to 6.4)	35/812; 4.3 (3.0 to 5.9)
Both urethral and rectal chlamydia	6/946; 0.6 (0.2 to 1.4)	5/812; 0.6 (0.2 to 1.4)

N = men tested; *n* = positive tests; MSM = men who have sex with men

chlamydia (Table 3). The proportion of men with rectal chlamydia when their partner had urethral chlamydia was significantly higher than the proportion of men with urethral chlamydia when their partner had rectal chlamydia (McNemar test; $p = 0.02$).

In a secondary analysis we excluded partnerships where either partner had symptomatic urethritis or proctitis. Of the 812 men in asymptomatic partnerships, 18 men had urethral chlamydia, of whom 8 (44%, 95% CI 22 to 69) had a partner with rectal chlamydia; and 35 men had rectal chlamydia, of whom 8 (23%, 95% CI 10 to 40) had a partner with urethral chlamydia (Table 4). The proportion of men with rectal chlamydia when their partner had urethral chlamydia was significantly higher than the proportion of men with urethral chlamydia when their partner had rectal chlamydia (McNemar test; $p = 0.005$). Table 5 includes data on 704 men who reported anal sex without condoms and proportions of chlamydia positivity are similar to those in Tables 3 and 4.

Discussion

Our data provide the first estimate of the concordance of chlamydia infection between the rectum and the urethra in same-sex male partnerships. The data suggest that the likelihood of chlamydia transmission between men is lower than that reported between men and women. In a study of 494 heterosexual partnerships that included symptomatic individuals, chlamydia was found in 68% of men with an infected female partner, and in 70% of women with an infected male partner [13]. These male–female concordance rates are analogous to our 30.4% urethral chlamydia positivity in MSM with a partner with rectal chlamydia, and our 46.7% rectal chlamydia positivity in MSM with a partner with urethral chlamydia, respectively. The chlamydia concordance in these heterosexual couples is significantly higher than chlamydia concordance between MSM partners in our study, suggesting that the transmission probability between MSM is lower than between heterosexual men and women. This may explain why chlamydia is not much more common in MSM than in heterosexuals whilst other STIs such as gonorrhoea and syphilis are many times more common in MSM [14]. However, the comparison

Table 3 Concordance of rectal chlamydia and urethral chlamydia between men in all 473 partnerships in which both men were screened for urethral and rectal chlamydia on the same day

	Urethra negative	Urethra positive	Total	Urethral chlamydia positivity % (95% CI)
Rectum negative	884	16	900	1.8 (1.0 to 2.9)
Rectum positive	32	14	46	30.4 (17.7 to 45.8)
Total	916	30	946	3.2 (2.1 to 4.5)
Rectal chlamydia positivity % (95% CI)	3.5 (2.4 to 4.9)	46.7 (28.3 to 65.7)	4.9 (3.6 to 6.4)	

(McNemar's test $p = 0.02$)
Each man is represented twice: once as a urethra and once as a rectum

Table 4 Concordance of rectal chlamydia and urethral chlamydia between men in 406 partnerships in which both men did not have symptoms of urethritis or proctitis

	Urethra negative	Urethra positive	Total number of tests	Urethral chlamydia positivity % (95% CI)
Rectum negative	767	10	777	1.3 (0.6 to 2.4)
Rectum positive	27	8	35	22.8 (10.4 to 40.1)
Total number of tests	794	18	812	2.2 (1.3 to 3.5)
Rectal chlamydia positivity % (95% CI)	3.4 (2.3 to 4.9)	44.4 (21.5 to 69.2)	4.3 (3.0 to 5.9)	

(McNemar's test $p = 0.005$)
Each man is represented twice: once as a urethra and once as a rectum

Table 5 Concordance of rectal chlamydia and urethral chlamydia between men in 352 partnerships who reported anal sex without condoms

	Urethra negative	Urethra positive	Total	Urethral chlamydia positivity % (95% CI)
Rectum negative	652	12	664	1.8 (0.9 to 3.1)
Rectum positive	27	13	40	32.5 (18.6 to 49.1)
Total	679	25	704	3.6 (2.3 to 5.2)
Rectal chlamydia positivity % (95% CI)	4.0 (2.6 to 5.7)	52.0 (31.3 to 72.2)	5.7 (4.1 to 7.7)	

(McNemar's test $p = 0.02$)
Each man is represented twice: once as a urethra and once as a rectum

between heterosexuals and MSM is complicated by the fact that MSM are likely to have more sexual partners and concurrent sexual partners, as highlighted by the difference in sexual partner numbers in our study compared to that found in heterosexual couples [13].

There was only one partnership in which both men had urethral chlamydia in the absence of either man having rectal chlamydia (Additional file 1: Table S1a), which suggests that urethra-to-urethra transmission is uncommon. Similarly, there were only two partnerships in which both men had rectal chlamydia in the absence of either man having urethral chlamydia (Additional file 1: Table S1b), which suggests that rectum-to-rectum transmission is also uncommon. These findings also support the notion that pharyngeal-to-urethra and pharynx-to-rectum for chlamydia transmission is likely to be uncommon [15, 16].

We conducted secondary analyses to assess the effect of any possible bias that may have resulted from symptomatic presentations or condom use. As expected, when symptomatic presentations were excluded, the transmission probabilities were somewhat lower because including symptomatic presentations may have biased towards transmission having had occurred. When we included only men who practised condomless anal sex, the transmission probabilities were somewhat higher (33-52%) but still lower than had been reported for heterosexuals.

Our data showed that 47% of partners of men with urethral chlamydia had rectal chlamydia while only 30% of partners of men with rectal chlamydia had urethral chlamydia. This difference remained significant when the analysis was restricted by symptoms and condom use. While this cross-sectional study cannot determine the direction of chlamydia transmission within each partnership, the results suggest that transmission from the urethra to the rectum may be more likely than transmission from the rectum to the urethra. These data do not reflect a difference in transmission efficiency during a single exposure, but instead describe the cumulative result of all exposures. We did not further investigate the causes for this difference, but it may be that the mechanics of anal sex more efficiently facilitates urethra-to-rectum transmission than rectum-to-urethra transmission. The difference in concordance should not be due to a difference in bacterial loads, as chlamydia loads have been shown to be higher in the rectum than in the urethra [17]. Interestingly, the aforementioned analysis in heterosexual partnerships found equal bidirectional transmission of chlamydia between men and women, where 68% of the male partners of infected women had chlamydia, and 70% of female partners of infected men had chlamydia [13].

A limitation of our analysis is that chlamydia in the pharynx was not screened for in our study. It is plausible that men can acquire urethral or rectal chlamydia through penile-oral sex, oral-anal contact, or the use of saliva as a lubricant for penile-anal sex [18]; however, direct evidence for these specific modes of transmission is limited, and there is disagreement in the published literature on the role of pharyngeal chlamydia in overall transmission. Studies have generally shown that rates of pharyngeal chlamydia in MSM are low. A study of attendees at sexual health clinic in Amsterdam found that 1.1% of MSM (95% CI 0.9 to 1.3) tested positive for pharyngeal chlamydia, [15] which is low compared with a positive rate of 9.8% for rectal chlamydia and 4.4% for urethral chlamydia [15]. They also assessed rates of spontaneous clearance, and found that at a median follow-up time of 12 days (range 7–58) pharyngeal chlamydia had spontaneously cleared in 37.2% of MSM [15]. A 2014 study from Melbourne showed that urethral chlamydia infection in MSM was strongly associated with insertive penile-anal sex without condoms, whereas urethral gonorrhoea and primary syphilis was not, leading the authors to hypothesise that pharyngeal infections were significant contributors to transmission for urethral gonorrhoea and primary syphilis, but not for urethral chlamydia [19]. This observation is further supported by a study from Seattle that showed that only 3% of urethral chlamydia cases were attributable to oral sex, compared with 34% of urethral gonorrhoea cases [20]. In contrast, findings from a study of MSM attending a sexual health clinic in San Francisco in 2007 support the role of oral sex as a risk factor for urethral chlamydia. They found that men who reported penile-oral sex only, not penile-anal sex, in the three months before testing had a urethral chlamydia positive rate of 4.8% (95% CI 2.9-7.4), which was not significantly different from the rate of urethral chlamydia of 7.0% (95% CI 5.6 to 8.6) amongst men who reported insertive penile-anal sex without condoms in the three months before testing [21]. Similarly, the Sydney-based "Health In Men" (HIM) study found that occasional (but not frequent) insertive oral sex was a risk factor for urethral chlamydia in MSM [18]. Whilst we were not able to assess the role of pharyngeal chlamydia infection directly, our study found relatively few men who had chlamydia of both the urethra and rectum (<10%). One explanation for this observation is that the pharynx is perhaps not commonly involved in chlamydia transmission in MSM, as pharyngeal chlamydia could potentially transmit to both a partner's urethra and rectum.

Our study has a number of other limitations. Firstly, we had no data on chlamydia infections in sexual partners other than the partner present on the day. Obviously, in every partnership at least one of the partners must have had sexual contact with a third party who had a chlamydia infection, but we are not able to determine in how many partnerships both partners separately acquired chlamydia from a third party, as this would require testing all third parties for chlamydia and conducting a molecular analysis of chlamydia serovars. A recently-published study of chlamydia concordance in heterosexual partnerships found that in 96.2% (51/53) of chlamydia-concordant partnerships both partners had the same chlamydia genotype (Schillinger et al., [22]). This finding suggests that concordance represents transmission within partnerships, but as described above, we may not be able to extrapolate from heterosexual partnerships to same sex male partnerships. By not accounting for instances where both partners acquired chlamydia from a third party, we may have over-estimated the likelihood of transmission between partners. Secondly, we did not collect data on the duration of the relationship, the frequency of sexual contact with that partner, whether their last sex act was with that partner, or whether they participated in group sex with that partner; hence it is not possible for us to estimate the per act transmission probability. Hence, in both our study and in the study by Quinn et al. of heterosexual partnerships, [13] chlamydia concordance reflects cumulative transmission rather than per-act transmission. Thirdly, we did not adjust for condom use because the number of men reporting consistent use of condoms for anal sex with their regular partner was quite small (171 of 946 men, 18%, for insertive anal sex; 172 of 946 men, 18%, for receptive anal sex). However, we did include a separate analysis of partnerships that reported anal sex without condoms with their regular partner, and found that the transmission estimates were similar (Table 5). Fourthly, our analysis included only men attending a single sexual health service with their male partner on the same day. It is likely that some men in partnerships did not present to our service on the same day as their partner and hence were not included in our study. We are not able to identify these partnerships, and their exclusion may have introduced a selection bias.

Conclusions

These data provide an estimate of the relative probability of transmission of chlamydia between the urethra and rectum, which will assist in the development of mathematical models. These models may then be used to assess novel public health interventions to combat the rising rates of chlamydia infections amongst MSM. However, further work is needed to clarify the role of pharyngeal chlamydia infections in overall transmission rates. These data also suggest that transmission of chlamydia between the urethra and rectum is less common than has been reported for transmission between the urethra and cervix in heterosexual couples [13], which may explain why the rate of chlamydia is not significantly higher among MSM than among heterosexuals, unlike the rates of other bacterial STIs. However, this inference needs to be interpreted with caution, due to significant behavioural differences between MSM couples and heterosexual couples.

Abbreviations

95% CI: 95% confidence interval; CASI: Computer-assisted self-interview; CSP: Casual sexual partner; IAI: Insertive anal intercourse; IQR: Interquartile range; MSHC: Melbourne sexual health centre; MSM: Men who have sex with men; RAI: Receptive anal intercourse; RSP: Regular sexual partner; STI: Sexually transmitted infection

Acknowledgements

The authors would like to acknowledge A. Afrizal for his assistance with the extraction of data from the MSHC database.

Funding

Funding for this project was, in part, supplied by a National Health and Medical Research Council (NHMRC) programme grant (number 568971). EPFC is supported by the Early Career Fellowships from the Australian NHMRC (number 1091226).

Authors' contributions

EPFC and CKF conceived the study. CJS undertook a preliminary analysis. VJC and EPFC extended the analysis for this paper including the stratification and application of statistical testing. VJC prepared the first draft, EPFC and CKF refined this and all authors contributed to and approved of the final version.

Competing interests

The authors declare that they have no competing interests.

Consent for publication

Not applicable.

Author details

[1]Melbourne Sexual Health Centre, Alfred Health, 580 Swanston St, Carlton, Melbourne, VIC 3052, Australia. [2]Central Clinical School, Faculty of Medicine, Nursing and Health Sciences, Monash University, Melbourne, Australia. [3]Melbourne School of Population and Global Health, University of Melbourne, Melbourne, Australia. [4]The Kirby Institute, The University of New South Wales, Sydney, Australia.

References

1. Newman L, Rowley J, Vander Hoorn S, Wijesooriya NS, Unemo M, Low N, Stevens G, Gottlieb S, Kiarie J, Temmerman M. Global Estimates of the Prevalence and Incidence of Four Curable Sexually Transmitted Infections in 2012 Based on Systematic Review and Global Reporting. PLoS One. 2015; 10(12):e0143304.
2. Torrone E, Papp J, Weinstock H. Prevalence of Chlamydia trachomatis genital infection among persons aged 14–39 years - United States, 2007–2012. MMWR Morb Mortal Wkly Rep. 2014;63(38):834–8.
3. The Kirby Institute. HIV, viral hepatitis and sexually transmissible infections in Australia Annual Surveillance Report 2014. In: Annual Surveillance Report 2014. Sydney: The Kirby Institute, UNSW Australia; 2014. p. 2052.
4. Ali H, Guy RJ, Fairley CK, Wand H, Chen MY, Dickson B, O'Connor CC, Marshall L, Grulich AE, Kaldor JM, et al. Understanding trends in genital Chlamydia trachomatis can benefit from enhanced surveillance: findings from Australia. Sex Transm Infect. 2012;88(7):552–7.
5. Chow EP, Tomnay J, Fehler G, Whiley D, Read TR, Denham I, Bradshaw CS, Chen MY, Fairley CK. Substantial increases in chlamydia and gonorrhea positivity unexplained by changes in individual-level sexual behaviors among men who have sex with men in an Australian sexual health service from 2007 to 2013. Sex Transm Dis. 2015;42(2):81–7.
6. Vodstrcil LA, Fairley CK, Fehler G, Leslie D, Walker J, Bradshaw CS, Hocking JS. Trends in chlamydia and gonorrhea positivity among heterosexual men

and men who have sex with men attending a large urban sexual health service in Australia, 2002–2009. BMC Infect Dis. 2011;11:158.
7. Mannion PK, Fairley CK, Fehler G, Tabrizi SN, Tan WS, Chen MY, Bradshaw CS, Chow EP. Trends in gonorrhoea positivity by nucleic acid amplification test versus culture among Australian heterosexual men with a low prevalence of gonorrhoea, 2007–2014. Sex Transm Infect. 2016;92(8):625–8.
8. Hocking J. Screening for chlamydia: does it work, results from accept. Sex Transm Infect. 2015;91 Suppl 2:A3.
9. Chow EP, Fehler G, Chen MY, Bradshaw CS, Denham I, Law MG, Fairley CK. Testing commercial sex workers for sexually transmitted infections in Victoria, Australia: an evaluation of the impact of reducing the frequency of testing. PLoS One. 2014;9(7):e103081.
10. Vodstrcil LA, Hocking JS, Cummings R, Chen MY, Bradshaw CS, Read TR, Sze JK, Fairley CK. Computer assisted self interviewing in a sexual health clinic as part of routine clinical care; impact on service and patient and clinician views. PLoS One. 2011;6(3):e18456.
11. Sexual transmitted infection testing guidelines for men who have sex with men 2010. [http://stipu.nsw.gov.au/wp-content/uploads/163932_STI_testing_guidelines_for_MSM_2010.pdf].
12. Morisette JT, Khorram S. Exact binomial confidence interval for proportions. Photogrammetr Eng Remote Sens. 1998;64:281–3.
13. Quinn TC, Gaydos C, Shepherd M, Bobo L, Hook 3rd EW, Viscidi R, Rompalo A. Epidemiologic and microbiologic correlates of Chlamydia trachomatis infection in sexual partnerships. JAMA. 1996;276(21):1737–42.
14. The Kirby Institute. HIV, viral hepatitis and sexually transmissible infections in Australia. Annual Surveillance Report 2015. In: Annual Surveillance Report 2015. Sydney: The Kirby Institute, UNSW Australia; 2015. p. 2052.
15. van Rooijen MS, van der Loeff MF, Morre SA, van Dam AP, Speksnijder AG, de Vries HJ. Spontaneous pharyngeal Chlamydia trachomatis RNA clearance. A cross-sectional study followed by a cohort study of untreated STI clinic patients in Amsterdam, The Netherlands. Sex Transm Infect. 2015;91(3):157–64.
16. Barbee LA, Khosropour CM, Dombrowski JC, Manhart LE, Golden MR. An estimate of the proportion of symptomatic gonococcal, chlamydial and non-gonococcal non-chlamydial urethritis attributable to oral sex among men who have sex with men: a case–control study. Sex Transm Infect. 2016;92(2):155–60.
17. Vodstrcil LA, McIver R, Huston WM, Tabrizi SN, Timms P, Hocking JS. The epidemiology of chlamydia trachomatis organism load during genital infection: a systematic review. J Infect Dis. 2015;211(10):1628–45.
18. Jin F, Prestage GP, Mao L, Kippax SC, Pell CM, Donovan B, Cunningham PH, Templeton DJ, Kaldor JM, Grulich AE. Incidence and risk factors for urethral and anal gonorrhoea and chlamydia in a cohort of HIV-negative homosexual men: the Health in Men Study. Sex Transm Infect. 2007;83(2):113–9.
19. Nash JL, Hocking JS, Read TR, Chen MY, Bradshaw CS, Forcey DS, Fairley CK. Contribution of sexual practices (other than anal sex) to bacterial sexually transmitted infection transmission in men who have sex with men: a cross-sectional analysis using electronic health records. Sex Transm Infect. 2014;90(1):55–7.
20. Barbee LA, Khosropour CM, Dombrowski JC, Manhart LE, Golden MR. An estimate of the proportion of symptomatic gonococcal, chlamydial and non-gonococcal non-chlamydial urethritis attributable to oral sex among men who have sex with men: a case–control study. Sex Transm Infect. 2015;0:1–6.
21. Bernstein KT, Stephens SC, Barry PM, Kohn R, Philip SS, Liska S, Klausner JD. Chlamydia trachomatis and Neisseria gonorrhoeae transmission from the oropharynx to the urethra among men who have sex with men. Clin Infect Dis. 2009;49(12):1793–7.
22. Schillinger JA, Katz BP, Markowitz LE, Braslins PG, Shrier LA, Madico G, Van Der Pol B, Orr DP, Rice PA, Batteiger BE. Genotype-specific concordance of chlamydia trachomatis genital infection within heterosexual partnerships. Sex Transm Dis. 2016;43(12):741–9.

Risk factors and molecular features of sequence type (ST) 131 extended-Spectrum-β-lactamase-producing *Escherichia coli* in community-onset female genital tract infections

Young Ah Kim[1], Kyungwon Lee[2,3] and Jae Eun Chung[4*]

Abstract

Background: *Escherichia coli (E. coli)* is known to cause urinary tract infection (UTI) and meningitis in neonates, as well as existing as a commensal flora of the human gut. Extended-spectrum β-lactamase (ESBL)-producing *E. coli* has increased in the community with the spread of CTX-M type ESBL-producing sequence type 131 (ST131)-O25-*H30Rx E. coli* clone. The role of ESBL-producing *E. coli* in female genital tract infection has not been elucidated. The clinical and molecular features of *E. coli* isolated from community-onset female genital tract infections were evaluated to elucidate the current burden in the community, focusing on the highly virulent and multidrug-resistant ST131 clone.

Methods: We collected and sequenced 91 non-duplicated *E. coli* isolates from the female genital tract of 514 patients with community-onset vaginitis. ESBL genotypes were identified by PCR and confirmed to be ESBL-producers by sequencing methods. ST131 clones were screened by PCR for O16-ST131 and O25b-ST131. Pulsed-field gel electrophoresis (PFGE) and PCR-based replicon typing (PBRT) were conducted in ESBL producers. Independent clinical risk factors associated with acquiring ESBL-producing *E. coli* and ST131 clone were analyzed using multivariate logistic regression analysis.

Results: Of the 514 consecutive specimens obtained from the infected female genital tract, 17.7% (91/514) had *E. coli* infection, of which 19.8% (18/91) were ESBL producers. CTX-M-15 was the most common type ($n = 15$). O25b-ST131 and O16-ST131 clones accounted for 15.4% (14/91) and 6.6% (6/91), respectively. In plasmid analysis, ten isolates succeeded in conjugation and plasmid types were IncFII ($n = 4$), IncFI ($n = 3$), IncI1-Iγ (n = 3) with one non-typable case. Compared to ESBL-nonproducing *E. coli*, ESBL-producing *E. coli* acquisition was strongly associated with recurrent vaginitis (OR 40.130; 95% CI 9.980–161.366), UTI (OR 18.915; 95% CI 5.469–65.411), and antibiotics treatment (OR 68.390; 95% CI 14.870–314.531).

Conclusion: A dominant clone of CTX-M type ESBL-producing *E. coli* in conjugative plasmids seems to be circulating in the community and considerable number of ST131 *E. coli* in the genital tract of Korean women was noted. Sustained monitoring of molecular epidemiology and control of the high-risk group is needed to prevent ESBL-producing *E. coli* from spreading throughout the community.

Keywords: Extended-spectrum beta-lactamase, *Escherichia coli*, Sequence type 131, Female genital tract infection

* Correspondence: jiupark@naver.com
[4]Department of Obstetrics and Gynecology, National Health Insurance Service Ilsan Hospital, Baekseok-dong 1232, Ilsandong-gu, Goyang 10444, South Korea
Full list of author information is available at the end of the article

Background

Escherichia coli (E. coli) is known to cause urinary tract infection (UTI), surgical site infection, and meningitis in neonates, as well as existing as a commensal flora of the human gut [1, 2]. The colonization of *E.coli* has been reported in both pregnant (24–31%) and non-pregnant (9–28%) women [3, 4]. The clinical risk factors for *E. coli* colonization or infection in the female genital tract is not fully understood, but postmenopausal changes including cessation of estrogen production, increased vaginal pH, disappearance of lactobacilli with the concurrent colonization of *Enterobacteriaceae* including *E. coli* is thought to play a role.[5] Pregnant women with *E. coli* infection prompt additional attention due to its consequences regarding the pregnancy outcome including the infection of the new born [5].

In the past decade, colonization or infection of extended-spectrum-β-lactamase (ESBL)-producing *E. coli* has remarkably increased in the community, mostly due to the spread of high virulent and multidrug-resistant sequence type 131 (ST131) *E. coli* clone [6–8]. According to recent epidemiologic studies based on community-onset UTI, the situation of Korea is not different [6–8]. The presence of ESBL-producing *E. coli* in female genital tract infections are scarcely identified within our knowledge.

In this prospective observational study, risk factors and molecular features of female genital tract infections by *E. coli* were evaluated. We focused on the highly virulent and multidrug-resistant ST131 clone because it could be another indicator of the spread in the community and an emerging public health threat.

Methods

For the prospective observational study, 91 non-duplicated *E. coli* isolates from the female genital tract specimens of 514 consecutive, sequentially encountered patients were analyzed. All specimen were retrieved from one community hospital in Gyeonggi-do province, South Korea (742 beds) under the diagnosis of community-onset vaginitis or cervicitis between June 2016 and April 2017. All patients had infection signs such as increased leucorrhoea, vaginal dyspareunia, intermittent pruritus, burning sensation, and foul odor. Sites of the acquisition were determined as described by Friedman with some modifications [9]. Community-onset was defined as diagnosis given within 48 h of admission, further categorized as community-onset healthcare-associated (COHA) and community-associated (CA) group. COHA infections had any one of the following histories: attended a hospital or hemodialysis clinic or received intravenous chemotherapy in the 30 days before the infection; hospitalized in an acute care hospital for 2 or more days in the 90 days, transfer-in from other healthcare facility before the infection. Others were defined as CA infection [9].

Species Identification and susceptibility testing were performed with Microscan Walk-away plus system (BeckmanCoulter, Inc., CA, USA) and MicroScan Neg Breakpoint Combo Type 44 (Siemens Healthcare Diagnostics Inc., West Sacramento, CA, USA). Antimicrobial susceptibility of the 91 *E. coli* isolates was tested and interpreted using CLSI criteria [10]. ESBL production was confirmed by ESBL double-disk synergy test [11], and ESBL genotype was determined by PCR and sequencing [12]. For the detection of ST131, all isolates were screened by PCR for O16-ST131, and O25b-ST131 [13]. Pulsed-field gel electrophoresis (PFGE) was performed as described in our previous study [14]. The patterns were analyzed using InfoQuest FP software (Bio-Rad) to generate a dendrogram based on the unweighted pair group method, with an arithmetic average (UPGMA) from the Dice coefficient with 1% band position tolerance and 0.5% optimization settings. A PCR based replicon typing (PBRT) were schemed in the 18 ESBL-producing *E. coli* isolates, targeting the replicons of the major plasmid families occurring in *Enterobacteriaceae* (HI2, HI1, I1-γ, X, L/M, N, FIA, FIB, FIC, W, Y, P, A/C, T, K, B/O) according to the protocol by Carattoli, et al. [15] Ten of the 18 isolates were successfully conjugated and PBRT was performed in these 10 transconjugants.

To find the independent clinical risk factors associated with acquiring the ESBL-producing *E. coli* and ST131 clone, medical records were reviewed for the patient's age, pregnancy status, pregnancy outcome, menopause status, underlying medical conditions such as Diabetes Mellitus(DM) and hypertension, use of the intrauterine device or pessary, nursing home residency, pelvic inflammatory disease(PID), types of vaginitis such as atrophic vaginitis or chlamydial infection, previous antimicrobial treatment within 1 month, history of UTI within 1 month, and history of recurrent vaginitis within 1 month.

Statistical analysis was performed using Chi-square test for the comparative analysis of categorical variables to determine the independent risk factors. Fisher's exact test was used when 25% of the cells had an expected frequency of less than 5. Odds ratio (OR) and 95% confidence interval (CI) values were calculated for binomial variables. Variables were first compared using univariate logistic regression, then a multivariate analysis using a backward selection with variables with a p-value < 0.1 in the univariate study was carried out. Multivariate logistic regression model was adjusted for age, pregnancy, intrauterine device use, menopause, admission from the nursing home, PID, recurrent vaginitis, UTI and previous antibiotic treatment within one month. Statistical significance was defined as $p < 0.05$. SPSS 17.0 (SPSS, Chicago, IL, USA) and SAS 9.4(SAS Institute Inc., Cary, NC) was used.

Results

Of the 514 consecutive specimens obtained from the infected female genital tract, 17.7% (91/514) had *E. coli* infection, of which 19.8% (18/91) were ESBL producers. All ESBL-producers had the CTX-M genotypes; CTX-M-15 was the most common type ($n = 15$), one of which also had CTX-M-27. CTX-M-55 producers were also detected ($n = 3$). Of the total 19 *E. coli* isolates, O25b-ST131 accounted for 15.4% (14/91) and O16-ST131 clones for 6.6% (6/91). Seven of the 18 ESBL producers were a ST131 clone with four being O25b-ST131 and three O16-ST131 (Table 1 and Additional file 1: Table S1). PFGE patterns of ESBL-producing *E. coli* showed three dominant clonal groups with the cut off 80% similarity, suggesting the clonal spread of ESBL-producing *E. coli* in the community (Fig. 1). In plasmid analysis, ten isolates succeeded in conjugation and plasmid types were IncFII ($n = 4$), IncFI ($n = 3$), IncI1-Iγ (n = 3) and one non-typable (Table 1). Antimicrobial susceptibility of the 91 *E. coli* isolates were analyzed. ST131 clone showed high resistance rates (RRs) to both 3rd generation cephalosporin and fluoroquinolones; 36% (O25b-ST131) versus 20% (non-ST131) to cefotaxime and 50% (O25b-ST131) versus 35% (non-ST131) to ciprofloxacin (Table 2 and Additional file 2: Table S2).

The median age of the patients with ESBL-producing *E. coli* was 45 years old (31–96) and accompanying diseases were recurrent vaginitis ($n = 4$), atrophic vaginitis ($n = 3$), pelvic inflammatory disease ($n = 3$), preterm labor ($n = 3$), and UTI ($n = 2$). They were treated with a variety of antimicrobial therapies, which included cephalosporin, carbapenems, piperacillin-tazobactam, and amikacin, alone or in combination and achieved a clinical cure. All three pregnancies with ESBL-producing *E. coli* female genital tract infection were prematurely terminated due to preterm labor (Table 1).

Independent clinical risk factors for acquiring the ESBL-producing *E. coli* over non-ESBL producing *E. coli* were preterm labor (OR, 10.911, 95% CI, 1.199–99.301; $P = 0.0339$), intrauterine device insertion (OR, 6.460; 95% CI, 1.004–41.568; $P = 0.0495$), history of recurrent vaginitis within one month (OR, 40.130; 95% CI, 9.980–161.366; $P \leq 0.0001$), history of UTI within one month (OR, 18.915; 95% CI, 5.469–65.411; $P \leq 0.0001$), and antibiotics treatment within one month (OR, 68.390; 95% CI, 14.870–314.531; $P \leq 0.0001$) (Table 3) .

Clinical characteristics were compared between the ST131 and non-ST131 clone. In the multivariate logistic regression analysis adjusting for the compounding variables, independent risk factors with statistical significance

Table 1 Clinical and molecular features of community-onset ESBL-producing *Escherichia coli* isolated from the infected female genital tract ($n = 18$)

No	Age	Specimen	Accompanying disease	Site of acquisition	ESBL genotype	Plasmid type	ST131 (O25b/O16)
C05	39	Cervix	Preterm labor	CA	CTX-M – 15	–	Non ST131
C08	45	Cervix	Malaria	CA	CTX-M – 15	–	Non ST131
C12	96	Cervix	Cervix cancer, pneumonia	COHA	CTX-M – 15	IncFI, IncI1-Iγ,	ST131 (O25b)
C15	32	Cervix	Preterm labor	CA	CTX-M – 55	IncFII	Non ST131
C24	42	Cervix	Pelvic inflammatory disease	CA	CTX-M – 15	–	Non ST131
C29	54	Cervix	Atrophic vaginitis	CA	CTX-M – 15	IncI1-Iγ,	ST131 (O25b)
C34	31	Cervix	Preterm labor	CA	CTX-M – 55	IncI1-Iγ,	ST131 (O16b)
C36	51	Cervix	Recurrent vaginitis, UTI	CA	CTX-M – 15	–	Non ST131
C39	86	Cervix	Endometritis	COHA	CTX-M – 15	IncFII	ST131 (O25b)
C43	32	Cervix	Recurrent vaginitis, UTI	COHA	CTX-M – 15	non-typable	ST131 (O25b)
C50	34	Cervix	Pelvic inflammatory disease	CA	CTX-M – 15 CTX-M-27	–	Non ST131
C60	68	Cervix	Atrophic vaginitis	CA	CTX-M – 15	–	ST131 (O16)
C71	45	Cervix	Atrophic vaginitis	CA	CTX-M – 15	–	Non ST131
C72	46	Cervix	Recurrent vaginitis	CA	CTX-M-15	IncFI	Non ST131
C73	45	Cervix	Recurrent vaginitis	CA	CTX-M – 15	–	Non ST131
C77	32	Cervix	Pelvic inflammatory disease	CA	CTX-M – 15	IncFII	ST131 (O16)
C79	42	Cervix	Pelvic inflammatory disease	CA	CTX-M – 15	IncFII	Non ST131
C96	86	Endometrium	Atrophic vaginitis	COHA	CTX-M – 55	IncFI	Non ST131

ESBL Extended-spectrum-β-lactamase, *n* Number, *UTI* Urinary tract infection, *CA* Community-associated, *COHA* Community-onset, healthcare-associated; –, unconjugative plasmid, *ST* Sequence type, *O25b* Serogroup O25b, *O16* Serogroup O16

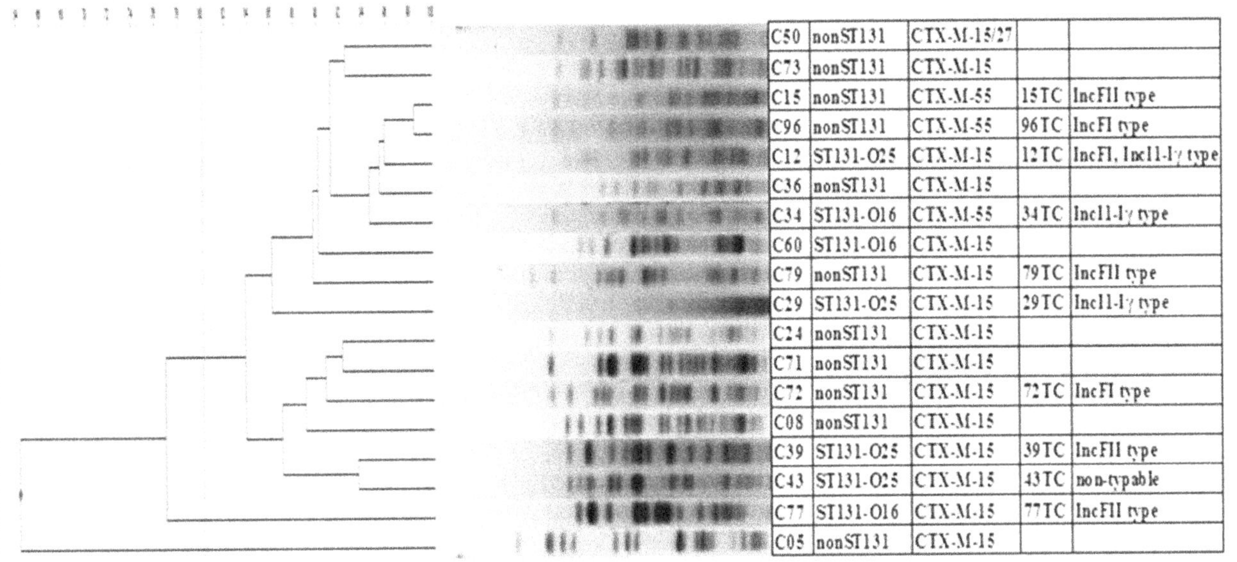

Fig. 1 Pulsed-field gel electrophoresis of *χbaI*-restricted DNA of community-onset ESBL-producing *Escherichia coli*, isolated from the infected female genital tract (*n* = 18)

Table 2 Antimicrobial resistance rates (%) of *Escherichia coli* isolates of patients with female genital tract infection

Antimicrobial agent	Total (*n* = 91)	ESBL (*n* = 18)	Non-ESBL (*n* = 73)	ST131[a] (*n* = 20)	O25b-ST131 (*n* = 14)	Non-ST131 (*n* = 71)
Ampicillin	67 (61/91)	100 (18/18)	59 (43/73)	85 (17/20)	79 (11/14)	62 (44/71)
Ampicillin/sulbactam	27 (25/91)	33 (6/18)	26 (19/73)	20 (4/20)	21 (3/14)	30 (21/71)
Piperacillin	65 (59/91)	100 (18/18)	56 (41/73)	85 (17/20)	79 (11/14)	59 (42/71)
Piperacillin/Tazobactam	0 (0/91)	0 (0/18)	0 (0/73)	0 (0/20)	0 (0/14)	0 (0/71)
Cefuroxime	25 (23/91)	94 (17/18)	8 (6/73)	40 (8/20)	36 (5/14)	21 (15/71)
Cefotaxime	25 (23/91)	94 (17/18)	7 (5/73)	40 (8/20)	36 (5/14)	20 (14/71)
Ceftazidime	24 (22/91)	94 (17/18)	7 (5/73)	40 (8/20)	36(5/14)	20 (14/71)
Cefoxitin	7 (6/91)	6 (1/18)	7 (5/73)	5 (1/20)	7 (1/14)	7 (5/71)
Cefepime	22 (20/91)	100 (18/18)	3 (2/73)	35 (7/20)	29 (4/14)	18 (13/71)
Aztreonam	22 (20/91)	94 (17/18)	4 (3/73)	35 (7/20)	29 (4/14)	18 (13/71)
Meropenem	0 (0/91)	0 (0/18)	0 (0/73)	0 (0/20)	0 (0/14)	0 (0/71)
Doripenem	0 (0/91)	0 (0/18)	0 (0/73)	0 (0/20)	0 (0/14)	0 (0/71)
Imipenem	0 (0/91)	0 (0/18)	0 (0/73)	0 (0/20)	0 (0/14)	0 (0/71)
Ciprofloxacin	36 (33/91)	67 (12/18)	29 (21/73)	40 (8/20)	50 (7/14)	35 (25/71)
Levofloxacin	30 (27/91)	61 (11/18)	22 (16/73)	40 (8/20)	50 (7/14)	27 (19/71)
Gentamicin	25 (23/91)	33 (6/18)	23 (17/73)	25 (5/20)	21 (3/14)	25 (18/71)
Tobramycin	18 (16/91)	22 (4/18)	16 (12/73)	15 (3/20)	14 (2/14)	18 (13/71)
Amikacin	1 (1/91)	0 (0/18)	1 (1/73)	0 (0/20)	0 (0/14)	1 (1/71)
Cotrimoxazole	40 (36/91)	44 (8/18)	38 (28/73)	45 (9/20)	43 (6/14)	38 (27/71)
Tigecycline	0 (0/91)	0 (0/18)	0 (0/73)	0 (0/20)	0 (0/14)	0 (0/71)
Colistin	0 (0/91)	0 (0/18)	0 (0/73)	0 (0/20)	0 (0/14)	0 (0/71)

[a]*ST131* Sequence type131 (both O25 and O16), *O25b* Serogroup O25b, *O16* Serogroup O16, ESBL, ESBL-producer; non-ESBL; non-ESBL producer

Table 3 Clinical risk factors of acquiring the ESBL-producing *Escherichia coli* and ST131 clone

Risk factors	ESBL vs non-ESBL				ST131 vs non-ST131			
	N (%)	OR	95% CI	*P*	N (%)	OR	95% CI	*P*
Preterm labor in pregnancy	3(16.7)	10.911	1.199–99.301	0.0339	–	–	–	–
Age								
30–39	6(33.3)				5(25.0)			
40–49	6(33.3)	1.057	0.289–3.861	0.9330	3(15.0)	0.828	0.170–4.026	0.5497
50–59	2(11.1)	0.385	0.075–1.967	0.2512	4(20.0)	5.541	0.130–236.943	0.8151
> = 60	4(22.2)	0.625	0.156–2.494	0.5054	8(40.0)	5.130	0.099–266.909	0.3716
Menopause	6(33.3)	0.0365	0.126–1.059	0.0636	12(60.0)	0.208	0.005–8.843	0.4118
IUD	3(16.7)	6.460	1.004–41.568	0.0495	1(5.0)	0.965	0.088–10.645	0.9770
Recurrent within 1 month	14(77.8)	40.130	9.980–161.366	< 0.0001	6(30.0)	1.883	0.105–33.820	0.6677
Nursing home T/I	3(16.7)	3.488	0.709–17.152	0.1242	3(15.0)	1.088	0.096–12.292	0.9459
PID	14(77.8)	0.489	0.113–2.122	0.3396	10(50.0)	0.744	0.164–3.378	0.7017
UTI[a]	9(50.0)	18.915	5.469–65.411	< 0.0001	11(55.0)	1.513	0.362–6.319	0.5506
Previous antibiotics[a]	15(83.3)	68.390	14.870–314.531	< 0.0001	6(30.0)	1.172	0.063–21.644	0.9149

ESBL, female genital tract infections with ESBL-producing *E. coli*; Non-ESBL, female genital tract infections with non-ESBL-producing *E. coli*; OR, odds ratio; 95% CI, 95% confidential interval; T/I, transfer-in; IUD, intrauterine device; PID, pelvic inflammatory disease; UTI, urinary tract infection; [a] within one month
Multivariate analysis adjusted for age, pregnancy, intrauterine device use, menopause, admission from the nursing home, PID, recurrent vaginitis, UTI and previous antibiotic treatment within one month

could not be found that were associated with acquiring the ST131 clone (Table 3).

Discussion

ESBL-producing *E. coli* was considered to be a crucial nosocomial pathogen when it was first isolated in the late 1980s [6–8]. With the occurrence of the ST131 clone, ESBL-producing *E. coli* in the community setting has been widely noted in recent studies [16–18]. Our previous study showed that 27% (58/213) of *E. coli* isolates from UTI patients belonged to the globally epidemic ST131 clone [6]. The Korean Antimicrobial Resistance Monitoring System (KARMS) reported the resistance rates of *E. coli* to cefotaxime to be 35% in 2015 [19]. Asymptomatic carriage of ESBL-producing *E. coli* among healthy individuals playing the role of reservoir are also known to have increased [20]. Fecal colonization with ESBL-producing *E. coli* are also on the rise [21].

Analysis of vaginal microbiome showed region-specific variation, setting the basis of the need for a region-specific data of the epidemic multi-drug resistant ST131 ESBL-producing *E. coli* clone [22, 23]. We evaluated the prevalence of ESBL-producing *E. coli*, focusing on the ST131 clone in female genital tract infections because it could be another indicator of the spread of highly virulent and multi-drug resistant *E. coli* in the community, which could be an emerging threat to the public health.

Of the 514 consecutive specimens obtained from the infected female genital tract, 17.7% (91/514) had *E. coli* infection, of which 19.8% (18/91) were ESBL producers. Fourteen of the 18 ESBL producers were community-associated(CA) without any history of hospitalization, suggesting the possibility of community based spread of ESBL-producing *E. coli* (Table 1).

CTX-M-15 was the most common type ($n = 15$) and this was in accordance of the previous isolates of CTX types in Korea in which either CTX-M-1 group (including CTX-M-15 or CTX-M-55) or CTX-M-9 group (including CTX-M-14 or CTX-M-27) prevailed [6, 7]. CTX-M-55 genotype is a variant of CTX-M-15 with a single amino acid substitution, which was known to frequent in China and considered as a potential threat to community spread [24]. Recently CTX-M-55-producing *Shigella* and *Salmonella* were isolated in Korea with *bla*$_{\text{CTX-M-55}}$ genes inserted into IncI1, IncA/C, and IncZ plasmid, downstream of IS*Ecp1*, IS*26*-IS*Ecp1* and IS*Ecp*-IS*5* sequences, which suggests CTX-M-55 dissemination to different bacterial species by lateral plasmid transfer [25]. In this study, ten of 18 ESBL-producing *E. coli* succeeded in conjugation, and plasmid types were IncFII ($n = 4$), IncFI ($n = 3$), IncI1-Iγ (n = 3) with one non-typable case. Most of ESBL-producing *E. coli* showed similar clonality in PFGE, which suggests that dominant clone of CTX-M type ESBL-producing *E. coli* in conjugative plasmids are circulating in the community.

O25b-ST131 and O16-ST131 clones accounted for 15.4% (14/91) and 6.6% (6/91), respectively, suggesting a high prevalence of ST131 *E. coli* clone in the female genital tracts of Korean women. The expansion of the ST131 *E. coli* clone with phylogenetic B2, serotype O25b, *fimH* type *H30* is suggested to reveal multidrug resistant property [8, 17]. In this study, O25b-ST131 clones showed high rates of multidrug-resistancy against the 3rd generation cephalosporins as well as fluoroquinolones (Table 2 and Additional file 2: Table S2).

Compared to the ESBL-nonproducing *E. coli* group, ESBL-producing *E. coli* group showed higher tendency of having clinical features such as history of recurrent vaginitis within 1 month (OR, 40.130; 95% CI, 9.980–161.366; $P \leq 0.0001$), history of UTI within 1 month (OR, 18.915; 95% CI, 5.469–65.411; $P \leq 0.0001$), and history or antibiotics treatment within 1 month (OR, 68.390; 95% CI, 14.870–314.531; $P \leq 0.0001$). *E. coli* is a well-known etiologic agent for UTI, so it is not surprising that female genital tract infection with ESBL-producing *E. coli* were strongly associated with UTI [6–8]. Previous antibiotic exposure might have resulted in the selection pressure of a resistant clone, concomitantly developing multidrug-resistancy [14, 26].

Aerobic vaginitis is a recently defined vaginitis type, which differs from the common bacterial vaginosis in terms of scarce presence of lactobacilli and positive cultured aerobic bacteria including group B streptococci, *E.coli*, and enterococci [5]. In postmenopausal women with atrophic vaginitis, the lack of estrogen results in deficiency of mucosal epithelial barrier, lactobacilli disappear from the vaginal flora decreasing the pH of the vagina, resulting in predominant colonization by *Enterobacteriaceae*, especially *E. coli.*, serving an adequate environment for aerobic vaginitis to set place [2, 27].

In cases of pregnancy, aerobic vaginitis is known to be associated with an increased risk of preterm labor and chorioamnionitis [5]. Although all three pregnancies infected by ESBL producers resulted in preterm labor in this study, due to the small number of included patients and the omission of cases without genital tract infection, the role of ESBL producers in poor pregnancy outcome should be interpreted with caution. Further studies including a larger number of pregnancies to elucidate the role of ESBL-producing *E. coli* in the genital tract infection is warranted.

Conclusions

In conclusion, a dominant clone of CTX-M type ESBL-producing *E. coli* in conjugative plasmids seems to be circulating in the community and considerable number of ST131 *E. coli* clone in the genital tracts of Korean women was noted. Sustained monitoring of molecular epidemiology and an adequate control of the clinically high-risk group is needed to prevent ESBL-producing *E. coli* from spreading throughout the community.

Acknowledgements

The authors thank Hae Yong Park from the department of policy research affairs, National Health Insurance Service Ilsan Hospital for the statistical support.

Funding

This study was funded by grants from the National health Insurance Service Ilsan Hospital (NHIMC2017CR001).

Authors' contributions

JEC handled the clinical part including taking the vaginal swab and reviewing the medical records. YAK worked on the microbiological part of this study. For the critical revision and approval of the final version, KL contributed. All three authors have read the final manuscript and hereby approve the manuscript.

Competing interests

The authors declare that they have no competing interests.

Author details

[1]Department of Laboratory Medicine, National Health Insurance Service Ilsan Hospital, Baekseok-dong 1232, Ilsandong-gu, Goyang 10444, South Korea. [2]Department of Laboratory Medicine, Yonsei University College of Medicine, 50-1 Yonsei-ro, Seodaemun-gu, Seoul 03722, South Korea. [3]Research Institute of Bacterial Resistance, Yonsei University College of Medicine, Seoul, South Korea. [4]Department of Obstetrics and Gynecology, National Health Insurance Service Ilsan Hospital, Baekseok-dong 1232, Ilsandong-gu, Goyang 10444, South Korea.

References

1. Gupta K, Stapleton AE, Hooton TM, Roberts PL, Fennell CL, Stamm WE. Inverse association of H2O2-producing lactobacilli and vaginal Escherichia coli colonization in women with recurrent urinary tract infections. J Infect Dis. 1998;178(2):446–50.
2. Han C, Wu W, Fan A, Wang Y, Zhang H, Chu Z, et al. Diagnostic and therapeutic advancements for aerobic vaginitis. Arch Gynecol Obstet. 2015; 291(2):251–7.
3. Obata-Yasuoka M, Ba-Thein W, Tsukamoto T, Yoshikawa H, Hayashi H. Vaginal *Escherichia coli* share common virulence factor profiles, serotypes and phylogeny with other extraintestinal *E. coli*. Microbiology. 2002;148: 2745–52.
4. Watt S, Lanotte P, Mereghetti L, Moulin-Schouleur M, Picard B, Quentin R. *Escherichia coli* strains from pregnant women and neonates: Intraspecies genetic distribution and prevalence of virulence factors. J Clin Microbiol. 2003;41(5):1929–35.
5. Donders G, Bellen G, Rezeberga D. Aerobic vaginitis in pregnancy. BJOG. 2011;118(10):1163–70.
6. Kim YA, Kim JJ, Kim H, Lee K. Community-onset extended-spectrum-β-lactamase-producing *Escherichia coli* sequence type 131 at two Korean community hospitals: the spread of multidrug-resistant *E. coli* to the community via healthcare facilities. Int J Infect Dis. 2017;54:39–42.
7. Cha MK, Kang C, Kim SH, Cho SY, Ha YE, Wi YM, et al. Comparison of the microbiological characteristics and virulence factors of ST131 and non-ST131 clones among extended-spectrum β-lactamase-producing *Escherichia coli* causing bacteremia. Diagn Microbiol Infect Dis. 2016;84: 102–4.
8. Colpan A, Johnston B, Porter S, Clabots C, Anway R, Thao L, et al. *Escherichia coli* sequence type 131 (ST131) subclone H30 as an emergent multidrug-resistant pathogen among US veterans. Clin Infect Dis. 2013;57:1256–65.
9. Friedman ND, Kaye KS, Stout JE, McGarry SA, Trivette SL, Briggs JP, et al. Health care–associated bloodstream infections in adults: a reason to change the accepted definition of community-acquired infections. Ann Intern Med. 2002;137:791–7.
10. Performance Standards for Antimicrobial Susceptibility Testing: 26th Informational Supplement. CLSI document M100S (ISBN 1-56238-923-8). Clinical and Laboratory Standards Institute, 2016.
11. Lee K, Cho SR, Lee CS, Chong Y, Kwon OH. Prevalence of extended broad-spectrum beta-lactamase in *Escherichia coli* and *Klebsiella pneumonia*. Korean J Infect Dis. 1994;26:341–8.

12. Ryoo NH, Kim E, Hong SG, Park YJ, Lee K, Bae IK, et al. Dissemination of SHV-12 and CTX-M-type extended-spectrum β-lactamase among clinical isolates of *Escherichia coli* and *Klebsiella pneumoniae* and emergence of GES-3 in Korea. J Antimicrob Chemother. 2005;56:698–702.
13. Johnson JR, Clermont O, Johnston B, Clabots C, Tchesnokova V, Sokurenko E, et al. Rapid and specific detection, molecular epidemiology, and experimental virulence of the O16 subgroup within *Escherichia coli* sequence type 131. J Clin Microbiol. 2014;52:1358–65.
14. Park YS, Bae IK, Kim J, Jeong SH, Hwang S, Seo Y, et al. Risk factors and molecular epidemiology of community-onset extended-spectrum β-lactamase-producing *Escherichia coli* bacteremia. Yonsei Med J. 2014;55: 467–75.
15. Carattoli A, Bertini A, Villa L, Falbo V, Hopkins KL, Threlfall EJ. Identification of plasmids by PCR-based replicon typing. J Microbiol Methods. 2005;63: 219–28.
16. Paterson DL, Bonomo RA. Extended-spectrum beta-lactamases: a clinical update. Clin Microbiol Rev. 2005;18:657–86.
17. Johnson JR, Johnston B, Clabots C, Kuskowski MA, Castanheira M. *Escherichia coli* sequence type ST131 as the major cause of serious multidrug-resistant *E. coli* infections in the United States. Clin Infect Dis. 2010;51:286–94.
18. Rogers BA, Sidjabat HE, Paterson DL. Escherichia coli O25b-ST131: a pandemic, multiresistant, community-associated strain. J Antimicrob Chemother. 2011;66:1–14.
19. Kim D, Ahn JY, Lee CH, Jang SJ, Lee H, Yong D, et al. Increasing resistance to extended-spectrum cephalosporins, fluoroquinolone, and carbapenem in gram-negative bacilli and the emergence of carbapenem non-susceptibility in *Klebsiella pneumoniae*: analysis of Korean antimicrobial resistance monitoring system (KARMS) data from 2013 to 2015. Ann Lab Med. 2017;37: 231–9.
20. Carlet J. The gut is the epicentre of antibiotic resistance. Antimicrob Resist Infect Control. 2012;271:1–7.
21. Karanika S, Karantanos T, Arvanitis M, Grigoras C, Mylonakis E. Fecal colonization with extended-spectrum beta-lactamase-producing Enterobacteriaceae and risk factors among healthy individuals: a systematic review and meta-analysis. Clin Infect Dis. 2016;63:310–8.
22. Hong KH, Hong SK, Cho SI, Ra E, Han KH, Kang SB, et al. Analysis of the vaginal microbiome by next-generation sequencing and evaluation of its performance as a clinical diagnostic tool in vaginitis. Ann Lab Med. 2016;36: 441–9.
23. Iredell J, Brown J, Tagg K. Antibiotic resistance in Enterobacteriaceae: Mechanisms and clinical implications. BMJ. 352:h6420. https://doi.org/10.1136/bmj.h6420.
24. Xia L, Liu Y, Xia S, Kudinha T, Xiao S-n, Zhong N-s, et al. Prevalence of ST1193 clone and an IncI1/ST16 plasmid in *E. coli* isolates carrying a blaCTX-M-55 gene from urinary tract infections patients in China. Sci Rep. 2017;7: 44866.
25. Kim JS, Kim S, Park J, Shin E, Yun Y, Lee D, et al. Plasmid-mediated transfer of CTX-M-55 extended-spectrum beta-lactamase among different strains of *Salmonella* and *Shigella* spp. in the Republic of Korea. Diagn Microbiol Infect Dis. 2017;89:86–8.
26. Vila J, Sáez-López E, Johnson JR, Römling U, Dobrindt U, Cantón R, et al. *Escherichia coli*: an old friend with new tidings. FEMS Microbiol Rev. 2016;40: 437–63.
27. Ravel J, Gajer P, Abdo Z, Schneider GM, Koenig SSK, McCulle SL, et al. Vaginal microbiome of reproductive-age women. Proc Natl Acad Sci US. 2011;108(Suppl 1):4680–7.

10

Sexually transmitted infections after bereavement

Emily Bond[1*†], Donghao Lu[1*†], Eva Herweijer[1], Karin Sundström[2], Unnur Valdimarsdóttir[1,3,4], Katja Fall[1,5], Lisen Arnheim-Dahlström[1], Pär Sparén[1] and Fang Fang[1]

Abstract

Background: Loss of a loved one has consistently been associated with various health risks. Little is however known about its relation to sexually transmitted infections (STIs).

Methods: We conducted a population-based cohort study during 1987–2012 using the Swedish Multi-Generation Register, including 3,002,209 women aged 10-44 years. Bereavement was defined as death of a child, parent, sibling or spouse ($N = 979{,}579$, 33 %). STIs were defined as hospital visits with an STI as main or secondary diagnosis. Poisson regression and negative binomial regression were used to estimate incidence rate ratios (IRRs) and 95 % confidence intervals (CIs) of STIs, comparing incidence rates of women who had experienced loss to those who had not.

Results: Bereaved women were at significantly higher risk of nearly all STIs studied. The relative risk of any STI was highest during the first year after loss (IRR: 1.45, 95 % CI: 1.27–1.65) and predominantly among women with subsequent onset of psychiatric disorders after bereavement (IRR: 2.61, 95 % CI: 2.00–3.34). Notably, a consistent excess risk, persisting for over five years, was observed for acute salpingitis (IRR: 1.28, 95 % CI: 1.13–1.44), a severe complication of bacterial STIs.

Conclusion: These data suggest that women who have experienced bereavement are at increased risk of STIs.

Keywords: Sexually transmitted infections, Bereavement, Psychological stress, Salpingitis, Condyloma, HPV vaccination

Background

That psychological stress has immune modulating effects is suggested by extensive experimental evidence from both animal [1] and human [2] studies. Experimental studies have further suggested that psychological stress increases susceptibility to viral infections [3]. On the contrary, epidemiological evidence for the potential impact of psychological stress, including various life stressors, on the susceptibility to infections remains weak [4]. However, multiple meta-analyses have shown that psychological stress might facilitate the recurrence of herpes simplex virus infection [5] and the progression of human immunodeficiency virus (HIV) infection [6], lending evidence to theories of psychological stress impairing our ability to control infection.

Sexually transmitted infections, including infections of human papillomavirus (HPV), are major, or even necessary, causes for many infection-related cancers [7, 8]. While the literature on the role of psychological stress in cancer development remains largely inconclusive [9, 10], three recent large population-based studies have suggested a higher risk of cervical cancer, and other HPV related cancers, among bereaved women [11–13]. Although the role of oncologic infections of HPV has been highlighted [13], little is known about whether the underlying mechanism linking bereavement to

* Correspondence: emily.bond@ki.se; donghao.lu@ki.se
†Equal contributors
[1]Department of Medical Epidemiology and Biostatistics, Karolinska Institutet, Nobels väg 12A, Box 281, Stockholm 17177, Sweden
Full list of author information is available at the end of the article

cervical cancer can be attributed to behavioral or biological changes.

To this end, in the present study, we aimed to complement these previous studies by elucidating whether there is an increased risk of sexually transmitted infections (STIs) after bereavement.

Methods

Study population

All women born in Sweden, who were at the age of 10–44 years during 1987–2012, who had at least one parent registered in the Swedish Multi-Generation Register (MGR), were included in the present study ($N = 3{,}002{,}209$) (Fig. 1). The MGR contains largely complete familial linkages for all Swedish residents born since 1932 onward [14].

Follow-up

All women were individually followed from January 1st 1987 or their tenth birthday, whichever came later, to an STI diagnosis, death, emigration, 45th birthday, HPV vaccination, or December 31st 2012, whichever came first, through cross-linkages to the Swedish Patient Register (for STI diagnosis), Cause of Death Register, Migration Register, as well as the Swedish Vaccination Register and the Prescribed Drug Register (collectively for HPV vaccination). Women receiving an HPV vaccination were further studied in a separate analysis.

The Patient Register collects hospital discharge records in Sweden since 1964/1965, and has a complete coverage for the entire country since 1987 [15]. Hospital-based outpatient specialist visits have been added in this register since 2001 with >80 % coverage of the entire country. The Patient Register does however not include visits to general practitioners. The 9th Swedish revision of the International Classification of Diseases (ICD-9) codes was used in this register between 1987 and 1996 and the 10th revision thereafter.

As previously described [16, 17], date for HPV vaccination was first retrieved from the Swedish Vaccination Register, and complemented by prescription date of HPV vaccination (Anatomical Therapeutic Chemical

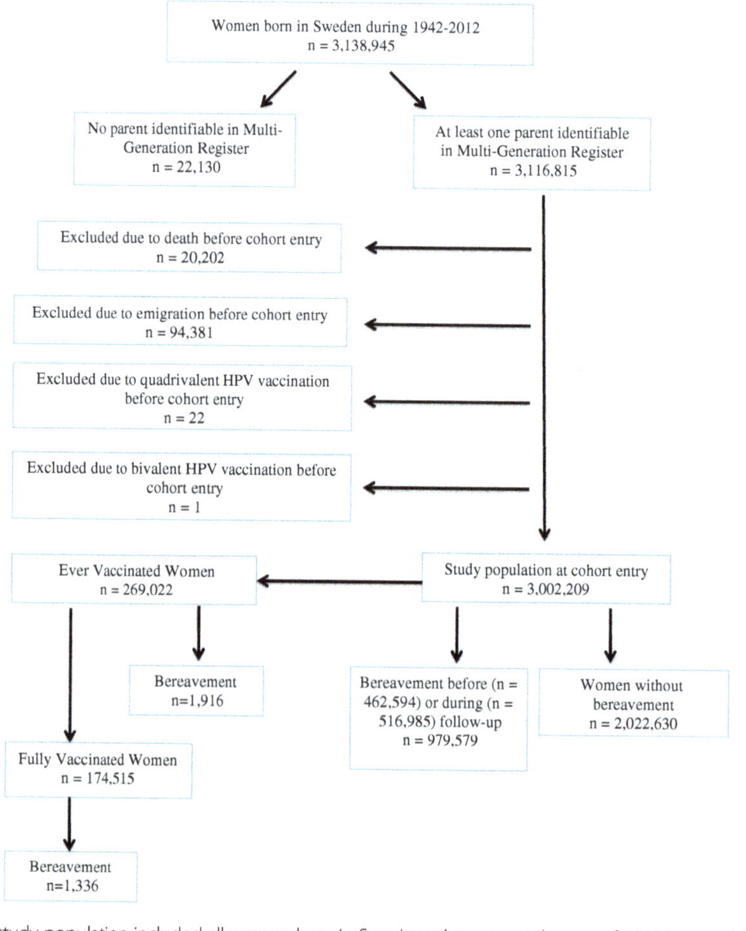

Fig. 1 Study population. The study population included all women born in Sweden who were at the age of 10–44 years during 1987–2012, and had at least one parent identifiable in the Multi-Generation Register. Women who received HPV vaccination during the study period were analyzed separately

(ATC) codes J07BM01 and J07BM02) according to the Prescribed Drug Register when needed. The Prescribed Drug Register records all prescribed drugs from all pharmacies in Sweden since July 2005 [18].

Women without bereavement contributed all person-time to the unexposed group, whereas the exposed women contributed person-time to the unexposed group before the bereavement and to the exposed group thereafter. If a woman had bereavement before entry to the cohort, she contributed person-time only to the exposed group. If a woman lost more than one family member, the first bereavement was counted.

Bereavement

We used the MGR to identify the first-degree relatives of all index women in our study population, including children, parents, and siblings. Spouses were defined through a registered common biological or adopted child in the MGR. We then linked all the family members to the Cause of Death Register and identified any death of these family members from January 1st 1961 until the end of study (December 31st 2012). Bereavement was first classified based on the relationship of the index women to the lost kin ("type of bereavement": loss of a child, spouse, parent, or sibling), and then categorized by cause of death ("cause of bereavement": self-harm, other injuries, cancer, or non-cancer diseases).

Sexually transmitted diseases and related outcomes

STIs were defined through hospital visits where STIs were recorded either as the main or a secondary diagnosis. The STIs studied in the present study included condyloma (i.e. Condyloma acuminatum), gonorrhea, chlamydia, syphilis, and genital herpes simplex (GHS) (Additional file 1: Table S1). Any STI was defined as the composite of the above STIs. The first STI diagnosis during follow-up was used as the outcome of interest for both the exposed and unexposed groups. As a result, bereaved women might have one STI diagnosis before bereavement and another STI diagnosis after bereavement. Concurrence of multiple STIs at the same hospital visit was possible and in such case, the specific STI recorded as the main diagnosis of the visit was used as the outcome of interest. Since we had complete data only on inpatient hospital records for the entire study period, we used the first inpatient hospital contact for STIs as the primary outcome. To assess the representativeness of our findings, we used any hospital contact (both inpatient and outpatient) as secondary outcome for the period of 2001–2010. As another secondary outcome, we complemented the definition of condyloma by using information from the Prescribed Drug Register as previously described [16, 17] for the period of July 2005 to December 2012. Briefly, prescriptions for the condyloma treatments, Aldara and Podophylotoxin (under age of 45 [16]), were identified with ATC codes D06BB10 and D06BB04 and used as alternative definitions of condyloma diagnosis.

Acute salpingitis, inflammation of the fallopian tubes, is not an STI by definition, but it largely shares risk factors with STIs [19]. Furthermore, it has been shown that the rates of acute salpingitis follow chlamydia epidemics very closely [20]. Although some of the STIs studied in the present study may also be diagnosed and treated in clinics outside hospitals (e.g., with general practitioners or youth clinics) and are therefore incompletely covered by the Patient Register, acute salpingitis is more consistently diagnosed and treated within hospital-based clinics.

We additionally studied infections of human immunodeficiency virus-1 (HIV) and hepatitis B (HBV) as STIs with other potential routes of transmission (including intravenous drug use) in addition to high risk sexual behavior.

Separate analysis of HPV vaccinated women

To better understand the potential impact of immune modulation on the studied associations, we conducted a separate analysis among women vaccinated with quadrivalent HPV vaccine for the period of June 2006 to December 2012. Our hypothesis was that the severe psychological stress induced by bereavement might compromise the host immunity in terms of its ability to mount an adequate response to vaccination – an exposure to HPV antigens unrelated to sexual behavior – and therefore result in a suboptimal vaccination efficacy. The quadrivalent HPV vaccine protects against HPV types 6, 11, 16 and 18 which cause about 90 % of condyloma [21]. In total, we identified 269,022 women who received at least one dose of quadrivalent vaccine ("ever vaccinated women") and 174,515 women who received all three doses of quadrivalent vaccine ("fully vaccinated women") (Fig. 1). For this analysis, ever vaccinated women were followed from the date of first dose and fully vaccinated women from the date of third dose.

Statistical analysis

We first calculated the unadjusted incidence rates (i.e., number of STIs divided by accumulated person-years) among women with and without bereavement separately. We then used log-linear Poisson regression models to estimate the incidence rate ratios (IRRs) and 95 % confidence intervals (CIs) of STIs of the bereaved women, compared to women without bereavement. If the Poisson model was found to be over-dispersed, negative binomial regression was used instead. All models were adjusted for age at follow-up (10-18 and 19-44 years for the analysis of vaccinated women; and 10–12, 13–15,

16–18, 19–21, 22–25, 26–29, 30–34, 35–39, and 40–44 years for the rest of the analyses), parental educational level and calendar period at follow-up (5-year groups). Information on parental educational level was obtained from linking the parents of the participants to the Swedish Education Register. Since we studied relatively young women (10–44 years), parental educational level was used as a proxy for the index woman's socioeconomic status. Three educational levels were defined, including low (<9 years or missing), middle (9 years plus 2-3 years of high school), and high (university or doctoral studies). These analyses were performed for both the primary outcome (i.e., inpatient hospital contact for STIs for the period of 1987–2012) and secondary outcome (i.e., any hospital contact for STIs for the period of 2001–2012; and any hospital contact plus prescription claim for condyloma for the period of 2005–2012).

To alleviate potential concern of unmeasured confounders, in a sensitivity analysis, we restricted the analyses to women with bereavement and compared the risk of STIs during the time period after bereavement with the risk during the time period before bereavement.

We further investigated the impact of type and cause of bereavement as well as time since bereavement (≤1 year, 2–4 years, or ≥5 years) in association with the inpatient hospital contact of any STI, acute salpingitis, and HIV or HBV (HIV/HBV). We further stratified the analyses of any STI, acute salpingitis, and HIV/HBV by age at follow-up (10–18, 19–29 and 30–44 years), calendar period of follow-up (1987–2000 and 2001–2012), and parental educational level.

Since mental illness is a known risk factor for high risk sexual behavior and STIs [22, 23], we ascertained the history of psychiatric disorders for all women according to the Patient Register (including both inpatient and outpatient hospital contact as well as main and secondary diagnoses for each visit), starting from 1981 to the end of 2012 (ICD-8/9 codes 290–319 during 1981–1996; and ICD-10 codes F00-F99 since 1997). Patients were classified as having preexisting psychiatric disorders during the entire follow-up if they had a diagnosis for any psychiatric disease before entry to the cohort or from the date of such diagnosis if after entry to the cohort. To examine whether preexisting psychiatric disorders might modify the association of bereavement with STIs, we first stratified the analyses by the history of psychiatric disorders. To examine whether psychiatric disorders might mediate the association, we additionally classified the bereaved women as with or without newly onset psychiatric disorders after bereavement, and compared their risk of STIs with women without bereavement. Bereaved women with preexisting psychiatric disorders were excluded from this analysis. Since HIV/HBV infections are highly related to substance abuse, we conducted specifically similar analyses for substance abuse (ICD-8, 304; ICD-9, 304 and 305X; ICD-10, F11-F16 and F18-F19).

Provided with a smaller number of participants, among HPV-vaccinated women, ever vaccinated or fully vaccinated, we only calculated the IRRs of condyloma and any STI. This analysis was performed only for secondary STI outcomes, i.e., both inpatient and outpatient hospital visits for any STI, and hospital visits plus prescribed drugs for condyloma. In organized vaccination programs, testing for prevalent HPV infection at the time of vaccination is not performed, and HPV status at vaccination is therefore unknown. Since an incubation period of three months has previously been observed for condyloma [17], in a sensitivity analysis, we excluded the first three months of follow-up.

Statistical analyses were conducted using SAS version 9.3 (SAS Institute, Inc.).

Results

The study included 3,002,209 women with an average follow-up of 14.4 years (Fig. 1). 979,579 of the entire cohort and 1916 of the vaccinated women experienced bereavement before or during follow-up.

Compared to the unexposed group, the exposed group had older age at cohort entry, lower parental education level, and less preexisting psychiatric diseases (Additional file 1: Table S2).

Overall, bereaved women had a higher risk of any STI, using either the primary (inpatient hospital visit; IRR: 1.16, 95 % CI: 1.08–1.24) or secondary (any hospital visit; IRR: 1.06, 95 % CI: 1.01-1.11) definition (Table 1). Individual STIs with significantly elevated risk among bereaved women included condyloma and chlamydia (Table 1). Bereaved women also had increased risks of acute salpingitis, HIV and HBV infections (Table 1).

Similar findings were noted when comparing the pre-bereavement to post-bereavement periods of the same women, although the magnitude of the associations was slightly diminished (Table 2).

Bereavement characteristics did not clearly modify the risks of any STI, acute salpingitis, or HIV/HBV infections, although slightly stronger associations with loss of a spouse or sibling, as well as bereavement due to self-harm or other injuries, were suggested for some STIs (Table 3). The strongest associations for any STI (IRR: 1.45, 95 % CI: 1.27–1.65) and acute salpingitis (IRR: 1.49, 95 % CI: 1.25-1.79) were seen during the first year after bereavement (Table 3).

The associations were not clearly modified by age at follow-up, calendar period of follow-up or parental educational level, except for a slightly stronger association for acute salpingitis among women at age 10-18 years (Table 4).

Table 1 Hospital contact of Sexually Transmitted Infections (STI), comparing bereaved women with non-bereaved women

	Inpatient hospital contact (1987–2012)					Any hospital contact (2001–2012)				
	No bereavement		Bereavement			No bereavement		Bereavement		
	N	Crude IR (100,000 PYs)	N	Crude IR (100,000 PYs)	IRR (95 % CI)	N	Crude IR (100,000 PYs)	N	Crude IR (100,000 PYs)	IRR (95 % CI)
Any STI	5903	17.00	1188	14.50	1.16 (1.08–1.24)	71061	453.00	9309	304.00	1.06 (1.01–1.11) [b]
Condyloma [a]	2833	8.14	700	8.54	1.18 (1.08–1.30)	42652	272.00	5334	174.00	1.06 (1.00–1.12) [b]
Gonorrhea	123	0.35	33	0.40	1.51 (0.97–2.28)	466	2.97	75	2.45	1.49 (1.14–1.92)
Chlamydia	952	2.74	136	1.66	1.23 (1.01–1.48)	10098	64.40	1185	38.60	1.14 (1.04–1.26) [b]
Syphilis	65	0.19	20	0.24	1.17 (0.66–2.01)	72	0.46	16	0.52	1.05 (0.57–1.84)
GHS	1946	5.59	302	3.68	1.06 (0.93–1.21)	17828	114.00	2709	88.30	1.04 (0.99–1.09) [b]
Acute salpingitis	11361	32.60	3540	43.20	1.28 (1.13–1.44)[b]	2929	18.70	1000	32.60	1.24 (1.15–1.34)
HIV	120	0.34	96	1.17	2.36 (1.76–3.17)	220	1.40	112	3.65	1.98 (1.53–2.53)
HBV	435	1.25	161	1.96	1.59 (1.30–1.94)	411	2.62	141	4.60	2.20 (1.78–2.71)

Notes:
The first hospital visit concerning an STI diagnosis during the unexposed follow-up and the first hospital visit concerning an STI diagnosis during the exposed follow-up were both counted in all analyses
CI confidence interval, *GHS* genital herpes simplex, *HBV* hepatitis B virus, *HIV* human immunodeficiency virus, *IR* incidence rate, *IRR* incidence rate ratio, *N* number, *PYs* person-years, *STI* sexually transmitted infection
IRR was adjusted for attained age (10–12, 13–15, 16–18, 19–21, 22–25, 26–29, 30–34, 35–39, and 40–44), calendar years (5-year group), and parental education levels (low/missing, medium, and high) as a proxy for socioeconomic status
[a] Any hospital contact for condyloma was further complemented by prescription claim
[b] Negative binomial regression was used instead due to over-dispersed Poisson regression

Table 2 Inpatient hospital contact of Sexually Transmitted Infections (STIs), comparing the post-bereavement to the pre-bereavement periods of women with bereavement

	Before bereavement		After bereavement		
	N	Crude IR (1000 PYs)	N	Crude IR (1000 PYs)	IRR (95 % CI)
Any STI	1428	0.26	1188	0.14	1.14 (1.05–1.25)
Condyloma [a]	831	0.15	700	0.09	1.15 (1.03–1.29)
Gonorrhea	21	0.00	33	0.00	2.71 (1.49–5.00)
Chlamydia	194	0.04	136	0.02	1.15 (0.90–1.46)
Syphilis	12	0.00	20	0.00	1.21 (0.55–2.76)
GHS	375	0.07	302	0.04	1.00 (0.84–1.18)
Acute salpingitis	3569	0.66	3540	0.43	1.09 (0.95–1.27)[b]
HIV	21	0.00	96	0.01	2.36 (1.46–3.99)
HBV	84	0.02	161	0.02	1.41 (1.06–1.89)

Notes:
The first hospital visit concerning an STI diagnosis before bereavement and the first hospital visit concerning an STI diagnosis after bereavement were both counted in all analyses
CI confidence interval, *GHS* genital herpes simplex, *HBV* hepatitis B virus, *HIV* human immunodeficiency virus, *IR* incidence rate, *IRR* incidence rate ratio, *N* number; PYs, person-years
IRR was adjusted for attained age (10–12, 13–15, 16–18, 19–21, 22–25, 26–29, 30–34, 35–39, and 40–44), calendar years (5-year group), and parental education levels (low/missing, medium, and high) as a proxy for socioeconomic status
[a] Any hospital contact for condyloma was further complemented by prescription claim
[b] Negative binomial regression was used instead due to over-dispersed Poisson regression

Apart from a null association between bereavement and any STI among women with preexisting psychiatric disorders, a positive association was noted for acute salpingitis and HIV/HBV, regardless of history of psychiatric disorders (Table 4). Similar result patterns were also noted for substance abuse (Table 4).

Bereaved women with a subsequent psychiatric disorder after bereavement had further increased risks of any STI, compared to bereaved women without psychiatric disorders after bereavement (Table 5). Similarly, more pronounced associations were noted among women with a subsequent diagnosis of substance abuse (Table 5).

Positive associations of any STI and condyloma were also suggested when only vaccinated women were analyzed, although not statistically significant (Table 6). Similar results were noted when the first three months of follow-up were excluded in this analysis (Additional file 1: Table S3).

Discussion

In this population-based cohort study, we found that bereavement, a severely stressful life event, was associated with increased risks of almost all studied STIs among young and middle aged women. The highest risk elevation was noted soon after bereavement and among women with subsequent psychiatric disorders after bereavement. Bereaved women were also more likely to develop acute salpingitis, a severe complication of bacterial STIs.

Sexual risk behavior has been shown to increase among parentally bereaved youth in some [24] but not

Table 3 Inpatient hospital contact of Sexually Transmitted Infections (STIs), by causes, types, and recentness of bereavement

	Any STI		Acute salpingitis		HIV/HBV	
	N	IRR (95 % CI)	N	IRR (95 % CI) [a]	N	IRR (95 % CI)
No bereavement	5903	1.0	11361	1.0	555	1.0
Type of bereavement						
Loss of a child	26	1.05 (0.69–1.51)	119	1.35 (1.03–1.76)	8	2.24 (1.01–4.22)
Loss of a spouse	28	1.81 (1.21–2.57)	94	1.48 (1.11–1.98)	18	6.88 (4.11–10.8)
Loss of a parent	924	1.13 (1.04–1.21)	2779	1.25 (1.10–1.42)	194	1.67 (1.39–2.00)
Loss of a sibling	210	1.24 (1.08–1.42)	548	1.41 (1.21–1.65)	37	1.83 (1.28–2.52)
Cause of bereavement						
Due to self-harm	160	1.16 (0.99–1.35)	510	1.54 (1.31–1.80)	42	2.49 (1.78–3.37)
Due to other injury	92	1.21 (0.98–1.48)	251	1.38 (1.14–1.66)	26	2.75 (1.80–4.00)
Due to cancer	314	1.09 (0.97–1.23)	935	1.18 (1.02–1.36)	59	1.36 (1.02–1.79)
Due to non-cancer diseases	622	1.18 (1.08–1.29)	1844	1.31 (1.15–1.50)	130	1.73 (1.40–2.12)
Time since bereavement						
First year	262	1.45 (1.27–1.65)	699	1.49 (1.25–1.79)	23	1.57 (0.99–2.37)
2–4 years	564	1.08 (0.98–1.18)	1628	1.16 (1.00–1.34)	74	1.70 (1.30–2.19)
≥ 5 years	362	1.07 (0.96–1.20)	1217	1.30 (1.13–1.51)	160	1.85 (1.51–2.25)

Notes:
The first hospital visit concerning an STI diagnosis during the unexposed follow-up and the first hospital visit concerning an STI diagnosis during the exposed follow-up were both counted in all analyses
CI confidence interval, *HBV* hepatitis B virus, *HIV* human immunodeficiency virus, *IRR* incidence rate ratio, *N* number, *STIs* sexually transmitted infections
IRR was adjusted for attained age (10–12, 13–15, 16–18, 19–21, 22–25, 26–29, 30–34, 35–39, and 40–44), calendar years (5-year group), and parental education levels (low/missing, medium, and high) as a proxy for socioeconomic status
[a] Negative binomial regression was used due to over-dispersed Poisson regression

all [25] studies. In contrast, an elevated risk of depression and substance abuse has been more consistently demonstrated among bereaved adults [26, 27] as well as parentally bereaved youth [28–30]. Increased sexual risk behavior has further been noted among patients with depression, including for example lower rates of contraceptive use [23, 31, 32]. Similarly, substance abuse has also been shown to correlate with sexual risk behavior [33]. Therefore, a possible link between bereavement and STIs might be posited, through altered sexual risk behaviors, either as a direct result of bereavement or secondary to psychiatric conditions consequent to bereavement. Such a link is supported by our finding that, as opposed to a loss of a child, sibling or parent, a slightly higher risk of any STI, and a considerably higher risk of HIV/HBV infection, was detected among women that had lost a spouse - a loss much more likely to lead to a change of sexual partner.

In the present study we observed a higher risk of STIs among bereaved women, regardless of whether or not they were treated in a hospital for psychiatric disorders, including substance abuse, after bereavement, suggesting that clinically diagnosed psychiatric disorders subsequent to bereavement might not be the only underlying pathways for the link of bereavement with STIs. However, since the risk increase was significantly higher among bereaved women with subsequent psychiatric disorders, these conditions appear to be important mediators of the studied association. Studies addressing specific behavior changes after bereavement are warranted to further elucidate these pathways.

In addition to the possible behavioral changes after bereavement, a direct biological impact of bereavement on immune modulation is also plausible [34, 35]. Little data is however available in this regard in terms of STIs. Animal studies have suggested that stress may increase susceptibility to chlamydia [36], and immunosuppression may increase the risk of chlamydia causing salpingitis [37]. Interestingly, the most consistent risk increase after bereavement noted in our study was for acute salpingitis, a severe complication of bacterial STIs. We also found a tendency toward an increased risk of condyloma among women after bereavement, even after HPV vaccination. This could potentially be explained by altered immune modulation after bereavement, leading to a suboptimal vaccine efficacy, or a higher risk of reactivation of pre-vaccination acquired infections. Taken together, our findings might imply that bereavement does not only impact the risk of primary infections through increased exposure and susceptibility, but also induce immunological changes affecting the clearing of the infection, leading to altered risk for complications of the acquired infections.

In previous studies we found an increased risk of cervical cancer in women who had lost a child during

Table 4 Inpatient hospital contact for Sexually Transmitted Infections (STIs), by age, calendar period, parental education level, and psychiatric history

	Any STI			Acute salpingitis			HIV/HBV		
	No bereavement	Bereavement	IRR (95 % CI)	No bereavement	Bereavement	IRR (95 % CI) [a]	No Bereavement	Bereavement	IRR (95 % CI)
Age at follow-up									
10 to 18 years	1181	71	1.15 (0.90–1.45)	1999	163	1.46 (1.24–1.71)	89	6	1.44 (0.56–3.05)
19 to 29 years	3709	494	1.15 (1.04–1.26)	5785	898	1.18 (1.08–1.28)	243	56	1.98 (1.46–2.65)
30 to 44 years	1013	623	1.18 (1.06–1.31)	3577	2479	1.19 (1.07–1.33)	223	195	1.73 (1.41–2.12)
Calendar period of follow-up									
1987 – 2000	4549	980	1.15 (1.06–1.24)	10291	3101	1.24 (1.08–1.42)	292	148	1.65 (1.32–2.05)
2001 – 2012	1354	208	1.19 (1.02–1.39)	1070	439	1.28 (1.13–1.44)	263	109	1.98 (1.54–2.53)
Parental education level									
Low/ Missing	1208	598	1.18 (1.06–1.31)	3173	2063	1.24 (1.00–1.54)	125	125	1.79 (1.37–2.34)
Middle	3002	428	1.15 (1.03–1.27)	5700	1151	1.32 (1.09–1.59)	260	99	2.03 (1.58–2.59)
High	1693	162	1.17 (0.99–1.38)	2488	326	1.25 (1.02–1.54)	170	33	1.48 (0.99–2.17)
History of psychiatric disorders									
No	5353	1121	1.19 (1.11–1.28)	10595	3318	1.28 (1.13–1.45)	352	174	2.08 (1.70–2.56)
Yes	550	67	0.88 (0.67–1.15)	766	222	1.26 (1.01–1.58)	203	83	1.95 (1.46–2.58)
History of substance abuse									
No	5827	1178	1.18 (1.10–1.26)	11253	3502	1.17 (1.13–1.22)	408	206	2.14 (1.77–2.59)
Yes	76	10	0.78 (0.36–1.51)	108	38	1.14 (0.75–1.69)	147	51	1.36 (0.95–1.92)

Notes:
The first hospital visit concerning an STI diagnosis during the unexposed follow-up and the first hospital visit concerning an STI diagnosis during the exposed follow-up were both counted in all analyses
CI confidence interval, *HBV* hepatitis B virus, *HIV* human immunodeficiency virus, *IRR* incidence rate ratio, *N* number, *STIs* sexually transmitted infections
IRR was adjusted for attained age (10–12, 13–15, 16–18, 19–21, 22–25, 26–29, 30–34, 35–39, and 40–44), calendar years (5-year group), and parental education levels (low/missing, medium, and high) as a proxy for socioeconomic status
[a] Negative binomial regression was used due to over-dispersed Poisson regression

Table 5 Inpatient hospital contact of Sexually Transmitted Infections (STIs), by subsequent psychiatric disorders or substance abuse after bereavement

	Any STI		Acute salpingitis		HIV & HBV	
	N	IRR (95 % CI)	N	IRR (95 % CI) [a]	N	IRR (95 % CI)
No bereavement	5903	1.0	11361	1.0	555	1.0
Newly diagnosed psychiatric disorder after bereavement						
No	1047	1.07 (1.00–1.15)	3202	1.21 (1.07–1.37)	113	0.85 (0.68–1.05)
Yes	74	2.95 (2.32–3.69)	116	2.09 (1.65–2.62)	61	12.0 (9.00–15.7)
Newly diagnosed substance abuse after bereavement						
No	1160	1.14 (1.06–1.21)	3472	1.26 (1.11–1.42)	150	1.06 (0.87–1.29)
Yes	18	5.12 (3.10–7.87)	30	3.56 (2.36–5.16)	56	76.5 (56.9–100.93)

Notes:
Bereaved women with preexisting psychiatric disorders were excluded from this analysis
The first hospital visit concerning an STI diagnosis during the unexposed follow-up and the first hospital visit concerning an STI diagnosis during the exposed follow-up were both counted in all analyses
CI confidence interval, *HBV* hepatitis B virus, *HIV* human immunodeficiency virus, *IRR* incidence rate ratio, *N* number
IRR was adjusted for attained age (10–12, 13–15, 16–18, 19–21, 22–25, 26–29, 30–34, 35–39, and 40–44), calendar years (5-year group), and parental education levels (low/missing, medium, and high) as a proxy for socioeconomic status
[a] Negative binomial regression was used due to over-dispersed Poisson regression

adulthood, as well as among women who had lost a parent during childhood [11, 12], potentially mediated through oncologic infections of HPV [13]. The present study lends further support to the potential pathways linking bereavement and cervical cancer, by demonstrating that the risks of STIs and their complications were higher among bereaved women. Hence, increased risk of primary infection together with impaired clearing of acquired infections, may work hand-in-hand to increase the risk of severe complications of STIs, potentially also including cervical cancer.

It is plausible that similar risk factors might lead to bereavement in early to mid-life and a higher risk of STIs. To address this concern, we adjusted for, and stratified by, several known risk factors for STIs in our analyses, such as age, socioeconomic status, and preexisting psychiatric disorders. Residual confounding could still exist since parental educational level might not be a perfect proxy for the women's socioeconomic status at early to mid-life. In a sensitivity analysis, we restricted the analysis among bereaved women only and compared the risk of STIs before and after bereavement. Even though this comparison had the inert disadvantage of having younger person-years and therefore a higher risk of STIs in the pre-bereavement period, compared to the post-bereavement period, bereavement was still associated with a higher risk of STIs. Comparing different time periods of the same women would largely argue against the possibility that our findings are solely explained by unmeasured confounding.

Since STIs were mainly retrieved from the Patient Register, not including patient visits to the general practitioners, maternity care clinics, and some youth clinics, our definition of STIs was not sensitive. This concern might be alleviated to some extent provided with the findings of condyloma where we used information from inpatient and outpatient hospital contacts as well as through prescription of condyloma medications – a

Table 6 Hospital contact of Sexually Transmitted Infections (STIs) after bereavement, among HPV vaccinated women

	No bereavement			Bereavement		
	N	Crude IR (1000 PYs)	IRR (95 % CI)	N	Crude IR (1000 PYs)	IRR (95 % CI)
Ever vaccinated						
Condyloma	1101	2.03	1.0	12	3.61	1.32 (0.71–2.23)
Any STI	2566	4.73	1.0	23	6.91	1.05 (0.68–1.55)
Fully vaccinated						
Condyloma	584	1.59	1.0	8	3.60	1.86 (0.85–3.50)
Any STI	1696	4.62	1.0	16	7.19	1.27 (0.74–2.00)

Notes:
The first hospital visit concerning an STI diagnosis during the unexposed follow-up and the first hospital visit concerning an STI diagnosis during the exposed follow-up were both counted in all analyses
CI confidence interval, *IR* incidence rate, *IRR* incidence rate ratio, *N* number, *PYs* person-years, *STIs* sexually transmitted infections
IRR was adjusted for attained age (10–18 and 19–44), calendar years (5-year group), and parental education levels (low/missing, medium, and high) as a proxy for socioeconomic status

definition with largely improved sensitivity [38] - and reassuringly found still an increased risk, although of smaller magnitude, after bereavement. In line with the clearer association of bereavement with inpatient care of STIs compared to any hospital care for STIs, the overall weaker association noticed for the comprehensive definition of condyloma compared to inpatient care-alone condyloma was expected. This observation should first argue against a pure explanation of altered healthcare seeking behavior among bereaved women leading to an increased detection of STIs, assuming that STIs in need of inpatient care are less prone to diagnostic bias. This observation might further indicate a specific impact of bereavement on severer cases of STIs compared to other cases. Such a possibility was further supported by findings on acute salpingitis which is more exclusively diagnosed and treated in hospital-based inpatient or emergency outpatient care, and was therefore more completely ascertained using our register-based definition.

Since the Patient Register has limited information about the clinical characteristics of the STI diagnoses, whether or not the association of bereavement with STIs would differ for new infection, persistent infection, and recurrence of previous infection needs to be investigated. In a previous study, we showed that bereavement was associated with infection of human papilloma virus (HPV), especially high viral load infection and recurrent infection [13].

Another limitation of the present study concerns the definition of psychiatric disorders, especially among the bereaved women. Since we identified only psychiatric disorders diagnosed through inpatient or outpatient care, whether or not the increased risk of STIs noted among bereaved women without subsequent psychiatric disorders was due to milder psychiatric conditions or symptoms not yet attended by specialist care needs to be further examined.

Since we identified spouses of the study women through a common child, women in childless marriages would have been classified as unexposed even if they did lose their spouses. Similarly, since we had no information on whether a woman resided with the father of her children, the impact of loss of a spouse would differ for different women according to whether or not they were living with the father of her children. These would however most likely have led to an underestimate of the real impact of loss of a spouse on STIs.

Lastly, residual confounding might still exist, even though multiple potential confounders have been adjusted for, such as age, calendar periods, and parental education level.

The strengths of the present study include the large sample size, the nationwide study design, the long and complete follow-up, as well as the prospectively and independently collected information on the exposure and outcomes.

This study contributes to the growing body of knowledge on how stressful life events affect our health. While the importance of counseling grieving family members to be mindful of their health might seem obvious, there is still a lot to be done. Our study indicates that sexual risk behavior should especially be taken into account when counseling adolescents who have lost a family member, especially those youth who develop psychiatric disorders at the wake of their loss.

Conclusions

Women who have lost a close relative are at increased risk of STIs. Bereaved women with subsequent psychiatric disorders may be at particularly high risk.

Abbreviations

ATC, anatomical therapeutic chemical; CI, confidence interval; GHS, genital herpes simplex; HBV, hepatitis B; HIV, human immunodeficiency virus; HPV, human papillomavirus; ICD, international classification of diseases; IRR, incidence rate ratio; MGR, multi-generation register; STI, sexually transmitted infections

Acknowledgements

We thank Pouran Almstedt for database management.

Funding

The study was partly supported by the Swedish Cancer Society (Grant No. CAN 2014/417), the Swedish Society for Medical Research and the Karolinska Institutet. The funding bodies had no direct part in the design of this project, nor in the collection, analysis and interpretation of data, or the writing process.

Availability of data and materials

The summary of data included in different registers used in the present study can be found on the homepages of the Swedish National Board of Health and Welfare (http://www.socialstyrelsen.se/register) as well as the Statistics Sweden (http://www.scb.se/sv_/Vara-tjanster/Bestalla-mikrodata/Vilka-mikrodata-finns/Individregister//). The authors confirm that, for approved reasons, some access restrictions apply to the data underlying the findings. The data used in this study are owned by the Swedish National Board of Health and Welfare and Statistics Sweden. According to Swedish law, the authors are not able to make the dataset publicly available.
Any researchers (including international researchers) interested in obtaining the data can do so by the following steps: 1) apply for ethical approval from their local ethical review boards; 2) contact the Swedish National Board of Health and Welfare and/or Statistics Sweden with the ethical approval and make a formal application of use of the registry data. Contact emails for request of register data: Swedish National Board of Health and Welfare: registerservice@socialstyrelsen.se, Statistics Sweden: Mikrodata.individ@scb.se. Please visit http://www.socialstyrelsen.se/register/bestalladatastatistik/

bestallaindividuppgifterforforskningsandamal (the Swedish National Board of Health and Welfare) and http://www.scb.se/sv_/Vara-tjanster/Bestalla-mikrodata/ (the Statistics Sweden) for detailed information about how to apply for access to registry data for research purposes.

Authors' contributions

EB and DL designed the study, collected and analyzed the data, and wrote the manuscript. EH collected and analyzed data. KS, UV, KF, LAD and PS aided in the design of the study and analysis of data. FF designed the study and analyzed data. All authors contributed to interpretation of data and critical revision of the manuscript. All authors read and approved the final manuscript.

Authors' information

E.B. MD, PhD, D.L., MD, E.H. PhD, K.S. MD, PhD, K.F. MD, PhD, L.A.D. PhD, Prof P.S. PhD, Prof U.V. PhD, F.F. M.D. PhD.

Competing interests

Dr. Sundström reports having received grants from Merck and Co, for register-based follow-up studies on HPV vaccination in Sweden.

Consent for publication

Not applicable.

Author details

[1]Department of Medical Epidemiology and Biostatistics, Karolinska Institutet, Nobels väg 12A, Box 281, Stockholm 17177, Sweden. [2]Department of Laboratory Medicine, Karolinska Institutet, H5, Division of Pathology, Karolinska Universitetssjukhuset Huddinge, Stockholm 14186, Sweden. [3]Center of Public Health Sciences, Faculty of Medicine, University of Iceland, Stapi v/Hringbraut, 101 Reykjavik, Iceland. [4]Department of Epidemiology, Harvard School of Public Health, 677 Huntington Avenue, Boston, MA 02115, USA. [5]Clinical Epidemiology and Biostatistics, School of Medical Sciences, Örebro University, Örebro, Sweden.

References

1. Schneiderman N, Ironson G, Siegel SD. Stress and health: psychological, behavioral, and biological determinants. Annu Rev Clin Psychol. 2005;1:607–28.
2. Glaser R, Kiecolt-Glaser JK. Stress-induced immune dysfunction: implications for health. Nat Rev Immunol. 2005;5(3):243–51.
3. Rozlog LA, Kiecolt-Glaser JK, Marucha PT, Sheridan JF, Glaser R. Stress and immunity: implications for viral disease and wound healing. J Periodontol. 1999;70(7):786–92.
4. Cohen S, Williamson GM. Stress and infectious disease in humans. Psychol Bull. 1991;109(1):5–24.
5. Chida Y, Mao X. Does psychosocial stress predict symptomatic herpes simplex virus recurrence? A meta-analytic investigation on prospective studies. Brain Behav Immun. 2009;23(7):917–25.
6. Chida Y, Vedhara K. Adverse psychosocial factors predict poorer prognosis in HIV disease: a meta-analytic review of prospective investigations. Brain Behav Immun. 2009;23(4):434–45.
7. Walboomers JM, Jacobs MV, Manos MM, Bosch FX, Kummer JA, Shah KV, Snijders PJ, Peto J, Meijer CJ, Munoz N. Human papillomavirus is a necessary cause of invasive cervical cancer worldwide. J Pathol. 1999;189(1):12–9.
8. Parkin DM, Bray F. Chapter 2: The burden of HPV-related cancers. Vaccine. 2006;24 Suppl 3:S3/11–25.
9. McGee R. Does stress cause cancer? There's no good evidence of a relation between stressful events and cancer. BMJ. 1999;319(7216):1015–6.
10. Janerich DT. Can stress cause cancer? Am J Public Health. 1991;81(6):687–8.
11. Fang F, Fall K, Sparen P, Adami HO, Valdimarsdottir HB, Lambe M, Valdimarsdottir U. Risk of infection-related cancers after the loss of a child: a follow-up study in Sweden. Cancer Res. 2011;71(1):116–22.
12. Kennedy B, Valdimarsdottir U, Sundstrom K, Sparen P, Lambe M, Fall K, Fang F. Loss of a parent and the risk of cancer in early life: a nationwide cohort study. Cancer Causes Control. 2014;25(4):499–506.
13. Lu D, Sundstrom K, Sparen P, Fall K, Sjolander A, Dillner J, Helm NY, Adami HO, Valdimarsdottir U, Fang F. Bereavement Is Associated with an Increased Risk of HPV Infection and Cervical Cancer: An Epidemiological Study in Sweden. Cancer Res. 2016;76(3):643–51.
14. Ekbom A. The Swedish Multi-generation Register. Methods Mol Biol. 2011;675:215–20.
15. Ludvigsson JF, Andersson E, Ekbom A, Feychting M, Kim JL, Reuterwall C, Heurgren M, Olausson PO. External review and validation of the Swedish national inpatient register. BMC Public Health. 2011;11:450.
16. Leval A, Herweijer E, Ploner A, Eloranta S, Fridman Simard J, Dillner J, Young C, Netterlid E, Sparen P, Arnheim-Dahlstrom L. Quadrivalent human papillomavirus vaccine effectiveness: a Swedish national cohort study. J Natl Cancer Inst. 2013;105(7):469–74.
17. Herweijer E, Leval A, Ploner A, Eloranta S, Simard JF, Dillner J, Netterlid E, Sparen P, Arnheim-Dahlstrom L. Association of varying number of doses of quadrivalent human papillomavirus vaccine with incidence of condyloma. JAMA. 2014;311(6):597–603.
18. Wettermark B, Hammar N, Fored CM, Leimanis A, Otterblad Olausson P, Bergman U, Persson I, Sundstrom A, Westerholm B, Rosen M. The new Swedish Prescribed Drug Register–opportunities for pharmacoepidemiological research and experience from the first six months. Pharmacoepidemiol Drug Saf. 2007;16(7):726–35.
19. Ross JD. Pelvic inflammatory disease. BMJ Clin Evid. 2013;2013:1-28.
20. Bjartling C, Osser S, Persson K. The frequency of salpingitis and ectopic pregnancy as epidemiologic markers of Chlamydia trachomatis. Acta Obstet Gynecol Scand. 2000;79(2):123–8.
21. Wiley DJ, Douglas J, Beutner K, Cox T, Fife K, Moscicki AB, Fukumoto L. External genital warts: diagnosis, treatment, and prevention. Clin Infect Dis. 2002;35 Suppl 2:S210–24.
22. Meade CS, Sikkema KJ. HIV risk behavior among adults with severe mental illness: a systematic review. Clin Psychol Rev. 2005;25(4):433–57.
23. Lehrer JA, Shrier LA, Gortmaker S, Buka S. Depressive symptoms as a longitudinal predictor of sexual risk behaviors among US middle and high school students. Pediatrics. 2006;118(1):189–200.
24. Hamdan S, Mazariegos D, Melhem NM, Porta G, Payne MW, Brent DA. Effect of parental bereavement on health risk behaviors in youth: a 3-year follow-up. Arch Pediatr Adolesc Med. 2012;166(3):216–23.
25. Muniz-Cohen M, Melhem NM, Brent DA. Health risk behaviors in parentally bereaved youth. Arch Pediatr Adolesc Med. 2010;164(7):621–4.
26. Stroebe M, Schut H, Stroebe W. Health outcomes of bereavement. Lancet. 2007;370(9603):1960–73.
27. Pilling J, Thege BK, Demetrovics Z, Kopp MS. Alcohol use in the first three years of bereavement: a national representative survey. Subst Abuse Treat Prev Policy. 2012;7:3.
28. Brent D, Melhem N, Donohoe MB, Walker M. The incidence and course of depression in bereaved youth 21 months after the loss of a parent to suicide, accident, or sudden natural death. Am J Psychiatry. 2009; 166(7):786–94.
29. Bylund Grenklo T, Kreicbergs U, Hauksdottir A, Valdimarsdottir UA, Nyberg T, Steineck G, Furst CJ. Self-injury in teenagers who lost a parent to cancer: a nationwide, population-based, long-term follow-up. JAMA Pediatr. 2013;167(2):133–40.
30. Hamdan S, Melhem NM, Porta G, Song MS, Brent DA. Alcohol and substance abuse in parentally bereaved youth. J Clin Psychiatry. 2013;74(8):828–33.
31. Hall KS, Moreau C, Trussell J, Barber J. Role of young women's depression and stress symptoms in their weekly use and nonuse of contraceptive methods. J Adolesc Health. 2013;53(2):241–8.
32. Stidham Hall K, Moreau C, Trussell J, Barber J. Young women's consistency of contraceptive use–does depression or stress matter? Contraception. 2013;88(5):641–9.
33. Keenan K, Grundy E, Kenward MG, Leon DA. Women's risk of repeat abortions is strongly associated with alcohol consumption: a longitudinal analysis of a Russian national panel study, 1994–2009. PLoS ONE. 2014;9(3):e90356.

34. Bartrop RW, Luckhurst E, Lazarus L, Kiloh LG, Penny R. Depressed lymphocyte function after bereavement. Lancet. 1977;1(8016):834–6.
35. Gerra G, Monti D, Panerai AE, Sacerdote P, Anderlini R, Avanzini P, Zaimovic A, Brambilla F, Franceschi C. Long-term immune-endocrine effects of bereavement: relationships with anxiety levels and mood. Psychiatry Res. 2003;121(2):145–58.
36. Belay T, Woart A. Cold-induced stress increases the intensity of Chlamydia genital infection in mice. J Microbiol Immunol Infect. 2013;46(5):330–7.
37. White HJ, Rank RG, Soloff BL, Barron AL. Experimental chlamydial salpingitis in immunosuppressed guinea pigs infected in the genital tract with the agent of guinea pig inclusion conjunctivitis. Infect Immun. 1979;26(2):728–35.
38. Leval A, Herweijer E, Arnheim-Dahlstrom L, Walum H, Frans E, Sparen P, Simard JF. Incidence of Genital Warts in Sweden Before and After Quadrivalent Human Papillomavirus Vaccine Availability. J Infect Dis. 2012;206(6):860–6.

11

Does typing of *Chlamydia trachomatis* using housekeeping multilocus sequence typing reveal different sexual networks among heterosexuals and men who have sex with men?

Bart Versteeg[1], Sylvia M. Bruisten[1,2], Arie van der Ende[2,3] and Yvonne Pannekoek[2,3*]

Abstract

Background: *Chlamydia trachomatis* infections remain the most common bacterial sexually transmitted infection worldwide. To gain more insight into the epidemiology and transmission of *C. trachomatis*, several schemes of multilocus sequence typing (MLST) have been developed. We investigated the clustering of *C. trachomatis* strains derived from men who have sex with men (MSM) and heterosexuals using the MLST scheme based on 7 housekeeping genes (MLST-7) adapted for clinical specimens and a high-resolution MLST scheme based on 6 polymorphic genes, including *ompA* (hr-MLST-6).

Methods: Specimens from 100 *C. trachomatis* infected men who have sex with men (MSM) and 100 heterosexual women were randomly selected from previous studies and sequenced. We adapted the MLST-7 scheme to a nested assay to be suitable for direct typing of clinical specimens. All selected specimens were typed using both the adapted MLST-7 scheme and the hr-MLST-6 scheme. Clustering of *C. trachomatis* strains derived from MSM and heterosexuals was assessed using minimum spanning tree analysis.

Results: Sufficient chlamydial DNA was present in 188 of the 200 (94 %) selected samples. Using the adapted MLST-7 scheme, full MLST profiles were obtained for 187 of 188 tested specimens resulting in a high success rate of 99.5 %. Of these 187 specimens, 91 (48.7 %) were from MSM and 96 (51.3 %) from heterosexuals. We detected 21 sequence types (STs) using the adapted MLST-7 and 79 STs using the hr-MLST-6 scheme. Minimum spanning tree analyses was used to examine the clustering of MLST-7 data, which showed no reflection of separate transmission in MSM and heterosexual hosts. Moreover, typing using the hr-MLST-6 scheme identified genetically related clusters within each of clusters that were identified by using the MLST-7 scheme.

Conclusion: No distinct transmission of *C. trachomatis* could be observed in MSM and heterosexuals using the adapted MLST-7 scheme in contrast to using the hr-MLST-6. In addition, we compared clustering of both MLST schemes and demonstrated that typing using the hr-MLST-6 scheme is able to identify genetically related clusters of *C. trachomatis* strains within each of the clusters that were identified by using the MLST-7 scheme.

Keywords: *Chlamydia trachomatis*, Multilocus sequence typing, MLST, High-resolution genotyping, Sexually transmitted infections, MSM

* Correspondence: y.pannekoek@amc.uva.nl
[2]Center for Infection and Immunity Amsterdam (CINIMA), Academic Medical Center, University of Amsterdam, Amsterdam, The Netherlands
[3]Department of Medical Microbiology, Academic Medical Center, Amsterdam, The Netherlands
Full list of author information is available at the end of the article

Background

Despite intensive efforts to reduce the spread of chlamydial infections, *Chlamydia trachomatis* remains the primary cause of bacterial sexually transmitted diseases worldwide [1]. These *C. trachomatis* infections can result in serious sequelae including epididymitis and pelvic inflammatory disease, leading to infertility in women and possibly also in men [2–4].

Molecular epidemiological studies are essential to understand the genetic population structure and to gain insight into the transmission of *C. trachomatis* [5, 6]. Until recently, the epidemiology of *C. trachomatis* was based on serotyping of the major outer membrane protein (MOMP) or sequence analysis of its encoding gene *ompA*. However, typing based on the *ompA*-gene only is not recommended as typing method for *C. trachomatis*, as whole-genome-sequencing (WGS) data revealed that it is an unstable and unreliable target due to extensive recombination [7]. Numerous sets of WGS data have become available for a variety of bacterial isolates including *C. trachomatis* [7]. Unfortunately, due to the complex intracellular lifecycle of *C. trachomatis* it remains technically challenging to perform WGS directly on clinical specimens. Instead, several multilocus sequence typing (MLST) schemes were successfully developed and validated to gain insight into the epidemiology and transmission of *C. trachomatis* [8–11]. An advantage of using MLST schemes to type *C. trachomatis* strains, is that it is a standardized and portable method to index variation among strains, which can easily be used in different laboratories on a global basis since it yields robust data [12–14].

In previous studies a clear separation of *C. trachomatis* strain types was seen for specimens derived from men who have sex with men (MSM) and from heterosexuals as defined by a high-resolution MLST scheme based on 6 polymorphic genes, including *ompA* (herein referred to as hr-MLST-6) [11, 15–17]. The hr-MLST-6 scheme was specifically designed for short-term epidemiology and outbreak investigations and was intended to be highly discriminating. In contrast, another MLST scheme was designed based on 7 housekeeping genes (herein referred to as MLST-7) [9]. The slow rate of molecular evolution within these housekeeping genes makes the MLST-7 scheme useful to answer evolutionary questions and to investigate the epidemiology of *C. trachomatis* over a longer time-frame. A limitation of the published MLST-7 scheme is that it consists of single PCRs, which has a decreased sensitivity making it less suitable for typing of *C. trachomatis* strains from direct clinical specimens and is therefore not applicable for large population studies. Typing of *C. trachomatis* using the MLST-7 scheme is therefore often dependent on an additional culture step possibly leading to biased study outcomes. Moreover, it is unknown whether the clear separation in transmission of *C. trachomatis* strain types for specimens derived from MSM and from heterosexuals can also be seen using the MLST-7 scheme.

The objective of this study was therefore to: (1) adapt the MLST-7 scheme to a nested assay to be suitable for direct typing of clinical specimens without the need for an additional cell culture step, (2) determine whether separate *C. trachomatis* transmission in MSM and from heterosexual hosts could also be seen using the MLST-7 scheme and (3) compare clustering of the *C. trachomatis* strain types according to both MLST schemes.

Methods

Clinical specimen selection

For this retrospective analysis, *C. trachomatis*-positive specimens and data were selected from a previous study [17]. All specimens and data were matched on sexgroup and a random selection was made using SPSS 21 (SPSS Inc., Chicago, IL, USA). In total, 100 specimens from MSM and 100 specimens from heterosexual women were selected. Rectal swab specimens from MSM were collected between July 2008 and August 2009. *C. trachomatis*-positive urogenital swab specimens from heterosexual women were collected between December 2011 and December 2012.

Ethics

The STI outpatient clinic of the Public Health Service of Amsterdam, the Netherlands uses an opting-out approach to recruit clients for scientific research. All clients of the STI clinic are notified that remainders of samples may be used for scientific research, after anonymisation and de-identification of client clinical data and samples. If clients objected, data and samples are discarded. Therefore, no additional informed consent was obtained for this study. This procedure was approved by the Medical Ethical Committee of the Academic Medical Center of the University of Amsterdam, the Netherlands (reference number W14-200 # 14.17.0247).

DNA Extraction and amplification

For DNA extraction 200 µl swab-containing transport medium of specimens that tested positive in a screening assay (Aptima combo TMA test, Hologic/Gen-Probe, San Diego, California, USA) was added to 500 µl lysis buffer (bioMérieux, Boxtel, the Netherlands), 1 µg glycogen (10 mg/ml; Roche Diagnostics, Almere, the Netherlands). DNA was subsequently precipitated by adding 700 µl of ice-cold isopropanol. The DNA precipitate was washed twice with 70 % ethanol and dissolved in 50 μl 10 mM Tris-buffer (pH 8.0). These DNA isolates were stored at −20 °C until further use.

Extracted DNA was tested to indicate the load of chlamydial DNA using an in-house *pmpH* real time PCR [11, 16, 17]. For DNA specimens that tested *pmpH* negative, DNA was re-extracted from the original Aptima *C. trachomatis* positive specimens and retested. All specimens that repeatedly tested negative for the *pmpH* target were excluded.

Primer selection for adaptation of MLST-7

Primers were designed and a nested PCR assay was developed to enable direct testing of clinical samples. MLST-7 regions were analyzed *in silico* using the Chlamydiales MLST database (http://pubmlst.org/chlamydiales/) Comparison of all available *C. trachomatis* sequences from the MLST database demonstrated that shortening of the original amplicons for 5 out of the 7 genes (*gatA, oppA_3, hflX, gidA* and *fumC*) to perform nested PCR would not result in loss of resolution as no known polymorphic sites for *C. trachomatis* were found in these 'deleted' regions. Therefore, new 'inner' PCR primers were designed for these 5 genes (Table 1). For two other genes (*hemN* and *enoA*) the original amplicon was extended to prevent loss of resolution and known polymorphic sites. Therefore, new 'outer'

Table 1 Primers used for the MLST-7 scheme for Chlamydia trachomatis[a]

Region	Locus tag[b]	Format	Direction	Sequence (5′ to 3′)	5′ position[c]	Fragment length (bp)[d]
gatA	CT0003	**Outer**	**Forward**	**GCTTTAGAATTARSARAWGCT**	2123	325
		Outer	**Reverse**	**GATCCTCCGGTATCYGATCC**	2615	
		Inner + Seq	Forward	ATGACGAACAGATTGGAGC	2186	
		Inner + Seq	Reverse	GGATTATTGGTAGGATGAA	2532	
oppA_3	CT0198	**Outer**	**Forward**	**ATGCGCAAGATATCAGTGGG**	222438	480
		Outer	**Reverse**	**AAAGCTCCRSTWGMTATMGGWAG**	223002	
		Inner + Seq	Forward	TCCTAGCATTAGCAACTTCT	222469	
		Inner + Seq	Reverse	TCTTTCCGTATCTGATGCTGCG	222970	
hflX	CT0379	**Outer**	**Forward**	**GCTTCTARAGTACTTTTAAATG**	432737	359
		Outer	**Reverse**	**TATTTRGAAATYTTTKCSAGYCG**	432758	
		Inner + Seq	Forward	AAGTATGCGGAAGTTTGCG	432768	
		Inner + Seq	Reverse	AATCAGGAGGTAGTGGTGGAGG	433106	
gidA	CT0498	**Outer**	**Forward**	**GGAGTCWCTACWAAAGAAGG**	577352	389
		Outer	**Reverse**	**TCGTAYTGYACATCRAAAGG**	577892	
		Inner + Seq	Forward	ACTTCTCTGGGGGACGATT	577449	
		Inner + Seq	Reverse	GACCGTTCACATAAACTTCTTG	577856	
enoA	CT0587	Outer	Forward	GCAAATACTTTACAGAGACCTT	662222	388
		Outer	Reverse	CGTCACAAATAGGTCGTCTC	662775	
		Inner + Seq	**Forward**	**CCTATGATGAATCTKATCAATGG**	662288	
		Inner + Seq	**Reverse**	**TCTTCTTCGGCTAGCCCATCT**	662698	
hemN	CT0746	Outer	Forward	GAATCTTGCCTTTCACAGTTGC	867674	448
		Outer	Reverse	ACTTCCACATCCCATTCTGC	868584	
		Inner + Seq	**Forward**	**AGATCTTCTTCWGGRGGWAGAGA**	867799	
		Inner + Seq	**Reverse**	**TTCYTTCAKAACSTAGGTTTT**	868269	
fumC	CT0855	**Outer**	**Forward**	**ATTAAAAAATGTGCTGCT**	1004691	451
		Outer	**Reverse**	**CCTTCAGGAACATTYAACCC**	1005242	
		Inner + Seq	Forward	ATTAAAAAATGTGCTGCT	1004691	
		Inner + Seq	Reverse	CCGCTCTAAACAATTATGCAACTG	1005159	

[a]The primers given in boldface were the original MLST primers taken from Pannekoek et al. [9]. All other primers were newly designed. Nested PCRs were performed for each region. The primers used for the outer PCRs are indicated with Outer, those used for the inner PCRs are indicated with Inner, and those used for sequencing are indicated with Seq

[b]Locus tags are given relative to the sequence of reference strain D/UW-3/CX (GenBank accession no. AE001273)

[c]Positions are given in base pairs relative to the sequence of reference strain D/UW-3/CX (GenBank accession no. AE001273)

[d]Fragment length is the number of base pairs sequenced with the primers excluded

PCR primers were designed, thus the same inner PCR product was obtained as published previously (Table 1) [9].

Nested PCR of MLST regions

For MLST-7, DNA extracts were amplified by nested PCR for all regions using the oligonucleotide primers shown in Table 1. Full hr-MLST-6 data was already available for all specimens from previous studies [17]. Also for this typing method a nested PCR was used to amplify the regions *ompA*, CT046 (*hctB*), CT058, CT144, CT172, and CT682 (*pbpB*). For both MLST schemes the inner PCR was performed with M13-tagged primers, identical to the standard inner primers. This allowed sequencing using universal M13 primers for high throughput purposes [11, 16, 17].

Sequencing analysis

The obtained sequences were analysed, assembled and trimmed using BioNumerics 7.5 (Applied Maths, Sint-Martens-Latem, Belgium). For MLST-7, cleaned primer-to-primer sequences were checked against the Chlamydiales MLST database (http://pubmlst.org/chlamydiales/). For hr-MLST-6, analysis was performed as described previously [17]. In brief, cleaned primer-to-primer sequences were checked against the *Chlamydia trachomatis* hr-MLST database (http://mlstdb.bmc.uu.se/).

Minimum spanning tree analysis

BioNumerics software (version 7.5, Applied Maths, Sint-Martens-Latem, Belgium) was used to construct a minimum spanning tree of fully typed specimens using STs of each of the MLST schemes. As algorithm we used the predefined template 'Minimum spanning tree for categorical data' plugin to generate an minimum spanning tree under the categorical coefficient of similarity and the priority rule of the highest number of single-locus variants (SLV), which calculates a standard minimum spanning tree. A large cluster was defined as a group of genetically related STs differing by not more than 1 locus from another ST within that group (SLV) and it had to include at least 5 % of the total number of specimens. Clusters containing less then 5 % of the total number of specimens were defined as small clusters.

Results

C. trachomatis typing using the MLST-7 scheme

Although in 188 of 200 *C. trachomatis*-positive specimens (94.0 %), sufficient chlamydial DNA was present, as assessed by qPCR, no amplicons were obtained using the MLST scheme, primers and cycle conditions as were previously described [9], indicating relative low sensitivity of the method. We therefore adapted the MLST-7 scheme to a nested assay and, using this adapted MLST-7 scheme, for 187 (93.5 %) specimens full MLST-7 profiles were obtained. Of these 187 typed specimens, 91 (48.7 %) specimens were from MSM and 96 (51.3 %) specimens were from heterosexuals (Additional file 1: Table S1). For the 187 fully typed specimens, we found 7 novel allele sequences: 3 for *oppA_3*, 1 for *gidA*, 1 for *enoA*, and 2 for *hemN*.

Among the 187 typed specimens, 21 unique MLST-7 STs could be assigned of which 18 (85.7 %) were novel to the Chlamydiales MLST database (http://pubmlst.org/chlamydiales/). Novel STs were found in 125 of 187 specimens (66.8 %). Of all identified STs, 8 (38.1 %) had multiple representatives (2 to 52 isolates) while 13 (61.9 %) were found in only a single isolate each (Table 2). Moreover, 4 STs (ST97, ST132, ST133, ST134; 19.0 %) were found in specimens from both MSM and heterosexuals and 6 STs (ST44, ST97 ST132, ST133, ST137, ST142; 28.6 %) were associated with multiple (2 to 5) *ompA* genovars (Table 2).

C. trachomatis typing using hr-MLST-6 scheme

Full hr-MLST-6 profiles were available for the 187 *C. trachomatis*-positive specimens that were also successfully typed using the adapted MLST-7 scheme (Additional file 2: Table S2). The hr-MLST-6 data from the 187 *C. trachomatis*-positive specimens have been described before in more detail [11, 15–17]. In brief, among the 187 typed specimens, 79 unique hr-MLST-6 STs could be assigned of which 22 (27.8 %) had multiple representatives (2 to 18 isolates) while 57 (72.2 %) were found in only a single isolate each (Table 3). Of all identified STs, 3 (ST12d, ST56a, ST90; 3.8 %) were found in specimens from both MSM and heterosexuals (Table 3).

Minimum spanning tree analysis of the MLST-7 scheme and the hr-MLST-6 scheme

A minimum spanning tree was generated based on the MLST-7 STs and 3 large clusters (A-C) could be identified (Fig. 1a). The number of specimens in these clusters ranged from 18 to 94 and included all typed specimens so no single isolates (singletons) or small clusters were identified. The minimum spanning tree showed mixed clusters of specimens from MSM and heterosexual individuals and a low genetic diversity among the *C. trachomatis* population. Cluster A contained 41 specimens from MSM (54.7 %) that were associated with 3 STs (Table 2). Two of those STs (ST131, ST148) were found in one MSM specimen each, whereas the remaining ST (ST132) was found in specimens from 52 individuals of whom 39 (75.0 %) where MSM. Cluster B contained 32 specimens from MSM (34.0 %) that were associated with 3 STs (ST97, ST133, ST134). Of those, ST97 was found in 42 specimens from individuals of whom 25 (59.5 %) were MSM, ST133 was found in specimens from 26 individuals of whom 6 were MSM and ST134 was found

Table 2 Results of *C. trachomatis* using the MLST-7 scheme based on seven housekeeping genes in comparison with *ompA*-typing and sexgroup

Sequence type	Number of strains	*gatA*	*oppA_3*	*hflX*	*gidA*	*enoA*	*hemN*	*fumC*	Cluster	*ompA* genovar (Number of strains)	Sexgroup[a] (number of strains)
8	1	2	1	1	2	4	2	3	B	F (1)	Hetero (1)
44	18	1	3	3	3	2	2	19	C	L2 (1), L2b (17)	MSM (18)
97	42	33	1	2	2	4	2	3	B	D (24), E(1), F(17)	Hetero (17), MSM (25)
106	1	2	3	2	5	3	2	3	A	J (1)	Hetero (1)
131	1	33	27	2	4	3	2	3	A	G (1)	MSM (1)
132	52	33	3	2	4	3	2	3	A	G (26), H (1), I (10), J (13), K(2)	Hetero (13), MSM (39)
133	26	33	1	1	2	4	2	3	B	D (3), E (21), F (2)	Hetero (20), MSM (6)
134	2	33	1	1	2	3	2	3	B	F (2)	Hetero (1), MSM (1)
135	19	33	4	1	2	4	2	3	B	E (19)	Hetero (19)
136	11	33	3	2	5	3	2	3	A	B (1), D (2), G (4), J (4)	Hetero (11)
137	1	33	3	2	40	3	2	3	A	G (1)	Hetero (1)
138	1	33	29	1	2	4	2	3	B	E (1)	Hetero (1)
139	1	33	1	1	2	32	2	3	B	E (1)	Hetero (1)
140	1	33	3	2	4	3	1	3	A	G (1)	Hetero (1)
141	4	33	3	2	5	3	1	3	A	D (3), I (1)	Hetero (4)
142	1	33	4	1	32	4	2	3	B	E (1)	Hetero (1)
143	1	33	3	2	5	3	25	3	A	K (1)	Hetero (1)
144	1	33	3	2	5	3	24	3	A	G (1)	Hetero (1)
145	1	33	3	2	4	24	2	3	A	H (1)	Hetero (1)
146	1	2	4	1	2	4	2	3	B	F (1)	Hetero (1)
147	1	33	28	2	4	3	2	3	A	J (1)	MSM (1)

[a]*Hetero* heterosexual, *MSM* men who have sex with men

in specimens from 2 individuals of whom 1 was MSM. Cluster C solely consisted of specimens from MSM which were all associated with the same ST (ST44).

A minimum spanning tree was also generated basted on the hr-MLST-6 STs and 8 large clusters (I-VIII) were identified (Fig. 1b). These clusters ranged from 13 to 27 specimens comprising 80.2 % of all specimens. The remaining 37 specimens were distributed over 20 singletons and 6 small clusters, ranging from 2 to 4 specimens. The minimum spanning tree showed a clear distinction between specimens from MSM and heterosexual individuals and high genetic diversity among the *C. trachomatis* population especially for strains from heterosexuals, as was also previously described by us [11, 15–17]. Of the 8 large clusters, 4 (III, IV, VI and VII) consisted predominantly of specimens from heterosexuals (82.6 to 100 %) whereas the other 4 large clusters (I, II, V and VIII) solely consisted of specimens from MSM (Table 3). Of the 4 clusters (III, IV, VI and VII) consisting predominantly of specimens from heterosexuals, only 2 clusters (IV and VI) contained MSM specimens. Cluster IV contained 4 specimens from MSM (17.4 %) that were associated with 4 STs (ST12d, ST90, ST91a). Of those 4 STs, ST12d was found in specimens from 13 individuals of whom 1 was MSM, ST90 was found in specimens from 2 individuals of whom 1 was MSM and ST91a was found in only one MSM specimen. Cluster VI contained 2 specimens from MSM which were associated with 1 ST (ST56a). This ST was found in specimens from 9 individuals of whom 2 were MSM.

Comparison of the two minimum spanning trees in Fig. 1 shows that the hr-MLST-6 scheme further diversified each of the clusters generated by using the adapted MLST-7 scheme. For example cluster A (11 STs; Fig. 1a) is subdivided into clusters I, II, and III, using the hr-MLST-6 scheme, and also the majority of the singletons and small clusters (Fig. 2) comprising 37 STs. Cluster B (9 STs; Fig. 1a) is further subdivided into clusters IV, V, VI, VII and some remaining singletons and small clusters (Fig. 2) comprising 39 STs. Cluster C (1 ST; Fig. 1a) is identical to cluster VIII (Figs. 1b and 2) but included 3 STs.

Discussion

In this study, we successfully adapted the MLST-7 scheme to a nested assay and applied it to direct clinical specimens.

Table 3 Results of *C. trachomatis* typing using the hr-MLST-6 scheme based on six polymorphic genes in comparison with *ompA*-typing and sexgroup

Sequence type	Number of strains	*ompA*	CT046	CT058	CT144	CT172	CT682	Cluster	*ompA* genovar (number of strains)	Sexgroup[a] (number of strains)
3	10	6	1	2	6	2	2	VII	E (10)	Hetero (10)
11	3	1	5	19	7	2	10		D (3)	MSM (3)
16	1	6	7	19	14	2	1	VI	E (1)	Hetero (1)
27	1	9	10	6	10	1	6		G (1)	Hetero (1)
30	1	12	10	7	1	3	8		K (1)	MSM (1)
32	1	12	10	7	1	4	8		K (1)	Hetero (1)
33	6	8	10	8	5	3	6	II	G (6)	MSM (6)
35	3	2	10	8	1	4	17		D (3)	Hetero (3)
52	17	8	20	8	5	3	6	II	G (17)	MSM (17)
59	1	6	7	19	7	2	1	VI	E (1)	Hetero (1)
69	1	6	5	19	6	2	2		E (1)	Hetero (1)
74	1	30	8	8	1	7	18		B (1)	Hetero (1)
90	2	24	5	19	1	1	4	IV	F (2)	Hetero (1), MSM (1)
101	1	36	38	5	12	7	18	III	I (1)	Hetero (1)
109	18	1	5	20	5	2	34	V	D (18)	MSM (18)
110	1	24	1	2	7	2	4	IV	F (1)	Hetero (1)
137	1	8	10	8	22	4	6		G (1)	Hetero (1)
143	1	28	44	13	17	13	28	VIII	L2b (1)	MSM (1)
153	2	6	35	19	7	2	1	VI	E (2)	Hetero (2)
165	1	35	12	5	1	9	8		H (1)	Hetero (1)
171	2	6	49	19	7	2	1	VI	E (2)	Hetero (2)
172	1	6	1	2	7	2	2	VII	E (1)	Hetero (1)
194	3	1	5	6	5	2	34	V	D (3)	MSM (3)
232	2	20	5	19	1	4	18		J (2)	Hetero (2)
240	1	24	5	19	12	1	4	IV	F (1)	Hetero (1)
265	1	10	10	4	1	3	7		G (1)	Hetero (1)
270	1	8	10	5	12	3	8		G (1)	Hetero (1)
272	1	36	10	5	12	24	18	III	I (1)	Hetero (1)
288	1	8	10	8	22	7	57		G (1)	Hetero (1)
301	1	8	20	8	5	1	6	II	G (1)	MSM (1)
303	1	8	20	8	5	3	34	II	G (1)	MSM (1)
304	1	8	20	8	5	4	6	II	G (1)	MSM (1)
305	1	6	25	2	6	2	2	VII	E (1)	Hetero (1)
307	2	53	29	8	5	3	58	I	J (2)	MSM (2)
318	1	1	45	20	5	2	34	V	D (1)	MSM (1)
324	1	1	55	20	5	2	34	V	D (1)	MSM (1)
338	1	6	67	2	7	2	60		E (1)	Hetero (1)
341	1	6	70	57	7	2	1		E (1)	Hetero (1)
345	2	53	74	8	5	3	6	I	J (2)	MSM (2)
353	1	8	81	8	5	3	6	II	G (1)	MSM (1)
395	1	2	83	4	1	3	17		D (1)	Hetero (1)
435	1	9	8	6	10	1	6		G (1)	Hetero (1)
448	1	6	1	2	11	2	2	VII	E (1)	Hetero (1)

Table 3 Results of *C. trachomatis* typing using the hr-MLST-6 scheme based on six polymorphic genes in comparison with *ompA*-typing and sexgroup *(Continued)*

449	1	6	1	19	1	1	1		E (1)	Hetero (1)
450	1	24	1	19	7	2	4	IV	F (1)	Hetero (1)
453	1	6	1	19	7	21	1	VI	E (1)	Hetero (1)
459	1	6	5	19	6	21	2		E (1)	Hetero (1)
462	1	6	5	19	7	2	56		E (1)	Hetero (1)
465	1	6	5	19	7	14	2		E (1)	Hetero (1)
466	1	24	5	19	7	21	4	IV	F (1)	Hetero (1)
482	1	9	10	6	10	1	8		G (1)	Hetero (1)
484	1	37	10	7	1	3	5		I (1)	Hetero (1)
498	1	6	24	19	14	2	1	VI	E (1)	Hetero (1)
502	1	6	45	19	6	1	2		E (1)	Hetero (1)
504	1	6	47	19	7	2	1	VI	E (1)	Hetero (1)
509	1	6	71	2	1	2	2	VII	E (1)	Hetero (1)
510	1	6	71	2	6	2	2	VII	E (1)	Hetero (1)
513	2	6	71	19	7	2	1	VI	E (2)	Hetero (2)
516	1	6	5	19	5	2	2		E (1)	Hetero (1)
517	2	36	38	5	12	3	18	III	I (2)	Hetero (2)
100b	3	36	10	5	12	7	18	III	I (3)	Hetero (3)
100c	1	37	10	5	12	7	18	III	I (1)	Hetero (1)
108c	9	53	29	8	5	3	6	I	J (9)	MSM (9)
12d	13	24	5	19	7	1	4	IV	F (13)	Hetero (12), MSM (1)
135a	1	20	10	5	12	4	18	III	J (1)	Hetero (1)
135b	2	36	10	5	12	4	18	III	I (2)	Hetero (2)
13b	1	24	5	19	15	1	4	IV	F (1)	Hetero (1)
148a	2	24	5	19	7	2	4	IV	F (2)	Hetero (1), MSM (1)
205b	1	20	10	6	22	4	8		J (1)	Hetero (1)
20a	1	2	10	4	1	4	17		D (1)	Hetero (1)
220a	1	12	10	4	1	3	8		K (1)	Hetero (1)
281a	1	20	10	8	1	4	18		J (1)	Hetero (1)
281b	1	63	10	8	1	4	18		J (1)	Hetero (1)
56a	9	6	1	19	7	2	1	VI	E (9)	Hetero (7), MSM (2)
58a	1	22	27	13	17	13	28	VIII	L2 (1)	MSM (1)
58b	16	28	27	13	17	13	28	VIII	L2b (16)	MSM (16)
77b	1	31	5	19	7	2	37		D (1)	Hetero (1)
91a	1	24	5	19	5	2	4	IV	F (1)	MSM (1)
97b	1	35	12	5	11	9	8		H (1)	Hetero (1)

[a] *Hetero* heterosexual, *MSM* men who have sex with men

Moreover, we demonstrated that using this adapted MLST-7 scheme no reflection of separate transmission between MSM and heterosexual hosts was seen. In addition, we compared clustering of both typing methods and demonstrated that typing using the hr-MLST-6 scheme is able to identify small genetically related clusters of *C. trachomatis* strains within each of the clusters that were identified by using the modified MLST-7 scheme (Fig. 2). These clusters seem to represent biovars.

We successfully modified the MLST-7 scheme that was previously published by us [9]. The sensitivity of the MLST-7 method was increased by modification into a

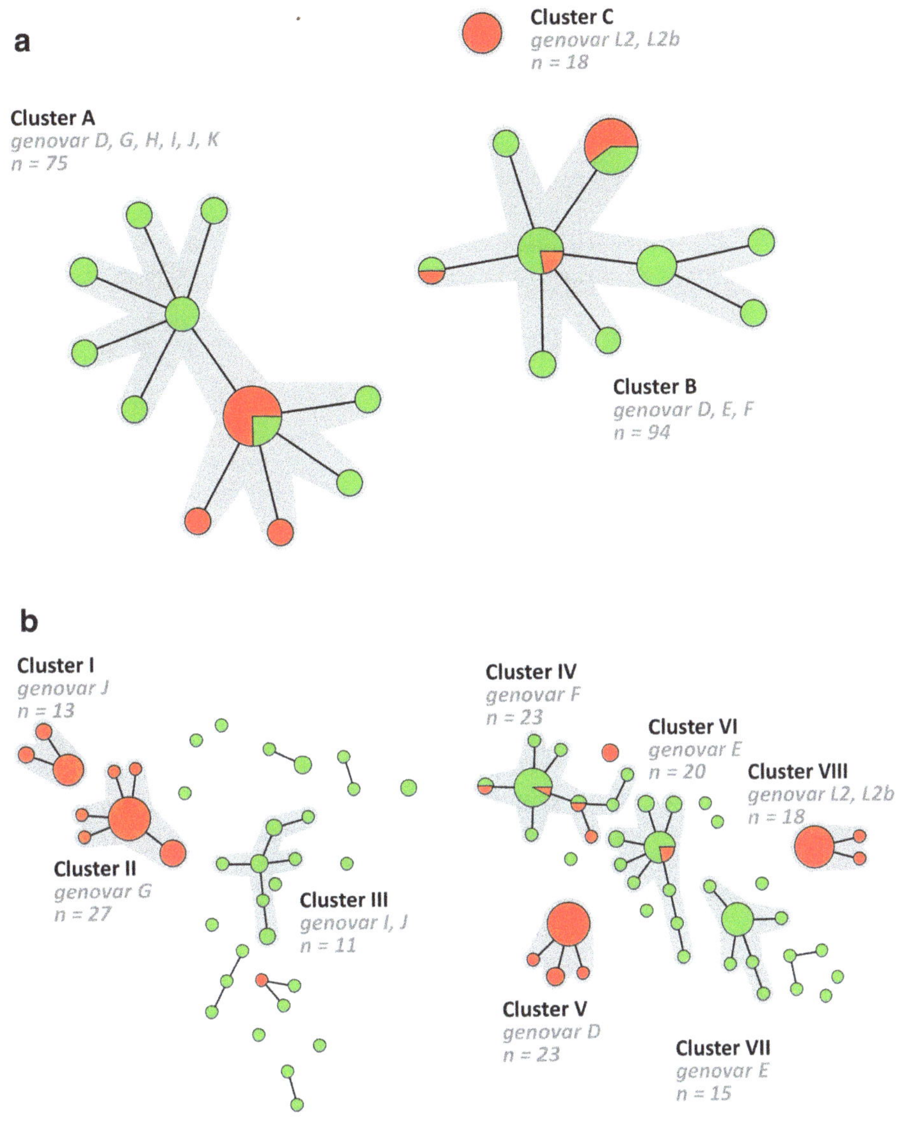

Fig. 1 Minimum spanning tree showing the clustering of 187 *Chlamydia trachomatis*-positive specimens from MSM and heterosexuals. Each circle represents one ST. Size of the circles is proportional to the number of identical ST profiles. Bold lines connect types that differ for one single locus. Halos indicate the distinct clusters. **a** Minimum spanning tree showing the clustering of the *C. trachomatis*-positive specimens according to the MLST-7 scheme; **b** Minimum spanning tree showing the clustering of the *C. trachomatis*-positive specimens according to the hr-MLST-6 scheme. The colour coding is: red, men who have sex with men ($n = 91$); green, heterosexuals ($n = 96$)

nested PCR format. This nested PCR format allowed detection of many novel sequence types because we were now able to test direct clinical specimens without the need for an additional cell culture step. In total, 187 of 188 samples could be fully typed using the modified MLST-7 scheme resulting in a high success rate of 99.5 %. Failure to generate an MLST-7 profile for one out of 188 samples after repeated testing is most likely the result of an insufficient amount of chlamydial DNA in this sample as it produced the highest cycling threshold value in the *pmpH* real time PCR.

The discriminatory capacity of the original MLST-7 scheme was maintained as no known polymorphic sites for *C. trachomatis* were lost due to shortening of some of the amplicons. Moreover for two genes (*hemN* and *enoA*) the amplicon was extended because new 'outer' PCR primers were designed which ensured that the same inner PCR product was obtained as published previously [9]. Designing 'inner' PCR primers for these two genes would have resulted in very short amplicons and loss of resolution as known polymorphic sites would have been lost. The maximum target length in our

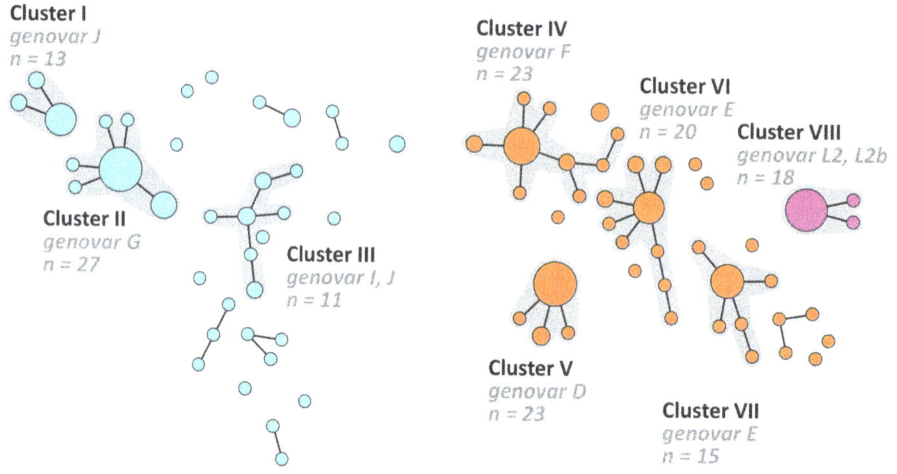

Fig. 2 Minimum spanning tree showing the diversification by hr-MLST-6 of the clusters that were generated using the MLST-7 scheme. Each circle represents one ST. Size of the circles is proportional to the number of identical ST profiles. Bold lines connect types that differ for one single locus. Halos indicate the distinct clusters. Colours indicate the MLST-7 clusters from Fig. 1a: blue, cluster A ($n = 75$); orange, cluster B ($n = 94$); fuchsia, cluster C ($n = 18$)

assay format was 480 bp, which allowed easy sequence analysis from single PCR fragments. It is unlikely that polymorphisms were missed by our adapted MLST-7 scheme. Even if there were so far unknown missed polymorphisms, we think that these would not dramatically increase the genetic diversity using the adapted MLST-7 scheme.

The MLST-7 scheme was developed according to the original MLST principle [13, 18, 19], which aims to index the diversity of nucleotide sequences of fragments of housekeeping genes. Housekeeping genes are presumed to be under neutral or nearly neutral selection pressure making them stable over time, which makes this method useful to answer evolutionary questions and to investigate the epidemiology of *C. trachomatis* over a longer period in time [18]. In comparison, the hr-MLST-6 scheme uses non-housekeeping genes that are under immune pressure or have variable repeat regions and are thus more polymorphic [11, 16]. This enabled us to demonstrate detailed genetic differences between *C. trachomatis* strains that were involved in transmission chains in human hosts in a short time-frame of only a few years [11, 15–17]. However, using the adapted MLST-7 scheme no reflection of separate transmission networks between MSM and heterosexual hosts was seen. Minimum spanning tree analysis of the MLST-7 scheme showed mixed clusters of specimens from MSM and heterosexual individuals with the exception of one cluster (Fig. 1a; cluster C) which solely included specimens from MSM. All these cluster C *C. trachomatis* specimens belonged to the lymphogranuloma venereum (LGV) biovar, which is known to show major genetic differences compared to the urogenital biovar types [20–23]. These results suggest that separate transmission chains in human hosts can only be observed over a small time-frame using highly discriminating genetic typing methods. Transmission chains between MSM and heterosexuals were not totally separated in our previous studies with larger trees, including randomly chosen samples [15–17]. This overlap was expected since there will also be individuals who identify themselves as MSM, but have had contact with heterosexual women (Fig. 1b).

Comparison of the clustering of both MLST schemes showed that both MLST schemes were able to resolve the *C. trachomatis* specimens in a number of STs and clusters. Minimum spanning tree analysis using data from the adapted MLST-7 scheme revealed 3 main groups of circulating *C. trachomatis* strains (Fig. 1), as was also previously described by us using the original MLST-7 scheme [9]. One group is composed solely of the LGV genovars. Another is composed of the clinically prevalent urogenital genovars, whereas the third contains the less frequently occurring urogenital genovars. Similar groupings are reported in previous studies using WGS analysis or MLST analysis based on housekeeping genes [7, 9, 10]. In comparison to MLST-7, minimum spanning tree analysis of the hr-MLST-6 scheme was able to further diversify each of these 3 main groups and clusters of circulating *C. trachomatis* strains in smaller genetically related clusters and thus allowed for more detailed analysis within these groups (Fig. 2). Using maximum likelihood analysis, we previously demonstrated that the hr-MLST-6 targets provided a tree similar to trees based on WGS, but with lower bootstrap support values [12]. Since we already observed clear differences in the diversification of strains between the MLST-7 and hr-MLST-6 scheme (Fig. 1), a similar tree based on the MLST-7 targets is expected to differ from a tree based on WGS by showing less genetic diversity.

Conclusions

We successfully adapted and applied the MLST-7 scheme to direct clinical specimens from MSM and heterosexuals. However, using this adapted MLST-7 scheme no distinct transmission of *C. trachomatis* could be observed in MSM and heterosexuals in comparison to the hr-MLST-6 scheme. In addition, we also compared clustering of both MLST schemes and demonstrated that typing using the hr-MLST-6 scheme is able to identify genetically related clusters of *C. trachomatis* strains within each of the clusters that were identified by using the MLST-7 scheme. Hr-MLST-6 may therefore also be a useful tool to for more detailed analysis of *C. trachomatis* strains within identified MLST-7 clusters.

Availability of data and materials

Data on all 187 samples typed with both the hr-MLST-6 en MLST-7 scheme are included in Additional file 1: Table S1 and Additional file 2: Table S2. Corresponding nucleotide sequences can be derived from the publicly available databases: http://mlstdb.bmc.uu.se/ (hr-MLST-6) and http://pubmlst.org/chlamydiales/ (MLST-7).

Competing interest

The authors declare that they have no competing interests.

Authors' contributions

SMB, AvdE and YP conceived the study, and participated in its design and coordination. BV performed the experiments. BV, SMB, AvdE, YP analysed the data. BV, SMB, AvdE, YP wrote the paper. All authors read and approved the final manuscript.

Acknowledgements

The authors thank Michelle Himschoot for technical assistance and expertise.

Author details

[1]Public Health Laboratory, Cluster Infectious Diseases, Public Health Service Amsterdam, Amsterdam, The Netherlands. [2]Center for Infection and Immunity Amsterdam (CINIMA), Academic Medical Center, University of Amsterdam, Amsterdam, The Netherlands. [3]Department of Medical Microbiology, Academic Medical Center, Amsterdam, The Netherlands.

References

1. WHO. Global incidence and prevalence of selected curable sexually transmitted infections: 2008. Reprod Health Matters. 2012;20:207–9.
2. Haggerty CL, Gottlieb SL, Taylor BD, Low N, Xu F, Ness RB. Risk of sequelae after Chlamydia trachomatis genital infection in women. J Infect Dis. 2010;201 Suppl 2:S134–55.
3. Land JA, Van Bergen JE, Morre SA, Postma MJ. Epidemiology of Chlamydia trachomatis infection in women and the cost-effectiveness of screening. Hum Reprod Update. 2010;16:189–204.
4. Rekart ML, Gilbert M, Meza R, Kim PH, Chang M, Money DM, et al. Chlamydia public health programs and the epidemiology of pelvic inflammatory disease and ectopic pregnancy. J Infect Dis. 2013;207:30–8.
5. Herrmann B, Torner A, Low N, Klint M, Nilsson A, Velicko I, et al. Emergence and spread of Chlamydia trachomatis variant, Sweden. Emerg Infect Dis. 2008;14:1462–5.
6. Jurstrand M, Christerson L, Klint M, Fredlund H, Unemo M, Herrmann B. Characterisation of Chlamydia trachomatis by ompA sequencing and multilocus sequence typing in a Swedish county before and after identification of the new variant. Sex Transm Infect. 2010;86:56–60.
7. Harris SR, Clarke IN, Seth-Smith HM, Solomon AW, Cutcliffe LT, Marsh P, et al. Whole-genome analysis of diverse Chlamydia trachomatis strains identifies phylogenetic relationships masked by current clinical typing. Nat Genet. 2012;44:413–9. S1.
8. Klint M, Fuxelius HH, Goldkuhl RR, Skarin H, Rutemark C, Andersson SG, et al. High-resolution genotyping of Chlamydia trachomatis strains by multilocus sequence analysis. J Clin Microbiol. 2007;45:1410–4.
9. Pannekoek Y, Morelli G, Kusecek B, Morre SA, Ossewaarde JM, Langerak AA, et al. Multi locus sequence typing of Chlamydiales: clonal groupings within the obligate intracellular bacteria Chlamydia trachomatis. BMC Microbiol. 2008;8:42.
10. Dean D, Bruno WJ, Wan R, Gomes JP, Devignot S, Mehari T, et al. Predicting phenotype and emerging strains among Chlamydia trachomatis infections. Emerg Infect Dis. 2009;15:1385–94.
11. Bom RJ, Christerson L, van der Loeff Schim MF, Coutinho RA, Herrmann B, Bruisten SM. Evaluation of high-resolution typing methods for Chlamydia trachomatis in samples from heterosexual couples. J Clin Microbiol. 2011;49:2844–53.
12. Herrmann B, Isaksson J, Ryberg M, Tangrot J, Saleh I, Versteeg B, et al. Global Multilocus sequence type analysis of Chlamydia trachomatis strains from 16 Countries. J Clin Microbiol. 2015;53:2172–9.
13. Maiden MC, Bygraves JA, Feil E, Morelli G, Russell JE, Urwin R, et al. Multilocus sequence typing: a portable approach to the identification of clones within populations of pathogenic microorganisms. Proc Natl Acad Sci U S A. 1998;95:3140–5.
14. de Vries HJ, van der Loeff Schim MF, Bruisten SM. High-resolution typing of Chlamydia trachomatis: epidemiological and clinical uses. Curr Opin Infect Dis. 2015;28:61–71.
15. Christerson L, Bom RJ, Bruisten SM, Yass R, Hardick J, Bratt G, et al. Chlamydia trachomatis strains show specific clustering for men who have sex with men compared to heterosexual populations in Sweden, the Netherlands, and the United States. J Clin Microbiol. 2012;50: 3548–55.
16. Bom RJ, van der Helm JJ, van der Loeff Schim MF, van Rooijen MS, Heijman T, Matser A, et al. Distinct transmission networks of Chlamydia trachomatis in men who have sex with men and heterosexual adults in Amsterdam, The Netherlands. PLoS One. 2013;8:e53869.
17. Versteeg B, van Rooijen MS, van der Loeff Schim MF, de Vries HJ, Bruisten SM. No indication for tissue tropism in urogenital and anorectal Chlamydia trachomatis infections using high-resolution multilocus sequence typing. BMC Infect Dis. 2014;14:464.
18. Jolley KA, Maiden MC. Using multilocus sequence typing to study bacterial variation: prospects in the genomic era. Future Microbiol. 2014;9:623–30.
19. Maiden MC, van Rensburg Jansen MJ, Bray JE, Earle SG, Ford SA, Jolley KA, et al. MLST revisited: the gene-by-gene approach to bacterial genomics. Nat Rev Microbiol. 2013;11:728–36.
20. Almeida F, Borges V, Ferreira R, Borrego MJ, Gomes JP, Mota LJ. Polymorphisms in inc proteins and differential expression of inc genes among Chlamydia trachomatis strains correlate with invasiveness and tropism of lymphogranuloma venereum isolates. J Bacteriol. 2012;194: 6574–85.
21. Borges V, Nunes A, Ferreira R, Borrego MJ, Gomes JP. Directional evolution of Chlamydia trachomatis towards niche-specific adaptation. J Bacteriol. 2012;194:6143–53.
22. Nunes A, Borrego MJ, Gomes JP. Genomic features beyond Chlamydia trachomatis phenotypes: what do we think we know? Infect Genet Evol. 2013;16:392–400.
23. Abdelsamed H, Peters J, Byrne GI. Genetic variation in Chlamydia trachomatis and their hosts: impact on disease severity and tissue tropism. Future Microbiol. 2013;8:1129–46.

12

Circumcision status at HIV infection is not associated with plasma viral load in men

Stephanie M. Davis[1,5*], Sherri Pals[1], Chunfu Yang[1], Elijah Odoyo-June[2], Joy Chang[1], Maroya Spalding Walters[1], Walter Jaoko[3], Naomi Bock[1], Larry Westerman[1], Carlos Toledo[1] and Robert C. Bailey[4]

Abstract

Background: Male circumcision provides men with approximately 60% protection from acquiring HIV infection via heterosexual sex, and has become a key component of HIV prevention efforts in sub-Saharan Africa. Possible mechanisms for this protection include removal of the inflammatory anaerobic sub-preputial environment and the high concentration of Langerhans cells on the inside of the foreskin, both believed to promote local vulnerability to HIV infection. In people who do acquire HIV, viral load is partially determined by infecting partner viral load, potentially mediated by size of infecting inoculum. By removing a portal for virion entry, prior male circumcision could decrease infecting inoculum and thus viral load in men who become HIV-infected, conferring the known associated benefits of slower progression to disease and decreased infectiousness.

Methods: We performed an as-treated analysis of plasma samples collected under a randomized controlled trial of male circumcision for HIV prevention, comparing men based on their circumcision status at the time of HIV acquisition, to determine whether circumcision is associated with lower viral load. Eligible men were seroconverters who had at least one plasma sample available drawn at least 6 months after infection, reported no potential exposures other than vaginal sex and, for those who were circumcised, were infected more than 6 weeks after circumcision, to eliminate the open wound as a confounder. Initial viral load testing indicated that quality of pre-2007 samples might have been compromised during storage and they were excluded, as were those with undetectable or unquantifiable results. Log viral loads were compared between groups using univariable and multivariable linear regression, adjusting for sample age and sexually transmitted infection diagnosis with 3.5 months of seroconversion, with a random effect for intra-individual clustering for samples from the same man. A per-protocol analysis was also performed.

Results: There were no viral load differences between men who were circumcised and uncircumcised at the time of HIV infection (means 4.00 and 4.03 $\log_{10}$ copies/mL respectively, $p = .88$) in any analysis.

Conclusion: Circumcision status at the time of HIV infection does not affect viral load in men.

Keywords: Circumcision, HIV prevention, Viral load, Clinical trials, Intervention

* Correspondence: smdavis@cdc.gov
[1]Division of Global HIV/AIDS and Tuberculosis, US Centers for Disease Control, Atlanta, GA, USA
[5]Division of Global HIV and TB, HIV Prevention Branch US Centers for Disease Control and Prevention, 1600 Clifton Rd. NE Mail Stop E-04, Atlanta, GA 30329, USA
Full list of author information is available at the end of the article

Background

Male circumcision (MC) has been shown in randomized controlled trials (RCTs) to confer approximately 60% protection to men from acquiring HIV infection via heterosexual sex [1–3]. It has become a key component of HIV prevention efforts in sub-Saharan Africa, with nearly 15 million voluntary medical male circumcisions (VMMC) performed since 2008 [4]. Widely-accepted possible mechanisms for the protective effect include: the removal of the inner foreskin's high concentration of Langerhans cells, through which HIV can access the immune system; the foreskin's vulnerability to microabrasions; the elimination of the anaerobic sub-preputial environment that supports a pro-inflammatory microbiome; and the greater incidence of genital ulcer disease (GUD) among uncircumcised men [5].

Nevertheless, many circumcised men will ultimately become HIV-infected. Determinants of plasma viral load (VL) set point among infected individuals are not entirely understood, but in addition to well-established associations like host immunogenetics [6] and viral genotype [7], it is associated with VL in "source" partners [8–10]. Although this relationship is sometimes attributed to viral genotype also, another suggested mechanism is that high source partner VL results in a higher infecting inoculum, which then results in higher VL in the newly-infected partner [11, 12]. (The majority of HIV infections resulting from heterosexual sex are believed to result from a single virion [9, 13], so the effect of inoculum size on VL is not hypothesized to result directly from a higher initial virion population. Instead, a larger inoculum may lead to increased host T-cell activation, which in turn enhances replication of the ultimately 'successful' virion [10]). Supporting evidence for inoculum size as an independent determinant of VL includes the association between source partner genital tract factors which would affect magnitude of viral shedding, such as bacterial vaginosis and genital herpes suppression, and VLs in seroconverting partners [12].

If source inoculum affects VL, the same mechanisms that confer partial protection against infection could operate in circumcised men who do become infected to decrease the proportion of virions breaching their skin, lowering inoculum and thus VL. Fig. 1 illustrates this proposed causal chain. If present, such an effect could confer substantial population-level benefit, as VL is a major determinant of both progression to clinical disease and infectiousness [14].

Evidence for the plausibility of this result comes from one study that found MC in genotype-confirmed male source partners was associated with lower HIV VLs among the female partners they infected [10, 15] (adjusted mean difference = –.63 $\log_{10}$ copies/mL, $p = .03$). The authors hypothesized the above mechanism in reverse: lower innocula transferred to female partners due to the removal of the male's infectious foreskin Langerhans cells via MC. This study did not find evidence of lower VL set points associated with MC among men infected by female source partners, but this outcome was limited by small sample size ($N = 55$) and the fact that participants were not randomized with respect to circumcision status.

We used stored plasma samples from the original RCT of MC for HIV prevention conducted in Kisumu, Kenya [2], to investigate whether MC status of male participants who became HIV-infected was associated with their VL.

Methods

Enrollment, randomization, sample collection and follow-up in the Kisumu-based RCT

Detailed methods of the RCT are described elsewhere [2] (ClinicalTrials.gov, NCT00059371). Briefly, it was conducted in Kisumu district, western Kenya. Male participants were recruited via newspapers, radio, fliers and street shows and enrolled between 2002 and 2005. Inclusion criteria included being an uncircumcised, HIV-negative, sexually active, 18–24-year-old Kisumu resident. Exclusion criteria included contraindications to, and absolute indications for, surgical MC. An opaque envelope system was used to produce 1:1 allocation between arms. Plasma HIV testing was performed and self-reported HIV exposure data collected at 1, 3, and 6 months after randomization, then at 6-month intervals. The trial was stopped early in December 2006 due to efficacy. Free MC was then offered to all interested

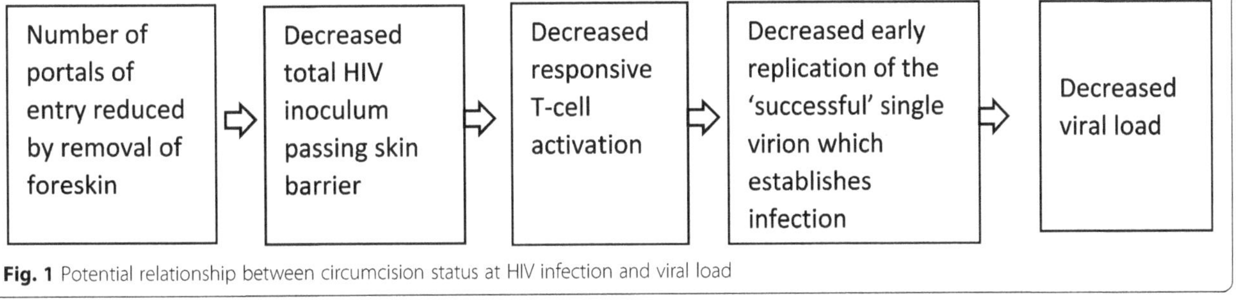

Fig. 1 Potential relationship between circumcision status at HIV infection and viral load

participants throughout the follow-up period, causing crossover from the control group. Semi-annual follow-up visits continued through September 2010. The dataset is publically available [16].

HIV testing and determination of seroconversion and infection dates

Two rapid tests were used at each visit, Determine HIV 1/2 (Abbott Diagnostic Division, Hoofddorp, Netherlands) and Unigold Recombigen (Trinity Biotech, Wicklow, Ireland). If one or both was positive, serum was sent for double enzyme-linked immunosorbent assay testing (Detect HIV 1/2, Adaltis Inc., Montreal, Canada and Recombigen HIV 1/2, Trinity Biotech, Wicklow, Ireland). If at least one ELISA was positive, final confirmatory testing was done by line immunoassay (INNO-LIA HIV 1/2, Immunogenetics NV, Ghent, Belgium). For participants confirmed as HIV positive, the first visit with at least one positive rapid test was designated the HIV seroconversion visit. We calculated the presumed infection date as the date midway between the final negative test and the HIV seroconversion visit.

Other data

Additional data collected at enrollment and in follow-up included MC procedure date, behavioral and other HIV risk factors, and sexually transmitted infection (STI) diagnoses. High-risk sexual behavior within the 6 months before a visit was defined as self-report of > 2 female sex partners, exchanging gifts or money for sex, or using a condom "less than half the time".

STI testing included serum rapid plasma reagin (RPR) (Becton Dickinson) with *T. pallidum* particle agglutination (TPHA) confirmation for syphilis and HSV-2 serology; and urine polymerase chain reaction (PCR) for *N. gonorrhoeae* and *C. trachomatis*. Men with urethral discharge also had urethral swabs for *N. gonorrhoeae* culture and PCR, *C. trachomatis* PCR (Roche Diagnostics), and *T. vaginalis* culture (In pouch test). Any genital ulcers were swabbed for *H. ducreyi* culture, and PCR and HSV-2 PCR testing using the Roche Multiplex PCR system. Men were defined as having an STI if any tests were positive except a positive RPR with negative TPHA. The study did not collect data on antiretroviral therapy (ART) initiation among participants; between 2005 and 2011, the Kenyan National HIV Treatment guidelines set a CD4 threshold for ART of <=200/mm^3.

Inclusion and exclusion criteria for HIV VL analysis

Individual inclusion criteria for this analysis were: seroconversion during the trial or follow-up; and having at least one available plasma sample drawn at least 6 months after infection date and, for those who became circumcised after infection, drawn 6 months after MC (to eliminate bias from the procedure causing transient VL increases). Individual exclusion criteria were: potential HIV exposures other than vaginal sex at any time (sex with men, intravenous drug use, or blood transfusion); a still-unhealed MC wound less than 3 weeks prior to infection; and for circumcised men, infection date fewer than 6 weeks after MC (unhealed wounds may have facilitated infection among men who resumed sex earlier).

Sample exclusion criteria were also applied. Samples drawn before Jan 1, 2007 were excluded from the final analysis because all but five (of 85) had undetectable or unquantifiable VLs, correlations described below between sample age and VL suggested older samples were subject to degradation, and none of these samples had second aliquots available for quality control. Finally, samples with undetectable or unquantifiable results were also ultimately excluded (see *Data Analysis* section for methods and reasoning). Among eligible men, the first eligible samples, up to three, were used.

Sample size

The anticipated sample size based on total available aliquots was 123 men (82 circumcised and 41 uncircumcised), which provided 80% power to detect a between-group difference in mean VL of .54 standard deviations, equivalent to .93 $\log_{10}$ copies/mL [12]. Power calculations were done using SAS 9.3 PROC POWER TWOSAMPLEMEANS with a two-sample t-test.

Sample storage and testing

Plasma samples were not tested at the time of collection, and were not thawed at any time before testing. They were stored at − 80 °C, initially at the Kenya Medical Research Institute in Kisumu, and permanently at the Chicago Developmental Center for AIDS Research. VL testing was performed by the International Laboratory Branch of the US Centers for Disease Control's Division of Global HIV and Tuberculosis in Atlanta, Georgia, using the Abbott HIV-1 Real Time HIV-1 assay on the Abbott m2000 instrument, with a lower limit of detection of 150 copies/mL with a 200 μL plasma input volume. All samples with an available second aliquot were retested and results compared against initial values, with a difference threshold of ≤0.5 $\log_{10}$ copies/mL for concurrence.

Data analysis

In the primary (as-treated) analysis, men were classified as circumcised or uncircumcised based on whether they had been circumcised through the RCT's services before infection. The secondary (per-protocol) analysis restricted the comparison to men remaining in their original randomization group. Analysis was performed using SAS 9.3 on $\log_{10}$-transformed VL results from the first round of testing.

Once a high proportion of samples with undetectable or unquantifiable (VL detected at a concentration below the quantifiability threshold, 2.18 log copies/mL) results was identified, methods for handling these values were devised. Prior to the second round of testing, it was pre-specified that all such samples would be retested if a second aliquot was available, and the values would be included in the analysis if at least 80% of their retested samples were again either undetectable or unquantifiable, increasing confidence that these represented true plasma values rather than degradation of the aliquots.

To compare characteristics between groups, we used Fisher's exact Chi-square test for categorical variables, and t-tests for continuous variables. Pearson correlation coefficients were used to examine the relationship between sample age and log VL.

PROC MIXED was used to test for differences in log VL between groups, with a random effect for individual to account for the correlation between samples from the same man, This approach yields results similar to an analysis on log VL means computed for each man and then compared between groups, but also allows for the use of sample-level covariates such as sample age.

Results

Specimen collection dates for included samples ranged from January 10, 2007 to September 30, 2010. VL results were concurrent between aliquots for all retested quantifiable samples, but samples with initially undetectable or unquantifiable VL results did not meet the prespecified criteria and were excluded, leaving 124 included samples representing 63 seroconverting participants (37 circumcised and 26 uncircumcised). Twenty-three men had only one sample. With the reduction in size, the analyzed sample had 80% power to detect a between-group difference of .73 standard deviations, or 1.26 $\log_{10}$ copies/mL. Log viral load results had a range of 2.33 to 6.21, with a median of 4.04 (IQR 3.57–4.53). For men with two or three results, the intraclass correlation between log viral loads was strong at 0.63. Table 1 compares key demographic and risk characteristics, and sample-level characteristics of draw timing and age at testing, for circumcised and uncircumcised participants. Groups were similar demographically. Circumcised men had a nonsignificant higher prevalence of risky behavior and lower prevalence of STI. Samples were similar in draw timing and age at testing.

A strong linear correlation was found between VL and sample age (Fig. 2; $r = -.48$, $p < .0001$, $R^2 = .23$); a quadratic term was tested for significance to assess for a nonlinear association, but was not significant and was therefore dropped. No significant correlation was found between VL and duration of infection at time of blood draw (Fig. 3; $r = .07$, $p = 0.40$).

No significant difference in log VL was found between circumcised and uncircumcised men in the as-treated (means 4.00 and 4.03 log copies/mL respectively, $p = .88$) or per-protocol (means 4.06 and 3.99 log copies/mL, $p = .76$) analyses. This remained true after adjusting for STI diagnosis within 3.5 months of seroconversion and age of sample, for both the as-treated (means 3.96 and 4.09 log copies/mL, $p = .47$) and the per-protocol (means 3.99 and 4.04 log copies/mL, $p = .80$) analysis.

Discussion

Our results do not support an effect of circumcision status larger than 1.26 $\log_{10}$ copies/mL at the time of seroconversion on VL after 6 months. This does not rule out a clinically significant effect: a 1 log difference in VL was found in Uganda to be associated with an adjusted

Table 1 Characteristics of circumcised and uncircumcised HIV-1 seroconverters and their samples (as-treated analysis)

Characteristic	Circumcised mean (SD) or % (n)	Uncircumcised mean (SD) or % (n)	*p*-value[a]
Individual-level (*N* = 37 circumcised, 26 uncircumcised)			
Mean age (years)	20.0 (1.5)	20.4 (1.6)	.32
Mean educational attainment (years)	9.3 (2.1)	10.0 (2.2)	.20
STI diagnosis within 3.5 months of seroconversion - % (n)	13.5 (5)	34.6 (9)	.08
High-risk sex within 6 months of seroconversion - % (n)	70.3 (26)	53.8 (14)	.20
Sample-level (*N* = 72 circumcised, 52 uncircumcised)			
Mean (days) between seroconversion and draw date	516.2 (210.7)	558.8 (330.3)	.42
Percent (n) drawn < 12 mo. post seroconversion	26.4 (19)	34.6 (18)	.28
Percent (n) drawn 12–17 mo. post seroconversion	31.9 (23)	23.1 (12)	
Percent (n) drawn > 18 mo. post seroconversion	27.8 (20)	19.2 (10)	
Percent (n) drawn > 24 mo. post seroconversion	13.9 (10)	23.1 (12)	
Mean age (days) of sample(s) at testing	2646.5 (367.5)	2702.4 (375.5)	.41

[a]Tests for continuous variables were done using t-tests; tests for categorical variables were done using exact Chi-square tests

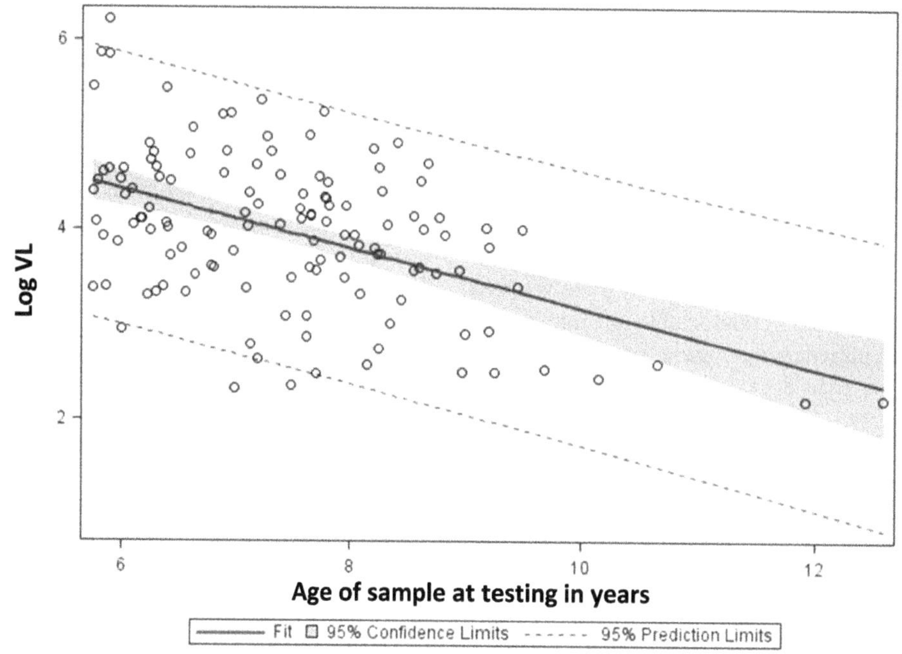

Fig. 2 Relationship between age of sample and $\log_{10}$ viral load

hazard ratio of 3.09 for death and 2.75 for progression to AIDS [17] and the 1 log difference between a VL of 10,000 and 100,000 copies/mL has been modeled to be associated with approximately a 5-year difference in asymptomatic survival [18]. However, this finding is consistent with the observational results reported by Lingappa et al. in participants from southern and eastern African countries, and represents gold-standard data due to randomization which is unlikely to become available from future studies. It also helps establish the assumptions needed for sample size planning for any observational studies further examining the issue. Given the

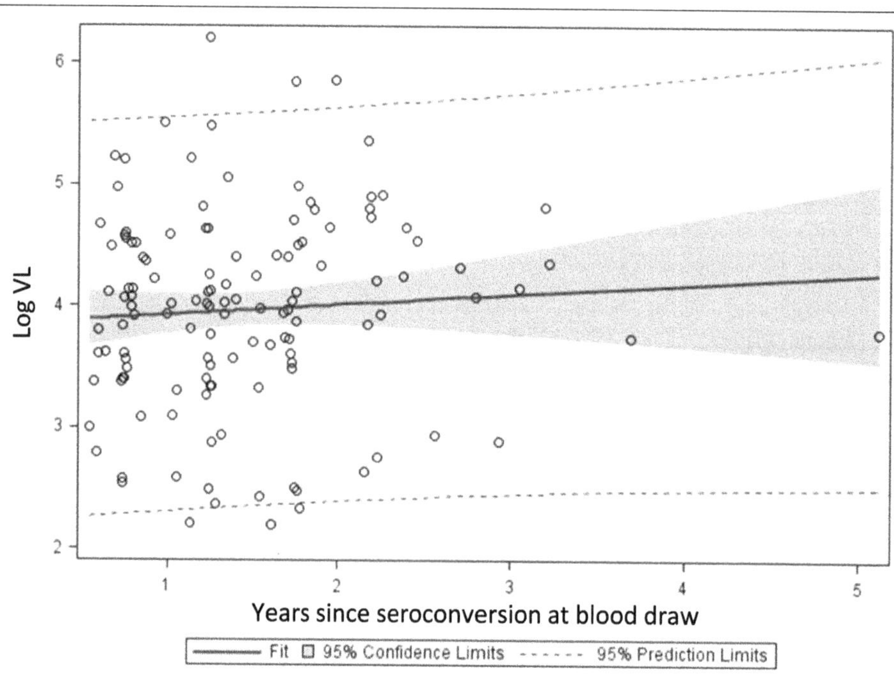

Fig. 3 Relationship between time since seroconversion and Log_{10} viral load

mechanistic biological nature of the proposed effect, results are also likely to be valid across populations.

If the lack of observed effect reflects biological fact, the explanation may lie in the set of portals of entry available to HIV virions on the male genitalia. In addition to the foreskin, the glans, urethral mucosa and possibly fossa navicularis are all portals across which translocation of cell-associated HIV-1 has been demonstrated in vivo [19]. Given the low per-act probability of female-to-male transmission through *any* of these portals (4 per 10,000 infectious exposures in a recent systematic review) [20], it seems to follow that the probability of transmission through any single portal is even lower, and thus that in any one act leading to infection, the most likely scenario is that only one portal is involved. Thus circumcision would remove one portal, decreasing infection risk, but would not affect the size of an inoculum passing through a different portal, thus not affecting VL if infectious becomes established. Others have found higher per-act transmission probabilities such as 0.38% in developing countries in the absence of commercial sex work or genital ulceration, [21] but also at this higher magnitude, a single portal seems likely to be involved in the majority of transmissions.

Conversely, the previously-observed lower VLs in women with circumcised male source partners are more likely to be related to total male viral shedding, which would be expected to come from multiple "portals of exit" during sex, including semen and penile mucosa. Shedding has been shown via coronal lavage to be reduced in HIV-infected men after healing from MC, compared to pre-MC levels [22].

It is also possible that infecting inoculum does not actually impact VL, though this would not explain Lingappa et al.'s [12] observed association between male infecting partner circumcision and lower female partner VL in their baseline data.

Finally, it is possible that there is a population-level effect of circumcision status at time of infection on men's VL, but that it is mediated by the known protective associations of MC with risk for genital ulcer disease (GUD) [23], thus decreasing VL indirectly through the same mechanisms postulated for a direct effect. Lingappa et al. [12] did not find an association between HSV-2 serology and VL set point, but thoroughly testing this possibility would require a much larger sample of circumcised and uncircumcised seroconverters with sufficient prevalence of GUD to estimate a true effect.

The major potential confounder is the effect of sample age on VL. Although controlling for this did not impact results, the effect of storage time on VL can have an unpredictable [24] component, which could have caused residual confounding. However, if substantial, this component should have eroded all observed associations; the observed correlations between VL and sample age, and between VLs from the same participant, should not have been seen.

Another potential confounder is ART initiation, which was not captured in the study data. However, between 2005 and 2011, Kenyan National HIV Treatment guidelines set a CD4 threshold for ART of $<=200/mm^3$ in the absence of clinical indications, and the maximum elapsed time of 5.1 years between calculated infection date and blood draw in our sample makes it unlikely that participants would have progressed to meet this criterion and start treatment. If any did, elimination of samples with undetectable viral load would also have been likely to exclude them. In other respects, although circumcised participants were somewhat more likely to report risky behavior, the difference was not significant, and VLs would not necessarily be higher in infections contracted through high-risk sex.

Finally, for participants with only one sample, stability of VL over time cannot be demonstrated; therefore, VL cannot necessarily be considered equivalent to VL set point.

Conclusions

Though circumcision in HIV-positive men has an observed association with HIV VL in female partners infected by them, this study provides no evidence that circumcision status at HIV seroconversion affects VL after 6 months in men.

Abbreviations

ART: Antiretroviral therapy; MC: Male circumcision; RCT: Randomized controlled trial; RPR: Rapid plasma reagin; STI: Sexually transmitted infection; TPHA: *T. pallidum* particle agglutination; VL: Viral load; VMMC: Voluntary medical male circumcision

Acknowledgements

Not applicable.

Funding

This research has been supported by the President's Emergency Plan for AIDS Relief (PEPFAR) through CDC. The original RCT of circumcision in Kisumu was funded by the Division of AIDS, NIAD, NIH, and storage of the samples was supported by the Chicago Developmental Center for AIDS Research.

Disclaimer

The findings and conclusions in this paper are those of the authors and do not necessarily represent the views of the US Centers for Disease Control and Prevention or NIH.

Authors' contributions

All authors have reviewed and approved the final manuscript. SD conceived of the analysis and drafted and revised the manuscript. SP performed all statistical calculations and figure development and revised the manuscript. CY and LW designed and supervised sample testing and revised the manuscript. EO and WJ led local protocol approval and revised the manuscript. MW contributed to analytic design and revised the manuscript. JC performed sample testing. NB and CT revised the manuscript. RB led the original trial, contributed to analytic design, and revised the manuscript.

Consent for publication
Not applicable.

Competing interests
The authors declare that they have no competing interests.

Author details
[1]Division of Global HIV/AIDS and Tuberculosis, US Centers for Disease Control, Atlanta, GA, USA. [2]Division of Global HIV/AIDS and Tuberculosis, US Centers for Disease Control, Kisumu, Kenya. [3]Department of Medical Microbiology, University of Nairobi, Nairobi, Kenya. [4]Division of Epidemiology and Biostatistics, University of Illinois Chicago School of Public Health, Chicago, IL, USA. [5]Division of Global HIV and TB, HIV Prevention Branch US Centers for Disease Control and Prevention, 1600 Clifton Rd. NE Mail Stop E-04, Atlanta, GA 30329, USA.

References
1. Auvert B, Taljaard D, Lagarde E, Sobngwi-Tambekou J, Sitta R, Puren A. Randomized, controlled intervention trial of male circumcision for reduction of HIV infection risk: the ANRS 1265 Trial. PLoS Med. 2005;2(11):e298.
2. Bailey RC, Moses S, Parker CB, Agot K, Maclean I, Krieger JN. Male circumcision for HIV prevention in young men in Kisumu, Kenya: a randomised controlled trial. Lancet. 2007;369(9562):643–56.
3. Gray RH, Kigozi G, Serwadda D, Makumbi F, Watya S, Nalugoda F. Male circumcision for HIV prevention in men in Rakai, Uganda: a randomised trial. Lancet. 2007;369(9562):657–66.
4. World Health Organization. Voluntary medical male circumcision for HIV prevention in 14 Priority Countries In Eastern And Southern Africa: July 2017 Progress Brief. Accessed online Feb 2, 2017 at http://www.who.int/hiv/pub/malecircumcision/vmmc-progress-brief-2017/en/.
5. Morris BJ, Wamai RG. Biological basis for the protective effect conferred by male circumcision against HIV infection. Int J STD AIDS. 2012;23(3):153–9. https://doi.org/10.1258/ijsa.2011.011228.
6. Saathoff E, Pritsch M, Geldmacher C, Hoffmann O, Koehler RN, Maboko L, et al. Viral and host factors associated with the HIV-1 viral load set point in adults from Mbeya region. Tanzania J Acquir Immune Defic Syndr. 2010; 54(3):324–30.
7. Hodcroft E, Hadfield JD, Fearnhill E, Phillips A, Dunn D, O'Shea D, et al, on behalf of the UK HIV Drug Resistance Database and the UK CHIC Study. The contribution of viral genotype to plasma viral set-point in HIV infection. PLoS Pathog. 2014 10(5): e1004112. doi: https://doi.org/10.1371/journal.ppat.1004112
8. Hollingsworth TD, Laeyendecker O, Shirreff G, Donnelly CA, Serwadda D, et al. HIV-1 transmitting couples have similar viral load set-points in Rakai. Uganda PLoS Pathology. 2010;6(5):e1000876. https://doi.org/10.1371/journal.ppat.1000876.
9. Tang J, Tang S, Lobashevsky E, Zulu I, Aldrovandi G, Allen S, et al. HLA allele sharing and HIV type 1 viremia in seroconverting Zambians with known transmitting partners. AIDS Res Hum Retrovir. 2004;20(1):19–25.
10. Hecht FM, Hartogensis W, Bragg L, Bacchetti P, Atchison R, Grant R, et al. HIV RNA level in early infection is predicted by viral load in the transmission source. AIDS. 2010;24(7):941–5.
11. Shaw GM, Hunter E. HIV transmission. Cold Spring Harb Perspect Med. 2012; 2(11):pii: a006965. https://doi.org/10.1101/cshperspect.a006965.
12. Lingappa JR, Thomas KK, Hughes JP, Baeten JM, Wald A, Farquhar C, et al. On behalf of Partners in Prevention HSV/HIV transmission study team. Partner characteristics predicting HIV-1 set point in sexually acquired HIV-1 among African seroconverters. AIDS Res Hum Retrovir. 2013;29(1):164–71.
13. Keele BF, Giorgi EE, Salazar-Gonzalez JF, Decker JM, Pham KT, Salazar MG, et al. Identification and characterization of transmitted and early founder virus envelopes in primary HIV-1 infection. Proc Natl Acad Sci U S A. 2008; 105(21):7552–7. https://doi.org/10.1073/pnas.0802203105. Epub 2008 May 19
14. Mellors JW, Rinaldo CR Jr, Gupta P, White RM, Todd JA, Kingsley LA. Prognosis in HIV-1 infection predicted by the quantity of virus in plasma. Science. 1996;272:1167–70.
15. Mackelprang RD, Carrington M, Thomas KK, Hughes JP, Baeten JM, Wald A, et al. Host genetic and viral determinants of HIV-1 RNA set point among HIV-1 seroconverters from sub-saharan Africa. J Virol. 2015;89(4):2104–11. https://doi.org/10.1128/JVI.01573-14. Epub 2014 Dec 3
16. Randomized Control Trial of Male Circumcision to Reduce HIV Incidence in Kisumu, Kenya. Accession number PB2012500016. National Technical Reports Library: https://ntrl.ntis.gov/NTRL/dashboard/searchResults.xhtml?searchQuery=Male%20circumcision
17. Eller MA, Opollo MS, Liu M, Redd AD, Eller LA, Kityo C, et al. HIV type 1 disease progression to AIDS and death in a rural Ugandan cohort is primarily dependent on viral load despite variable subtype and T-cell immune activation levels. J Inf Dis. 2014;211(10):1574–84.
18. Fraser C, Hollingsworth D, Chapman R, de Wolf F, Hange WP, et al. Variation in HIV-1 set-point viral load: epidemiological analysis and an evolutionary hypothesis. PNAS. 2007;104(44):17441–6.
19. Ganor Y, Zhou Z, Bodo J, Tudor D, Leibowitch J, Mathez D, et al. The adult penile urethra is a novel entry site for HIV-1 that preferentially targets resident urethral macrophages. Nature. 2013;6:4.
20. Patel P, Borkowf CB, Brooks JT, Lasry A, Lansky A, Mermin J. Estimating per-act HIV transmission risk: a systematic review. AIDS. 2014;28(10):1509–19. https://doi.org/10.1097/QAD.0000000000000298.
21. Boily M-C, Baggaley RF, Wang L, Masse B, White RG, Hayes R, et al. Heterosexual risk of HIV-1 infection per sexual act: a systematic review and meta-analysis of observational studies. Lancet Infect Dis. 2009 Feb;9(2):118–29. https://doi.org/10.1016/S1473-3099(09)70021-0.
22. Odoyo-June E, Rogers JH, Jaoko W, Bailey RC. Changes in plasma viral load and penile viral shedding after circumcision among HIV-positive men in Kisumu, Kenya. J Acquir Immune Defic Syndr. 2013;64(5):511–7. https://doi.org/10.1097/QAI.0b013e3182a7ef05.
23. Mehta SD, Green SJ, Maclean I, Hu H, Bailey RC, Gillevet PM, Spear GT. Microbial diversity of genital ulcer disease in men enrolled in a randomized trial of male circumcision in Kisumu, Kenya. PLoS One. 2012;7(7):e38991. https://doi.org/10.1371/journal.pone.0038991.
24. Sebire K, McGavin K, Land S, Middleton T, Birch C. Stability of human immunodeficiency virus RNA in blood specimens as measured by a commercial PCR-based assay. J Clin Microbiol. 1998;36(2):493–8.

13

Time to clearance of *Chlamydia trachomatis* RNA and DNA after treatment in patients coinfected with *Neisseria gonorrhoeae*

Carolien M. Wind[1,2], Maarten F. Schim van der Loeff[3,4], Magnus Unemo[5], Rob Schuurman[6], Alje P. van Dam[7,8] and Henry J. C. de Vries[1,2,4*]

Abstract

Background: Performing a test of cure (TOC) could demonstrate success or failure of antimicrobial treatment of *Chlamydia trachomatis* infection, but recommendations for the timing of a TOC using nucleic acid amplification tests (NAATs) are inconsistent. We assessed time to clearance of *C. trachomatis* after treatment, using modern RNA- and DNA-based NAATs.

Methods: We analysed data from patients with a *C. trachomatis* and *Neisseria gonorrhoeae* coinfection who visited the STI Clinic Amsterdam, The Netherlands, from March through October 2014. After treatment with ceftriaxone plus either azithromycin or doxycycline, patients self-collected anal, vaginal or urine samples during 28 consecutive days. Samples were analysed using an RNA-based NAAT (Aptima Combo 2) and a DNA-based NAAT (Cobas 4800 CT/NG). We defined clearance as three consecutive negative results, and defined "blips" as isolated positive results following clearance.

Results: We included 23 patients with *C. trachomatis* and *N. gonorrhoeae* coinfection. All patients cleared *C. trachomatis* during follow-up, and we observed no reinfections. The median time to clearance (range) was 7 days (1–13) for RNA, and 6 days (1–15) for DNA. Ninety-five per cent of patients cleared RNA at day 13, and DNA at day 14. The risk of a blip after clearance was 4.4 % (RNA) and 1.7 % (DNA).

Conclusions: If a TOC for anogenital chlamydia is indicated, we recommend performing it at least 14 days after initiation of treatment, when using modern RNA- and DNA-based assays. A positive result shortly after 14 days probably indicates a blip, rather than a treatment failure or a reinfection.

Keywords: *Chlamydia trachomatis*, *Neisseria gonorrhoeae*, Antimicrobial resistance, Nucleic acid amplification test, Test of cure

Background

Chlamydia trachomatis is the most common bacterial sexually transmitted infection (STI) globally, leading to late sequelae like pelvic inflammatory disease and infertility [1, 2]. Currently, the first-choice treatment for anogenital chlamydia consists of a single 1000 mg dose of azithromycin, or 100 mg doxycycline twice daily for 7 days [3, 4]. No resistance of *C. trachomatis* to either of these drugs has been reported, and a recent randomized controlled trial suggested no inferiority of azithromycin (97 % effective) compared to doxycycline (100 % effective) in urogenital chlamydia infections [5]. However, some studies voice concern about the efficacy of azithromycin as first-choice treatment for anorectal chlamydia [6–9]. Persisting *C. trachomatis* infections could be detected by performing a test of cure (TOC) after treatment. Current chlamydia treatment guidelines recommend a TOC between 3 and 4 weeks after initiation of treatment, in certain patient groups or when symptoms persist [4, 7, 10].

* Correspondence: h.j.devries@amc.uva.nl
[1]STI Outpatient Clinic, Department of Infectious Diseases, Public Health Service Amsterdam, PO Box 2200, 1000 CE Amsterdam, The Netherlands
[2]Department of Dermatology, Academic Medical Center, University of Amsterdam, Amsterdam, The Netherlands
Full list of author information is available at the end of the article

However, up to 90 % of chlamydia infections are asymptomatic, which could lead to persisting infections remaining undetected [4, 11, 12]. Previous reports on the appropriate timing of a TOC using molecular methods are inconsistent, and show (intermittent) persistence of *C. trachomatis* nucleic acids between 0 and 42 % up to 51 days after treatment [9, 13–19]. Recently, we performed a prospective cohort study on time to clearance for *N. gonorrhoeae*, using modern RNA- and DNA-based nucleic acid amplification tests (NAATs) [20]. Thirty-seven per cent of the included patients were also coinfected with *C. trachomatis*. As this study has results of 28 consecutive days for both RNA and DNA, we evaluated the appropriate timing of TOC for anogenital *C. trachomatis* infections in these coinfected patients.

Methods

Study population and procedure

In a previously performed cohort study we included patients with anogenital *N. gonorrhoeae* infection, who visited the STI Outpatient Clinic in Amsterdam, The Netherlands, from March through October 2014 [20]. We collected follow-up data and samples for only one infected anatomical site. The Academic Medical Center Amsterdam medical ethics committee approved the original cohort study (NL45935.018.13), and all patients provided written informed consent. For the current analysis, only patients coinfected with *C. trachomatis* were included from the cohort.

All patients had received routine treatment for *N. gonorrhoeae* and *C. trachomatis* coinfection, consisting of a single intramuscular dose of 500 mg ceftriaxone, plus one oral dose of azithromycin 1000 mg in case of urogenital infection, or doxycycline 100 mg twice daily for at least 7 days in case of anorectal infection. Participants self-collected urine, anal or vaginal NAAT samples: one for RNA-based and one for DNA-based NAAT. Samples were collected pre-treatment and subsequently daily for 28 consecutive days after treatment. We requested participants to abstain from sexual contact or use condoms, refrain from vaginal or rectal douching and keep a study diary. At the end-of-study visit (within 35 days of inclusion) a nurse collected samples from the designated anatomical site for both NAATs.

NAAT testing for *C. trachomatis*

Samples for the RNA-based NAAT were tested using the Aptima Combo 2 assay for *C. trachomatis* and *N. gonorrhoeae* (Hologic, San Diego, California). Test sensitivity is 93–98 % and specificity is >99 % [21–23]. Equivocal results were retested using the Aptima CT assay (Hologic). We considered repeatedly equivocal results as positive and excluded samples with repeatedly invalid results.

Samples for DNA-based NAAT were tested using the Cobas 4800 CT/NG assay for *C. trachomatis* and *N. gonorrhoeae* (Roche, Basel, Switzerland), and reported as either negative or positive with corresponding cycle threshold (Ct) value. Test sensitivity is 87–97 % and specificity is >99 % [22–24]. Pre-treatment samples with discrepant RNA and DNA results were retested, using the Aptima CT assay (Hologic) for RNA samples, and the Abbott RealTime CT/NG assay (Abbott, Abbott Park, Illinois) for DNA samples.

Statistical analysis

The primary endpoint, clearance of *C. trachomatis* using RNA- or DNA-based NAAT, was defined as three or more consecutive negative results following a positive result. We allowed one missing sample between the last positive and the first negative result. Reinfection was defined as positive test results on three or more consecutive days after clearance; tests had to be positive for both RNA and DNA on at least 1 day. To analyse differences we compared patients grouped by anatomical site using Chi-square, Fisher's exact or Kruskal-Wallis testing. Time to clearance was analysed with Kaplan-Meier curves, log-rank testing and Cox regression analysis. If we could not determine the exact day of clearance due to missing samples, the patient was excluded from this analysis.

The secondary endpoint, intermittent presence of RNA or DNA ("blip"), was defined as a positive test following clearance, not due to reinfection. Only positive results after the three consecutive negative tests results, used to define clearance, were eligible as a blip. We used logistic regression with generalized estimated equation (GEE) models to identify characteristics associated with blips. All analyses were performed using Stata (version 13; StataCorp, College Station, Texas).

Results

Participants

Out of 462 patients with anogenital gonorrhoea diagnosed at our STI clinic from March through October 2014, 77 were included in the original cohort. Twenty-six patients (34 %) had a coinfection with *C. trachomatis* of whom three were lost to follow-up. The remaining 23 patients were included in the current analysis.

Baseline characteristics

We included nine women, all with endocervical infections, and 14 men, of whom seven had a urethral and seven a rectal infection; 71 % were men who have sex with men (MSM, Table 1). The median age was 24 years (interquartile range [IQR]: 20–35 years); women were

Table 1 Baseline characteristics of 23 patients with *Chlamydia trachomatis* and *Neisseria gonorrhoeae* coinfection at inclusion

Characteristics	Total N (%)[a]	Urethra N (%)[a]	Rectum N (%)[a]	Endocervix N (%)[a]	*P*
Total	23	7 (30.4)	7 (30.4)	9 (39.1)	
Gender					
Male	14 (60.9)	7 (100.0)	7 (100.0)	0 (0.0)	
Female	9 (39.1)	0 (0.0)	0 (0.0)	9 (100.0)	
Median age, in years (IQR)	24 (20–35)	29 (24–35)	40 (24–44)	20 (19–23)	0.003
Ethnicity					1.00
Dutch	11 (47.8)	3 (42.9)	4 (57.1)	4 (44.4)	
Non-Dutch	12 (52.2)	4 (57.1)	3 (42.9)	5 (55.6)	
Sexual risk group					
MSM	10 (43.5)	3 (42.9)	7 (100.0)	0 (0.0)	
Hetero male	4 (17.4)	4 (57.1)	0 (0.0)	0 (0.0)	
Female	9 (39.1)	0 (0.0)	0 (0.0)	9 (100.0)	
HIV positive	5 (21.7)	1 (14.3)	4 (57.1)	0 (0.0)	0.02
Using cART	4 (80.0)	0 (0.0)	4 (100.0)	-	0.20
CD_4^+ cell count (cells/mm^3)					1.00
350–499	1 (20.0)	0 (0.0)	1 (25.0)	-	
≥ 500	4 (80.0)	1 (100.0)	3 (75.0)	-	
Previous chlamydia episode	12 (52.2)	3 (42.9)	4 (57.1)	5 (55.6)	1.00
Chlamydia in preceding 6 months	3 (13.0)	0 (0.0)	1 (14.3)	2 (22.2)	0.75
Symptoms or signs at examination[b,c]	13 (56.5)	6 (85.7)	3 (42.9)	4 (44.4)	0.23
Median time to inclusion, days (IQR)	8 (0–12)	0 (0–0)	10 (7–13)	9 (8–12)	0.003
Treatment at inclusion[d]					0.001
Ceftriaxone + azithromycin	16 (69.6)	7 (100.0)	1 (14.3)	8 (88.9)	
Ceftriaxone + doxycycline	7 (30.4)	0 (0.0)	6 (85.7)	1 (11.1)	

IQR interquartile range, *MSM* men who have sex with men, *HIV* human immunodeficiency virus, *cART* combination antiretroviral therapy

[a]Unless otherwise indicated

[b]Symptoms included: discharge, itch, burning, frequent or painful urination, bleeding, abdominal pain, pain during sex, anal cramps or pain, and changed defecation

[c]Signs included: red urethra, discharge, bleeding, fragile mucosa, swelling or anal ulcerations

[d]1 patient was negative for *Chlamydia trachomatis* at the initial visit and therefore received ceftriaxone mono-therapy. The test at inclusion was positive and doxycycline was started 6 days after inclusion; therefore the start of the study for the *C. trachomatis* analysis in this patient was day 6, and the treatment was ceftriaxone + doxycycline

significantly younger (median 20 years) compared to men (median 32 years, $P < 0.001$). Five men (22 %) were HIV-positive, and four (80 %) were on antiretroviral therapy, of whom three had CD_4^+ cell counts of ≥500 cells/mm^3. A previous chlamydia infection was reported by 12 patients (52 %), and 13 (57 %) currently experienced symptoms. The median time between diagnosis and inclusion was 8 days (range 0–12). At inclusion 16 patients (70 %) received ceftriaxone with azithromycin, and seven (30 %) received ceftriaxone with doxycycline.

Behaviour after inclusion

The median number of collected samples was 28 (range 25–28, Table 2). Forty-eight per cent of patients missed at least one sample. Rectal or vaginal douching was reported by four of 16 patients with rectal or endocervical chlamydia (25 %). Sexual contact at some point during the 28 days of follow-up was reported by 12 patients (52 %), and condomless sex by five patients (22 %).

Clearance of *C. trachomatis* RNA and DNA

During the 28 days of follow-up all patients cleared *C. trachomatis* RNA, and none experienced a reinfection (Table 2). Because of missing samples in the days around clearance, we could not determine the exact day of clearance for two patients. The median time to clearance for the remaining 21 patients was 7 days (range 1–13), and 95 % of patients had cleared RNA at day 13 (Fig. 1a). One patient was post-hoc excluded from the DNA analysis because of a negative pre-treatment DNA result for *C. trachomatis*. All other patients cleared *C. trachomatis*

Table 2 Behaviour after inclusion and clearance of *Chlamydia trachomatis* based on RNA and DNA testing, by anatomical site

Characteristics	Total n (%)[a]	Urethra n (%)[a]	Rectum n (%)[a]	Endocervix n (%)[a]	*P*
Patients	23	7 (30.4)	7 (30.4)	9 (39.1)	
Behaviour after inclusion					
Median no. of samples collected (range)	28 (25–28)	28 (26–28)	28 (26–28)	27 (25–28)	0.01
Patients with missed samples	11 (47.8)	1 (14.3)	2 (28.6)	8 (88.9)	0.009
Median no. of missed samples (IQR)	1 (1–3)	2 (2–2)	1.5 (1–2)	1 (1–3)	0.86
Rectal/vaginal douching	4 (25.0)[g]	-	3 (42.9)	1 (11.1)	0.26
Sexual contact	12 (52.2)	3 (42.9)	4 (57.1)	5 (55.6)	1.00
Condomless sex	5 (21.7)	1 (14.3)	2 (28.6)	2 (22.2)	1.00
RNA clearance[b]					
Clearance during follow-up	23 (100.0)	7 (100.0)	7 (100.0)	9 (100.0)	
Day of clearance definable[c]	21 (91.3)	7 (100.0)	6 (85.7)	8 (88.9)	1.00
Median time to clearance, days (range)	7 (1–13)	5 (1–13)	6.5 (5–9)	8 (6–13)	0.20
Blips[d]					
Samples at risk for blip	411	140	126	145	
Number of blips	18	0	12	6	
Number of patients	8 (34.8)	0 (0.0)	3 (42.9)	5 (55.6)	0.09
Median time to first blip from being at risk, days (range)	1 (1–16)	-	1 (1–2)	4.5 (1–16)	0.61
DNA clearance[b,e]					
Clearance during follow-up	22 (100.0)	6 (100.0)	7 (100.0)	9 (100.0)	
Day of clearance definable[f]	21 (95.5)	6 (100.0)	7 (100.0)	8 (88.9)	
Median time to clearance, days (range)	6 (1–15)	6 (1–14)	5 (2–9)	7.5 (5–15)	0.08
Blips[f]					
Samples at risk for blip	403	117	138	144	
Number of blips	7	0	0	7	
Number of patients	5 (22.7)	0	0	5 (55.6)	0.01
Median time to first blip from being at risk, days (range)	3 (2–8)	-	-	3 (2–8)	
Mean Ct-value (range)	38.6 (35.3–41.7)	-	-	38.6 (35.3–41.7)	

RNA ribonucleic acid, *DNA* deoxyribonucleic acid; *IQR* inter-quartile range; *Ct* cycle threshold
[a]Unless otherwise indicated
[b]Based on a definition of 3 consecutive negative tests following a positive test
[c]For 2 patients the exact day of clearance could not be defined due to missing samples in the period of clearance
[d]Blip was defined as a positive test following clearance. Samples from all 23 patients were included; for those without an exact day of clearance due to missing samples, all samples after the first three consecutive negative results were considered at risk for blips
[e]One patient was excluded from this analysis because the sample at inclusion was negative for *Chlamydia trachomatis* DNA
[f]For 1 patient the exact day of clearance could not be defined due to missing samples in the period of clearance
[g]Rectal/vaginal douching was only reported on by the 16 patients with rectal/endocervical infection

DNA during follow-up, and there were no reinfections. We could not determine the exact day of clearance for one patient (Table 2). The median time to clearance of the 21 patients was 6 days (range 1–15), and 95 % of patients had cleared DNA at day 14 (Fig. 1b).

Because of the small sample size the power to detect associations with clearance is very limited. Cox regression analyses showed no significant associations with clearance, and Kaplan-Meier curves with log-rank testing showed no significant difference in clearance by anatomical site or treatment.

Blips after clearance of *C. trachomatis*

After clearance of RNA, eight patients experienced 18 blips (Table 2). After clearance of DNA, five patients experienced seven blips, of which three (all vaginal samples) coincided with RNA blips (Table 2). Among the patients with blips, sex after clearance was reported by five (RNA) and three (DNA) patients. We observed both RNA and DNA blips among vaginal samples, while we observed only RNA blips among rectal samples, and no blips among urine samples.

When analysing all samples after clearance (411 for RNA and 403 for DNA), the median number of days at

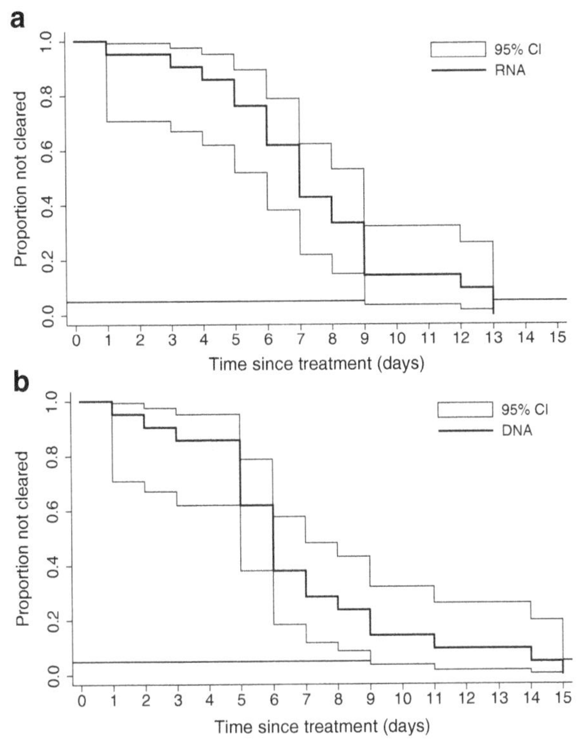

Fig. 1 Time to clearance of *Chlamydia trachomatis* RNA (**a**) and DNA (**b**). The horizontal line represents 95 % clearance. *RNA*, ribonucleic acid; *DNA*, deoxyribonucleic acid

risk per patient was 19 (range 12–25) for RNA, and 20 (range 11–25) for DNA. The overall risk of finding a blip after clearance was 4.4 % per day for RNA and 1.7 % per day for DNA. DNA blips had significantly higher Ct-values (mean: 38.6, range: 35.3–41.7) compared to pre-treatment samples (mean: 31.6, range: 27.8–39.3, $P < 0.001$). Only two RNA blips and two DNA blips were observed within 24 h of reported sex, of which one was a blip in both RNA and DNA testing (Fig. 2).

Although the sample size was relatively small, we determined characteristics associated with blips using GEE logistic regression. RNA blips were significantly associated with HIV-positivity (odds ratio [OR]: 8.0, 95 % confidence interval [95 %-CI]: 2.3–28.1, $P = 0.001$), a chlamydia infection in the previous 6 months (OR: 6.6, 95 %-CI: 1.8–24.7, $P = 0.005$), and with absence of symptoms or signs (OR: 0.17, 95 %-CI: 0.03–0.97, $P = 0.05$). In multivariable analysis, HIV-status and previous chlamydia infection remained significantly associated (OR: 7.1, 95 %-CI: 2.5–19.9, $P < 0.001$, and OR: 5.9, 95 %-CI: 2.2–16.3, $P = 0.001$, respectively). As there were seven DNA blips, the power for this analysis was limited; only sexual contact in the 24 h before sampling was significantly associated in univariable analysis (OR: 6.8, 95 %-CI: 1.3–36.7, $P = 0.03$).

Discussion

In this study we analysed the time to clearance of anogenital *C. trachomatis* after treatment in patients coinfected with *N. gonorrhoeae*, using modern RNA- and DNA-based NAATs and daily collected samples. The median time to clearance was 7 days for RNA and 6 days for DNA. Ninety-five per cent of patients had cleared *C. trachomatis* RNA and DNA after 13 and 14 days, respectively.

Several previous studies reported on in vivo clearance of *C. trachomatis* after treatment, but used different molecular testing methods, and a sampling frequency of no more than twice a week. Some studies observed clearance of DNA within 3 weeks using ligase chain reaction or in-house PCR methods [13, 14], while other studies reported 5–25 % DNA persistence after 3–4 weeks [9, 15, 16, 25]. The exact time to clearance of RNA, when tested by NAAT, was also previously unknown. Sena et al. reported 12 % RNA persistence after 4 weeks in men, while Dukers et al. reported 42 % intermittent positive results up to 51 days [9, 19]. In addition, a recent study reported 24 % positivity in 180 patients after 6 months, but no data on re-exposure or reinfections were reported [26]. Since none of these previous studies reported results from consecutive days, the exact time to clearance could not be determined, and prolonged persistence could not be distinguished from blips. In addition, none reported data on events that could have caused reinfection, like was done in the current study. Although no previous studies have been performed on the clearance of *C. trachomatis* in patients coinfected with *N. gonorrhoeae*, our results confirm the assumption that *C. trachomatis* RNA and DNA are cleared after 2 weeks [14, 17, 25].

Intermittent positive results or blips have been previously described by several studies; between 5 and 18 % of patients had a positive test result following a previous negative result after treatment [9, 14, 17–19]. We report an overall risk of blips after clearance of almost 2 % for DNA and 4 % for RNA, and no treatment failures or reinfections. The slightly higher sensitivity of the RNA test could explain the higher frequency of RNA blips, compared to DNA blips. The fact that all but one of the pretreatment samples initially diagnosed by RNA testing were also positive for DNA, makes it unlikely that the different sensitivity is of clinical importance in diagnosing chlamydia. On the other hand, when performing a TOC, higher sensitivity could result in more positive results. The implications of this should be clarified in larger studies. Unfortunately, NAAT testing only gives information about the presence of genetic material, but not on the viability of the pathogen or whether this is still infectious. Therefore blips could be the result of deposition of viable or non-viable genetic material by a

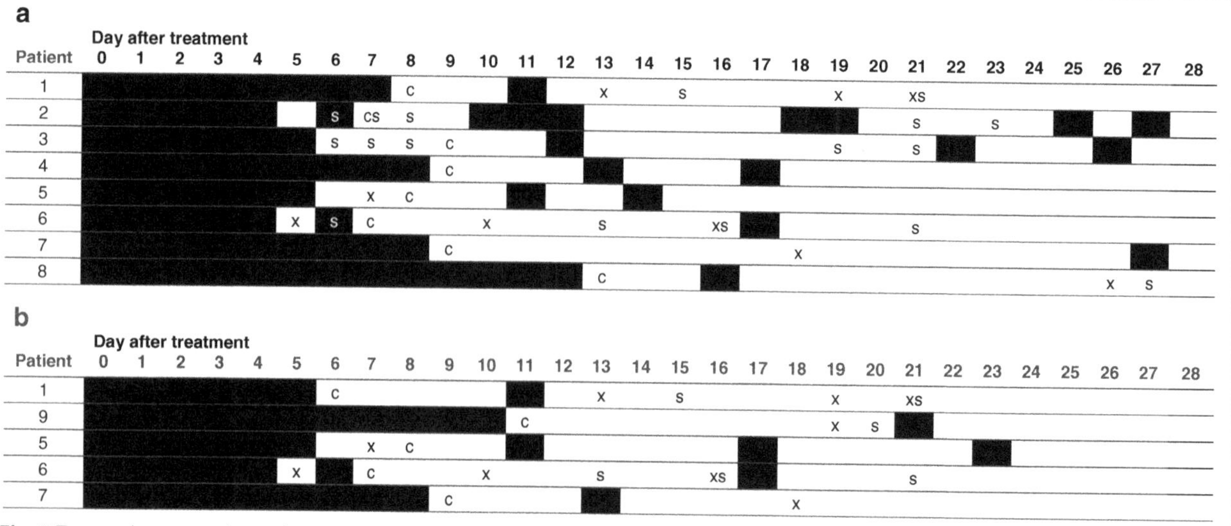

Fig. 2 Test results, reported sexual contact and blips of *Chlamydia trachomatis* RNA (**a**) or DNA (**b**) per day of follow-up after treatment in patients with blips. Black squares: positive for *C. trachomatis* (before clearance, or blip); white squares: negative for *C. trachomatis*; c: clearance; x: missing sample; s: sexual contact reported on this day (after sampling)

sexual partner, release of genetic material by degrading cells, or possibly the presence of elementary bodies that hold genetic components of *C. trachomatis* [18, 27]. The origin of blips needs to be further examined in future research. Due to the small sample size we could not identify characteristics associated with the occurrence of blips. However, the occurrence of blips, as well as reinfections, could explain the higher positivity rates reported by some studies, especially in those with very long follow-up and limited sampling [9, 15, 18, 19, 26].

Our study has several limitations. It was performed at a single centre in a high-incidence population, which may limit the generalizability. We selected patients from a cohort infected with *N. gonorrhoeae*, so this concerns a population coinfected with *N. gonorrhoeae* and *C. trachomatis*, which may influence both time to clearance and the occurrence of blips. Because all patients were coinfected with *N. gonorrhoeae*, they were also treated with ceftriaxone. Since ceftriaxone is not effective against chlamydia, it is unlikely that treatment with ceftriaxone influenced the clearance of *C. trachomatis*. Nevertheless, confirmation of our results in chlamydia monoinfected patients is warranted.

Conclusions

Our results are the first to show that *C. trachomatis* RNA and DNA are cleared within 14 days of initiating treatment, using daily testing. Despite the small sample size, our results suggest that if a TOC is indicated in patients with *C. trachomatis* and *N. gonorrhoeae* coinfection, it is best performed after at least 2 weeks. Positive results obtained more than 2 weeks after initiation of treatment should be evaluated carefully, as these probably represent blips, and do not necessarily indicate treatment failure or reinfection. To exclude blips as the cause of a positive TOC, we recommend to obtain a new sample for retesting.

Abbreviations

95 %-CI: 95 % confidence interval; DNA: Deoxyribonucleic acid; GEE: Generalized estimated equation; HIV: Human immunodeficiency virus; IQR: Interquartile range; MSM: Men who have sex with men; NAAT: Nucleic acid amplification test; OR: Odds ratio; PCR: Polymerase chain reaction; RNA: Ribonucleic acid; STI: Sexually transmitted infection; TOC: Test of cure;

Acknowledgments

We thank all participants of the cohort for their effort. We also thank Myra van Leeuwen, Claudia Owusu and Princella Felipa for their assistance in recruiting the participants. We thank Fred Zethof for performing the Aptima Combo 2 assays, Davy Janssen for performing the Cobas 4800 assays and Paul Smits for performing the Abbott NG/CT assays.

Funding

This study was funded by the Public Health Service Amsterdam.

Authors' contributions

CMW, MFSL, MU, APD and HJCV designed the study. CMW coordinated the study implementation, included patients and collected samples. APD and RS supervised the laboratory testing. CMW analysed the data. MFSL provided statistical advice for the data analysis. All authors interpreted the data. CMW wrote the first draft of the manuscript. All authors critically reviewed the manuscript and approved the final version.

Competing interests

Hologic provided Aptima test materials and kits in kind. Roche provided Cobas test materials and kits in kind.

Consent for publication

Not applicable.

Author details
[1]STI Outpatient Clinic, Department of Infectious Diseases, Public Health Service Amsterdam, PO Box 2200, 1000 CE Amsterdam, The Netherlands. [2]Department of Dermatology, Academic Medical Center, University of Amsterdam, Amsterdam, The Netherlands. [3]Department of Infectious Diseases, Public Health Service Amsterdam, PO Box 22001000 CE Amsterdam, The Netherlands. [4]Center for Infection and Immunity Amsterdam, Academic Medical Center, University of Amsterdam, Amsterdam, The Netherlands. [5]WHO Collaborating Centre for Gonorrhoea and Other STIs, National Reference Laboratory for Pathogenic Neisseria, Department of Laboratory Medicine, Microbiology, Örebro University, SE-701 85 Örebro, Sweden. [6]Department of Medical Microbiology, University Medical Centre Utrecht, PO Box 855003508 GA Utrecht, The Netherlands. [7]Public Health Laboratory, Public Health Service Amsterdam, Amsterdam, The Netherlands. [8]Department of Medical Microbiology, Onze Lieve Vrouwe Gasthuis General Hospital, Amsterdam, The Netherlands.

References

1. Newman L, Rowley J, Vander Hoorn S, Wijesooriya NS, Unemo M, Low N, et al. Global estimates of the prevalence and incidence of four curable sexually transmitted infections in 2012 based on systematic review and global reporting. PLoS One. 2015;10:e0143304.
2. European Centre for Disease Prevention and Control. Annual Epidemiological Report 2014 - Sexually Transmitted Infections, Including HIV and Blood-Borne Viruses. Stockholm: ECDC; 2015.
3. Centers for Disease Control and Prevention. Sexually transmitted diseases treatment guidelines 2015. MMWR Recomm Rep. 2015;64(No. RR-3):1–137.
4. Lanjouw E, Ouburg S, de Vries HJ, Stary A, Radcliffe K, Unemo M. 2015 European guideline on the management of *Chlamydia trachomatis* infections. Int J STD AIDS Published (Online first) 24 november 2015. doi: 10. 1177/0956462415618837.
5. Geisler WM, Uniyal A, Lee JY, Lensing SY, Johnson S, Perry RC, et al. Azithromycin versus Doxycycline for Urogenital *Chlamydia trachomatis* Infection. N Engl J Med. 2015;373:2512–21.
6. Hocking JS, Kong FY, Timms P, Huston WM, Tabrizi SN. Treatment of rectal chlamydia infection may be more complicated than we originally thought. J Antimicrob Chemother. 2015;70:961–4.
7. Horner PJ. Azithromycin antimicrobial resistance and genital *Chlamydia trachomatis* infection: duration of therapy may be the key to improving efficacy. Sex Transm Infect. 2012;88:154–6.
8. Kong FY, Hocking JS. Treatment challenges for urogenital and anorectal *Chlamydia trachomatis*. BMC Infect Dis. 2015;15:293.
9. Dukers-Muijrers NH, Morre SA, Speksnijder A, van der Sande MA, Hoebe CJ. *Chlamydia trachomatis* test-of-cure cannot be based on a single highly sensitive laboratory test taken at least 3 weeks after treatment. PLoS One. 2012;7, e34108.
10. Geisler WM. Diagnosis and Management of Uncomplicated *Chlamydia trachomatis* Infections in Adolescents and Adults: Summary of Evidence Reviewed for the 2015 Centers for Disease Control and Prevention Sexually Transmitted Diseases Treatment Guidelines. Clin Infect Dis. 2015;61 Suppl 8: S774–84.
11. Rebe K, Lewis D, Myer L, de Swardt G, Struthers H, Kamkuemah M, et al. A cross sectional analysis of Gonococcal and chlamydial infections among Men-Who-have-Sex-with-Men in Cape Town, South Africa. PLoS One. 2015; 10:e0138315.
12. Tongtoyai J, Todd CS, Chonwattana W, Pattanasin S, Chaikummao S, Varangrat A, et al. Prevalence and correlates of *chlamydia trachomatis* and *Neisseria gonorrhoeae* by anatomic site among urban Thai Men Who have Sex with Men. Sex Transm Dis. 2015;42:440–9.
13. Claas HC, Wagenvoort JH, Niesters HG, Tio TT, Van Rijsoort-Vos JH, Quint WG. Diagnostic value of the polymerase chain reaction for Chlamydia detection as determined in a follow-up study. J Clin Microbiol. 1991;29:42–5.
14. Gaydos CA, Crotchfelt KA, Howell MR, Kralian S, Hauptman P, Quinn TC. Molecular amplification assays to detect chlamydial infections in urine specimens from high school female students and to monitor the persistence of chlamydial DNA after therapy. J Infect Dis. 1998;177:417–24.
15. Morre SA, Sillekens PT, Jacobs MV, de Blok S, Ossewaarde JM, van Aarle P, et al. Monitoring of *Chlamydia trachomatis* infections after antibiotic treatment using RNA detection by nucleic acid sequence based amplification. Mol Pathol. 1998;51:149–54.
16. Whittington WL, Kent C, Kissinger P, Oh MK, Fortenberry JD, Hillis SE, et al. Determinants of persistent and recurrent *Chlamydia trachomatis* infection in young women: results of a multicenter cohort study. Sex Transm Dis. 2001; 28:117–23.
17. Jang D, Sellors J, Howard M, Mahony J, Frost E, Patrick D, et al. Correlation between culture testing of swabs and ligase chain reaction of first void urine from patients recently treated for *Chlamydia trachomatis*. Sex Transm Infect. 2003;79:237–9.
18. Renault CA, Israelski DM, Levy V, Fujikawa BK, Kellogg TA, Klausner JD. Time to clearance of *Chlamydia trachomatis* ribosomal RNA in women treated for chlamydial infection. Sex Health. 2011;8:69–73.
19. Sena AC, Lensing S, Rompalo A, Taylor SN, Martin DH, Lopez LM, et al. *Chlamydia trachomatis*, *Mycoplasma genitalium*, and *Trichomonas vaginalis* infections in men with nongonococcal urethritis: predictors and persistence after therapy. J Infect Dis. 2012;206:357–65.
20. Wind CM, Schim van der Loeff MF, Unemo M, Schuurman R, van Dam AP, de Vries HJC. Test of cure for anogenital gonorrhoea using modern RNA-based and DNA-based nucleic acid amplification tests - a prospective cohort study. Clin Infect Dis. 2016;62:1348-55.
21. Schachter J, Moncada J, Liska S, Shayevich C, Klausner JD. Nucleic acid amplification tests in the diagnosis of chlamydial and gonococcal infections of the oropharynx and rectum in men who have sex with men. Sex Transm Dis. 2008;35:637–42.
22. Van Der Pol B, Liesenfeld O, Williams JA, Taylor SN, Lillis RA, Body BA, et al. Performance of the cobas CT/NG test compared to the Aptima AC2 and Viper CTQ/GCQ assays for detection of *Chlamydia trachomatis* and *Neisseria gonorrhoeae*. J Clin Microbiol. 2012;50:2244–9.
23. Taylor SN, Liesenfeld O, Lillis RA, Body BA, Nye M, Williams J, et al. Evaluation of the Roche cobas(R) CT/NG test for detection of *Chlamydia trachomatis* and *Neisseria gonorrhoeae* in male urine. Sex Transm Dis. 2012; 39:543–9.
24. Geelen TH, Rossen JW, Beerens AM, Poort L, Morre SA, Ritmeester WS, et al. Performance of cobas(R) 4800 and m2000 real-time assays for detection of *Chlamydia trachomatis* and *Neisseria gonorrhoeae* in rectal and self-collected vaginal specimen. Diagn Microbiol Infect Dis. 2013;77:101–5.
25. Hillis SD, Coles FB, Litchfield B, Black CM, Mojica B, Schmitt K, et al. Doxycycline and azithromycin for prevention of chlamydial persistence or recurrence one month after treatment in women. A use-effectiveness study in public health settings. Sex Transm Dis. 1998;25:5–11.
26. Kapil R, Press CG, Hwang ML, Brown L, Geisler WM. Investigating the epidemiology of repeat *Chlamydia trachomatis* detection after treatment by using *C. trachomatis OmpA* genotyping. J Clin Microbiol. 2015;53:546–9.
27. Bragina EY, Gomberg MA, Dmitriev GA. Electron microscopic evidence of persistent chlamydial infection following treatment. J Eur Acad Dermatol Venereol. 2001;15:405–9.

14

A novel point-of-care testing strategy for sexually transmitted infections among pregnant women in high-burden settings

Steven G. Badman[1*], Lisa M. Vallely[1], Pamela Toliman[2], Grace Kariwiga[3], Bomesina Lote[4], William Pomat[2], Caroline Holmer[5], Rebecca Guy[1], Stanley Luchters[6,7], Chris Morgan[6], Suzanne M. Garland[8,9], Sepehr Tabrizi[8], David Whiley[10], Stephen J. Rogerson[11], Glen Mola[12], Handan Wand[1], Basil Donovan[1,13], Louise Causer[1], John Kaldor[1] and Andrew Vallely[1]

Abstract

Background: Sexually transmitted and genital infections in pregnancy are associated with an increased risk of adverse maternal and neonatal health outcomes. High prevalences of sexually transmitted infections have been identified among antenatal attenders in Papua New Guinea. Papua New Guinea has amongst the highest neonatal mortality rates worldwide, with preterm birth and low birth weight major contributors to neonatal mortality. The overall aim of our study was to determine if a novel point-of-care testing and treatment strategy for the sexually transmitted and genital infections *Chlamydia trachomatis* (CT), *Neisseria gonorrhoeae* (NG), *Trichomonas vaginalis* (TV) and Bacterial vaginosis (BV) in pregnancy is feasible in the high-burden, low-income setting of Papua New Guinea.

Methods: Women attending their first antenatal clinic visit were invited to participate. CT/NG and TV were tested using the GeneXpert platform (Cepheid, USA), and BV tested using BVBlue (Gryphus Diagnostics, USA). Participants received same-day test results and antibiotic treatment as indicated. Routine antenatal care including HIV and syphilis screening were provided.

Results: Point-of-care testing was provided to 125/222 (56 %) of women attending routine antenatal care during the three-month study period. Among the 125 women enrolled, the prevalence of CT was 20.0 %; NG, 11.2 %; TV, 37.6 %; and BV, 17.6 %. Over half (67/125, 53.6 %) of women had one or more of these infections. Most women were asymptomatic (71.6 %; 47/67). Women aged 24 years and under were more likely to have one or more STI compared with older women (odds ratio 2.38; 95 % CI: 1.09, 5.21). Most women with an STI received treatment on the same day (83.6 %; 56/67). HIV prevalence was 1.6 % and active syphilis 4.0 %.

Conclusion: Point-of-care STI testing and treatment using a combination of novel, newly-available assays was feasible during routine antenatal care in this setting. This strategy has not previously been evaluated in any setting and offers the potential to transform STI management in pregnancy and to prevent their associated adverse health outcomes.

Keywords: Antenatal, Pregnancy outcome, Molecular testing, Syndromic management, Low-middle-income country, Genexpert, Point-of-care, STIs

* Correspondence: sbadman@kirby.unsw.edu.au
[1]The Kirby Institute, University of New South Wales, Sydney, Australia
Full list of author information is available at the end of the article

Background

Previous studies among antenatal women in low-resource settings have found high prevalences of sexually transmitted and genital infections, particularly *Chlamydia trachomatis* (CT), *Neisseria gonorrhoeae* (NG), *Trichomonas vaginalis* (TV) and Bacterial vaginosis (BV), that are readily curable with cheap antibiotics [1]. Untreated, these bacteria are associated with an increased risk of preterm birth, low birth weight, premature rupture of membranes and other adverse maternal and neonatal health outcomes [1].

Papua New Guinea (PNG) has among the highest neonatal mortality rates worldwide, with an estimated 23 neonatal deaths per 1,000 livebirths [2]. Preterm birth and low birth weight are major contributors to neonatal mortality; in PNG an estimated 16 % of all infants are of low birth weight [3]. In addition, an estimated 15 infants per 1,000 births are stillborn [4]. Preliminary results from the country's first bio-behavioural survey of STIs in pregnancy ($n = 765$) identified high prevalences of CT (23.1 %), NG (13.8 %), and TV (24.1 %) [5]. Overall, 44 % of pregnant women had at least one of these infections [5]. Around 80 % of women with laboratory-confirmed CT, NG or TV were asymptomatic and therefore would not have been detected and treated using national STI syndromic management guidelines that are based on clinical criteria alone, consistent with WHO recommendations for routine care in low-income settings [6, 7].

The lack of affordable, timely, easy-to-use and accurate STI tests that can be used at point-of-care has meant that for the last two decades routine practice in many low and middle-income countries (LMIC) has been based on syndromic management. Recent advances in STI diagnostics however may herald a new era in STI diagnosis and management in such settings, although this as yet is untested in a LMIC setting such as PNG.

The GeneXpert platform (Cepheid, Sunnyvale CA, USA) provides fully automated, easy-to-use point-of-care molecular tests for CT, NG and TV that are as accurate as laboratory-based nucleic acid amplification tests (NAATs) [8]. This robust and portable platform has already revolutionized the diagnosis and management of tuberculosis in a number of LMIC [9] and is now being used in PNG. Disposable single-use cartridges hold the reagents for the simultaneous detection of CT and NG, with a separate cartridge used for TV detection. Test results are available in 90 (CT/NG) and 60 (TV) minutes, allowing for immediate management.

The platform requires specific training in test procedures, some infrastructure including reliable electrical power or a backup generator, as well as modifications to service provision and patient flow to allow for immediate treatment and contact tracing.

The diagnosis of BV has until recently relied on skilled microscopic examination and scoring of Gram stained vaginal smears using Nugent or Amsel scores. The BVBlue test (OSOM BVBlue Test, Gryphus Diagnostics, USA) is a recently developed chromogenic test for the diagnosis of BV that detects increased vaginal fluid sialidase activity in 10 min. It is the first robust point-of-care test available for BV and has a sensitivity of 90 % and specificity of 95 % compared to Nugent or Amsel scoring [10].

In this paper we present findings from the first feasibility study of antenatal point-of-care testing and treatment of CT, NG, TV and BV using a combination of GeneXpert CT/NG, TV and the BVBlue Test, provided in a routine antenatal clinic setting. This research was conducted in preparation for a large-scale field trial to evaluate this same strategy to improve pregnancy outcomes in PNG and other high-burden, LMIC settings.

Methods

Study design and procedures

A descriptive feasibility study was undertaken at a government-run urban antenatal clinic in Alotau, Milne Bay Province, PNG, between August and December 2014. All nursing staff at the clinic (Nursing Officers, Midwives and Community Health Workers) were trained in all aspects of the study, including the point-of-care testing.

Women aged 18 years or over and attending their first antenatal visit were invited to participate. Following written informed consent, women were enrolled consecutively and assigned a unique alphanumeric study identity (ID) number. Nursing staff conducted a short face-to-face interview with each participant, during which socio-demographic and sexual behaviour data were collected.

Women received routine antenatal and provider-initiated HIV and syphilis screening, and haemoglobin estimation. HIV testing was conducted using HIV rapid tests at point-of-care (Alere Determine HIV-1/2; followed by confirmatory Chembio Stat-Pak HIV-1/2), as per national guidelines. Syphilis testing used a rapid point-of-care screening test (SD Bioline anti-TP 3.0, Alere, Germany) followed by a confirmatory laboratory-based rapid plasma reagin (RPR) test. Women with a positive anti-TP plus a reactive RPR (any titre) test were considered to have active syphilis.

Following instructions from the nursing staff, participants provided two self-collected, mid-cavity, vaginal swabs for on-site testing: CT/NG and TV using the GeneXpert platform; and BV using the BVBlue rapid test assay. Testing was conducted by nursing staff supported by the in-country investigator team. Women diagnosed with any of these four infections were offered same-day antibiotic treatment in accordance with PNG STI management guidelines; risk-reduction counselling, and contact tracing was provided as necessary.

Data management and statistical methods

Study-specific case record forms (CRFs) were used to record socio-demographic, sexual behaviour, obstetric and clinical information. STI test results were automatically recorded in the GeneXpert laptop database by participant study ID number and were similarly recorded in a paper-based laboratory test log. CRF data were entered by study ID into a study-specific database without personal identifiers. Each day, all CRFs and test result log entries were reviewed for completion and consistency by the lead investigators. Clinical and STI test result data were entered into a study-specific Excel database and all electronic database entries validated against participant study folders for accuracy.

Data were summarised as frequencies and percentages. Fisher's exact test was used to compare statistical differences in outcomes of interest between younger and older women (e.g. STI prevalences). Data were analysed using Stata IC v14.0 (StataCorp LP, Texas, USA). Due to the modest sample size, it was not possible to conduct multivariate analysis to examine independent risk factors.

Results

Clinic staff were able to conduct point-of-care testing with minimal supervision after one day of intensive training. Interest in the study was high with nearly women who attended antenatal clinic requesting to participate. Due to a clinic schedule that allocates one weekday to new antenatal attendances (resulting in 20–25 new visits on a single day); the availability of limited testing facilities (one single, four-module GeneXpert machine) and the requirement to provide same-day test results, we were unfortunately unable to enrol all those who asked to join. As such, 125 of the 222 (56 %) who attended the clinic were enrolled. Given these limitations women were enrolled as they presented to clinic, i.e. on a first come, first served basis and were not selected in any way by clinic staff or the research team. The integration of study procedures into routine antenatal clinic activities resulted in an average of two hours additional waiting time per woman.

Among the 125 women recruited, the median age was 24 years; around 75 % (81/107) of women attended in the first or second trimester of pregnancy; and almost half were primigravid (59/125; 47 %; Table 1).

Province of birth was considered significant so as to identify what proportion of women had been born in the study province (Milne Bay) and what proportion were not, in order to look at differences in STI prevalence among these groups. 'Other province' includes all other provinces in PNG (there are 22 in total). Due to small numbers for each individual province we aggregated these and present this as 'Other province' rather than individual provinces.

Six women (6/125; 5 %) had a previous history of miscarriage, stillbirth or neonatal death. Based on point-of-care test results, more than half of women (67/125; 53.6 %) had any of CT, NG, TV or BV, among whom 71.6 % (48/67) were asymptomatic. Overall, the prevalence of CT was 20.0 %; NG, 11.2 %; TV, 37.6 %; and BV, 17.6 %. The prevalence of HIV was 1.6 %, and 4.0 % of the women had active syphilis. Women aged 24 years or under were significantly more likely to have any of CT, NG, TV or BV, compared with older women (63.6 % vs. 42.4 %; odds ratio [OR] 2.38, 95 % confidence interval [CI]: 1.09, 5.21). Younger women with genital symptoms were six times more likely to have an infection compared with older women who had genital symptoms (25.8 % vs. 5.1 %; OR 6.48, 95 % CI: 1.70, 36.0). There were no significant differences between younger and older women in sexual behavioural characteristics, past history of an STI, or current genital symptoms. Among the 67 women who had one or more of CT, NG, TV or BV, there were no significant differences in sexual behavioural characteristics between younger and older women.

Among the 34 women who reported genital symptoms at enrolment, around half (19/34; 55.9 %) had any of CT, NG, TV or BV. Among the six women who reported a previous adverse pregnancy outcome, four had a history of stillbirth, of whom two had TV, and one had CT, TV and BV in the current study. All women received their test results the same day. Of those with any STI or genital infection, 83.6 % (56/67) received same-day treatment.

The remaining 12.4 % (11/67) had to leave prior to receiving treatment due to family commitments or the need to travel significant distances back to their homes by foot or by bus. All women had received treatment within one week. Partners in attendance at the clinic were treated the same day. All women and their partners diagnosed with an infection received treatment in accordance with PNG national guidelines [11]. Given the resource limitations of this study, test of cure follow-up was not possible. It will however be a part of future large scale antenatal trials.

Discussion

Antenatal point-of-care STI testing and treatment using a combination of novel, newly-available diagnostic tests proved feasible when integrated as part of routine antenatal care in this setting. This is the first study in any setting to evaluate the feasibility of this approach. The

Table 1 Socio-demographic characteristics, sexual behaviour, obstetric history, genital symptoms and point-of-care test results

		Total *N* (%)	≤24 years *N* = 66 (%)	≥25 years *N* = 59 (%)	*p* value
Socio-demographic characteristics					
Age, median (IQR:18-41years)		24 years	21 years	30 years	
Province of birth	Milne Bay Province	100 (80.0)	54 (81.8)	46 (78.0)	
	Other province	25 (20.0)	12 (18.2)	13 (22.0)	
Marital Status	Married	108 (86)	51 (77.3)	57 (96.6)	
	Single	17 (13.6)	15 (22.7)	2 (3.4)	$p = 0.002$
Level of education (*N* = 124)	Never attended school	4 (3.2)	0 (0)	4 (6.7)	$p = 0.032$
	Only primary school	39 (31.2)	18 (27.3)	21 (35.6)	
	Secondary school	81 (65.3)	47 (71.2)	34 (57.6)	
	Tertiary education	24 (19.2)	9 (13.6)	15 (25.4)	
Obstetric history					
Parity (*N* = 124)	Primigravid	59 (47.6)	48 (72.8)	11 (18.6)	
	Para 1–3	46 (37.0)	17 (25.8)	29 (49.2)	$p < 0.0001$
	Para 4 or more	19 (15.3)	0 (0.0)	19 (32.2)	$p = 0.008$
Previous miscarriage/stillbirth/perinatal/neonatal death (*N* = 125)		6 (4.8)	3 (4.5)	3 (5.1)	
Estimated gestational age at enrolment based on LMP (*N* = 107)	12 weeks or less	13 (11.2)	5 (7.6)	8 (13.6)	
	13–26 weeks	68 (63.5)	38 (57.6)	30 (50.1)	
	27–36 weeks	24 (22.4)	9 (13.7)	15 (25.4)	
	More than 36 weeks	2 (1.9)	1 (1.5)	1 (1.7)	
Sexual behaviour					
Age at sexual debut, median (IQR: 13–31years)		19 years	18 years	20 years	
Lifetime number of sexual partners (*N* = 119)	1 partner	37 (31.1)	20 (30.3)	17 (28.8)	
	2–3 partners	51 (42.9)	29 (43.9)	22 (37.2)	
	4–6 partners	21 (17.6)	11 (16.6)	10 (16.9)	
	7 or more partners	10 (8.4)	4 (6.1)	6 (10.2)	
Sexual partners in previous month (*N* = 124)	0	31 (25.0)	18 (27.3)	13 (22.0)	
	1	80 (64.5)	41 (62.1)	39 (66.1)	
	2 or more partners	13 (10.5)	6 (9.1)	7 (11.9)	
Number of times had vaginal sex in the last month (*N* = 122)	0	36 (29.5)	22 (33.3)	14 (23.7)	
	1–2 times	28 (23.0)	11 (16.7)	17 (28.8)	
	3 times or more	32 (26.2)	17 (25.6)	15 (25.4)	
	More than once/unknown	26 (21.3)	15 (22.7)	11 (18.6)	
Condom use last sex (N = 124)	Yes	29 (23.4)	12 (18.2)	17 (28.8)	
	No	95 (76.6)	54 (81.8)	41 (69.5)	
Ever had sex for gifts/favours/money		31 (24.8)	16 (24.2)	15 (25.4)	
Reported genital symptoms at enrolment					
Previous STI/genital infection		28 (22.4)	15 (22.8)	13 (22.0)	
Current genital symptoms	Any symptom	34 (27.2)	20 (30.3)	14 (23.7)	
	Vaginal discharge[a]	24 (19.2)	16 (24.2)	8 (13.6)	
	Genital sores	1 (0.8)	1 (1.5)	0 (0.0)	
	Abdominal pain[a]	8 (6.4)	4 (6.1)	4 (6.8)	
	Itching[a]	19 (15.2)	10 (15.1)	9 (15.3)	

Table 1 Socio-demographic characteristics, sexual behaviour, obstetric history, genital symptoms and point-of-care test results *(Continued)*

	Other symptoms[b]	6 (4.8)	4 (6.1)	2 (3.4)	
STI test results					
	Any STI	67 (53.6)	42 (63.6)	25 (42.4)	$p = 0.017$
	1 STI	39 (31.2)	22 (33.3)	17 (28.8)	
	2 or more STIs	28 (22.4)	20 (30.3)	8 (13.6)	$p = 0.025$
	HIV	2 (1.6)	2 (3.0)	0 (0.0)	
	Active syphilis[c]	5 (4.0)	3 (4.5)	2 (3,4)	
	C. trachomatis (CT)	25 (20)	18 (27.3)	7 (11.9)	$p = 0.032$
	N. gonorrhoeae (NG)	14 (11)	12 (18.2)	2 (3.4)	$p = 0.009$
	T. vaginalis (TV)	47 (37.6)	31 (47.0)	16 (27.1)	$p = 0.022$
	Bacterial vaginosis (BV)	22 (17.6)	11 (16.7)	11 (18.7)	
	Genital symptoms and 1 or more STI detected	19 (15.2)	16 (24.3)	3 (5.1)	$p = 0.002$
	Genital symptoms but no STI detected	15 (12.0)	4 (6.1)	11 (18.6)	$p = 0.031$

[a]14 women had multiple symptoms/[b] discharge, pus, "wetness"/[c]anti-TP+ and RPR+, all titres

high interest shown in study participation and 100 % completion of study procedures among those enrolled suggest the intervention has a high level of acceptability, but needs to be formally established. An important limitation was our inability to meet antenatal testing demand: we were only able to recruit around 56 % of those who attended yet nearly all women expressed an interest in joining the study. Future intervention studies and demonstration projects should consider setting up more than one four-module GeneXpert machine per clinic in situations of high workload.

High prevalences of STIs and genital infections were observed among pregnant women in this setting, particularly those aged 24 years or under. These findings are consistent with our earlier research among antenatal women in PNG [12, 13]. A minority of women (34/125; 27.2 %) in the current study reported genital symptoms at enrolment, of whom around half had CT, NG, TV or BV; whilst more than 70 % of women with one or more of these curable infections were asymptomatic. These findings suggest that STI syndromic management, based on clinical presentation alone, is a poor strategy for the detection and treatment of STIs among pregnant women in this setting and underline the need for robust, easy-to-use, timely, and accurate point-of-care tests.

In this pilot study, the cost-effectiveness of this new and broad based POC testing approach was not examined in detail. A cluster randomised trial of antenatal point-of-care testing and treatment to improve pregnancy outcomes is due to start in PNG in 2016 [13]. This trial will establish the efficacy, acceptability, cost-effectiveness and health system requirements of the proposed test and treat strategy, and will inform future international policy and practice on the diagnosis and management of STIs in pregnancy.

Conclusions

With increased Genexpert device availability this integrated point of care testing strategy has the potential to change the way STI's in pregnancy are managed and reduce the number of associated adverse health outcomes for antenatal women in Papua New Guinea.

Abbreviations

BV, Bacterial vaginosis; CT, Chlamydia trachomatis; CRF, Case record form; HIV, Human Immunodeficiency Virus; LMIC, Low middle income country; NAAT, Nucleic acid amplification test; NHMRC, National Health and Medical Research Council; NG, Neisseria gonorrhoeae; PNG, Papua New Guinea; POC, Point of care; RPR, Rapid plasma reagin; STI, Sexually transmitted infection; TV, Trichomonas vaginalis; WHO, World Health Organisation

Acknowledgments

We are extremely grateful to all the women who took part in this research and to their families and communities for supporting this project. We would especially like to thank the clinic staff involved in this work, without whom this study would not have been possible: Ester Gibson, Rose Joshua, Jane Raurela, Hadassha Dugutara, Leanne Raurela, Janet Adrian, Hilda Henry, Noreen Tabua, Faith Malesa, Catherine Wallace, Amos Giarua, Angela Kamnanaya and Jenny Poela. We also acknowledge the invaluable support and guidance provided by the Milne Bay Provincial Health Authority and Alotau General Hospital, in particular: Billy Naidi, Dr Jacob Morewaya and Dr Noel Yaubihi.

Funding

This study was funded under a Program Grant from the National Health and Medical Research Council, Australia.

Authors' contributions

SB, AV, LV and PT were the primary investigator team and provided point-of-care training and supervision of this research over the duration of the study. GK, WP, GM provided provincial and national level assistance in the formation of this study and liaison with key in-country stakeholders. SL, CM, SG, SR, BD, LC, RG, CH and JK provided guidance with the study design and related technical issues. BL is the senior clinic manager and provided direction to clinic staff, supporting the integration of POC testing into the clinic workflow.

DW and ST advised on laboratory techniques. HW supported the statistical analysis of data. All authors reviewed and approved the final manuscript.

Competing interests
The authors declare that they have no competing interests.

Consent for publication
Not applicable.

Author details
[1]The Kirby Institute, University of New South Wales, Sydney, Australia. [2]Papua New Guinea Institute of Medical Research, Goroka, Papua New Guinea. [3]Department of Obstetrics & Gynaecology, Alotau General Hospital, Milne Bay Province, Alotau, Papua New Guinea. [4]Alotau Urban Clinic, Alotau, Milne Bay Province, Papua New Guinea. [5]University of Technology, Sydney, Australia. [6]The Burnet Institute, Melbourne, Australia. [7]Melbourne School of Population and Global Health, University of Melbourne, Melbourne, VIC, Australia. [8]Department of Microbiology and Infectious Diseases, The Royal Women's Hospital, Parkville, VIC, Australia. [9]Department of Obstetrics and Gynaecology, University of Melbourne, Murdoch Children's Research Institute, Parkville, VIC, Australia. [10]University of Queensland, Herston, QLD, Australia. [11]Department of Medicine, University of Melbourne, Melbourne, Australia. [12]Department of Obstetrics & Gynaecology, School of Medicine and Health Sciences, University of Papua New Guinea, National Capital District, Papua New Guinea. [13]Sydney Sexual Health Centre, Sydney, Australia.

References
1. Mullick S, Watson-Jones D, Beksinska M, Mabey D. Sexually transmitted infections in pregnancy: prevalence, impact on pregnancy outcomes, and approach to treatment in developing countries. Sex Transm Infect. 2005;81: 294–302.
2. UNICEF, WHO, Bank W, UnitedNations. Levels & Trends in Child Mortality: Estimates Developed by the UN Inter-agency Group for Child Mortality Estimation. New York: UNICEF; 2012.
3. NDoH, National Health Information Systems. Sector Performance Annual Review 2013. Papua New Guinea: National Department of Health; 2014.
4. UNFPA, ICM, WHO. The State of the Worlds Midwifery. A universal pathway. A woman's right to health. New York: United Nations; 2014.
5. Vallely A: Sexually transmitted infections in Papua New Guinea: Achievements, challenges and the way forward. In: 2014 Australasian Tropical Health Conference. Cairns; 2014
6. WHO. Guidelines for the Management of Sexually Transmitted Infections, vol. WHO/RHR/01.10. Geneva: World Health Organization; 2001.
7. WHO. Global strategy for the prevention and control of sexually transmitted infections: 2006–2015: breaking the chain of transmission. Geneva: World Health Organization; 2007.
8. Tabrizi SN, Unemo M, Golparian D, Twin J, Limnios AE, Lahra M, Guy R, Investigators T. Analytical evaluation of GeneXpert CT/NG, the first genetic point-of-care assay for simultaneous detection of Neisseria gonorrhoeae and Chlamydia trachomatis. J Clin Microbiol. 2013;51(6):1945–7.
9. WHO Guidelines Approved by the Guidelines Review Committee. In: Policy Statement: Automated Real-Time Nucleic Acid Amplification Technology for Rapid and Simultaneous Detection of Tuberculosis and Rifampicin Resistance: Xpert MTB/RIF System. edn. Geneva: World Health Organization. Copyright (c) World Health Organization 2011.; 2011.
10. Bradshaw CS, Morton AN, Garland SM, Horvath LB, Kuzevska I, Fairley CK. Evaluation of a point-of-care test, BVBlue, and clinical and laboratory criteria for diagnosis of bacterial vaginosis. J Clin Microbiol. 2005;43(3):1304–8.
11. Mola GDL: Manual of Standard Managements in Obstetrics and Gynaecology for Doctors, HEOs and Nurses in Papua New Guinea, Sixth Edition edn; 2010
12. Wangnapi RA, Soso S, Unger HW, Sawera C, Ome M, Umbers AJ, Ndrewei N, Siba P, Li Wai Suen CS, Vallely A et al. Prevalence and risk factors for Chlamydia trachomatis, Neisseria gonorrhoeae and Trichomonas vaginalis infection in pregnant women in Papua New Guinea. Sex Transm Infect. 2015;91(3):194–200.
13. Vallely AJ: Point-of-care testing and treatment of sexually transmitted infections to improve pregnancy outcomes in high-burden settings..In: World STI & HIV Congress 2015. Brisbane, Australia; 2015

Retesting and repeat positivity following diagnosis of *Chlamydia trachomatis* and *Neisseria gonorrhoea* in New Zealand

Sally B. Rose[1*], Susan M. Garrett[1], James Stanley[2] and Susan R. H. Pullon[1]

Abstract

Background: Testing for reinfection at 3 to 6 months following treatment for *Chlamydia Trachomatis* or *Neisseria gonorrhoea* is recommended in best practice sexual health management guidelines. This study aimed to describe rates of retesting and repeat positivity following diagnosis of chlamydia or gonorrhoea in a defined geographic region of New Zealand.

Methods: Retrospective cohort study in Wellington, New Zealand involving analysis of laboratory data for chlamydia and gonorrhoea tests performed in primary care and sexual health clinics (July 2012–July 2015). Outcome measures: rate of retesting and rate of repeat positivity 6 weeks to 6 months after a positive result (index event). Kaplan-Meier curves were used to plot time from first index event to retest. Logistic regression modelling was used to determine the odds of retesting and repeat positivity between 6 weeks and 6 months of follow-up, adjusting for potential confounders (age, gender, ethnicity and socioeconomic deprivation).

Results: Overall 29.4% (1919/6530) of the cohort was retested between 6 weeks and 6 months, with 18% (347/1919) of those retested returning positive results. Lower odds of retesting were observed for males (OR 0.4, 95% CI 0.34–0.48), and individuals of NZ Maori (OR 0.72, 0.61–0.85) and Pacific ethnicities (OR 0.49, 0.39–0.62, reference European). Factors associated with higher odds of repeat positivity on retesting included male gender (OR 2.0, 1.14–2.82), age 15–19 years (OR 1.78, 1.32–2.41, reference 20–24 years), chlamydia/gonorrhoea co-infection (OR 2.39, 1.32–4.35, reference chlamydia only), Maori (OR 1.6, 1.18–2.17) and Pacific ethnicities (OR 1.88, 1.22–2.9, reference European).

Conclusions: We observed low adherence to STI retesting guidelines, and marked gender and ethnic disparities in rates of retesting and repeat positivity. Low retesting rates are suggestive of low levels of awareness of this aspect of patient management, and an absence of a systematic approach to retesting. High rates of repeat positivity reinforce the importance of advising patients about reducing their risk of reinfection, including notification and treatment of all recent sexual partners. Greater priority needs to be placed on increasing retesting and reducing rates of reinfection, with strategies implemented to improve these important aspects of patient care and population STI control.

Keywords: *Chlamydia trachomatis*, *Neisseria gonorrhoea*, Sexually transmitted infections, Partner notification, Test of reinfection

* Correspondence: sally.rose@otago.ac.nz
[1]Department of Primary Health Care and General Practice, University of Otago, Wellington, PO Box 7343, Wellington South 6242, New Zealand
Full list of author information is available at the end of the article

Background

Individuals diagnosed with *Chlamydia trachomatis* or *Neisseria gonorrhoea* are a known risk group for subsequent reinfection [1]. Chlamydia remains the most commonly diagnosed bacterial sexually transmitted infection (STI) worldwide [2], despite the widespread availability of highly sensitive diagnostic technologies and highly effective single dose treatment for uncomplicated infection. Modelling studies suggest reinfection is likely to play a significant role in sustaining the global chlamydia epidemic [3], in turn highlighting the critical role that treating sexual partners plays in STI control.

Chlamydial infection occasionally persists due to treatment failure, but repeat positivity upon retesting is most often due to reinfection from an untreated sexual partner or an infected new partner [4, 5]. Undetected and untreated repeat infection can result in more serious long-term reproductive sequelae than an initial infection, with an estimated four-fold increased risk of pelvic inflammatory disease, a two-fold risk of ectopic pregnancy and a resultant higher risk of infertility [1, 5]. Treating partners together with early detection and treatment of reinfection are therefore important to minimize harm and onward transmission [6].

Testing for reinfection (rather than test of cure) at 3 months following treatment for both chlamydia and gonorrhoea is recommended in STI management guidelines [5, 7, 8]. If retesting at 3 months is not possible, some guidelines recommend retesting whenever care is next sought in the 12 months following treatment [5]. A test of cure is no longer routinely recommended for these bacterial infections due to the high efficacy of first line treatments, but is advised in more limited circumstances including pregnancy, when second line treatments were used, treatment compliance is in question, or symptoms persist [5, 9, 10]. Testing sooner than three to 5 weeks post-treatment for chlamydia or gonorrhoea is not recommended to avoid detection of residual nonviable organisms that can give a false-positive result [5, 7].

New Zealand has comparatively high rates of chlamydia with the burden of infection carried by young people (under 25 years), and particularly young Maori (the indigenous people of New Zealand) and Pacific peoples [11]. In 2014, chlamydia rates in New Zealand were 2092 and 3062 per 100,000 population for ages 15–19 and 20–24 respectively [11]. By comparison, 2014 chlamydia rates in the US were 1804 and 2485 per 100,000 for ages 15–19 and 20–24 [12], and in the UK, rates were 1708 and 2189 per 100,000 population for the same age-groups [13]. While there is no national screening programme in New Zealand, opportunistic chlamydia screening is recommended for females under 25 years meeting various risk criteria, and others deemed 'at risk' (e.g. two or more partners in the past 12 months, a recent partner change or inconsistent use of condoms) [9, 10]. Partner notification is recommended as part of chlamydia and gonorrhoea management using 'patient referral' as the preferred method, whereby patients are advised of the need to notify their sexual contacts of the past 2-months. If patient safety is a concern, 'provider referral' should be offered (the clinician notifies contacts with the patient's consent) [9, 10]. New Zealand Sexual Health Society guidelines also recommend testing for reinfection at 3 months [9], and Ministry of Health chlamydia management guidelines recommend testing within three to 6 months [10]. The present study was designed to assess the extent to which guideline recommendations regarding retesting are met in a defined geographical region of New Zealand. Retesting rates within 6 months of a chlamydia or gonorrhoea diagnosis in primary care and sexual health clinics were analysed and demographic characteristics (age, ethnicity, gender) assessed to identify factors associated with receipt of retesting and repeat positivity.

Methods

This study was reviewed and approved by the Southern Health and Disability Ethics Committee, New Zealand on July 16th 2015 (Ref 15/STH/109).

Design and setting

This retrospective cohort study analysed data obtained from one diagnositic laboratory pertaining to chlamydia and gonorrhoea tests requested by primary care and sexual health service providers in the greater Wellington region of New Zealand (population approximately 450,000). The laboratory provides all community testing services for the region and uses the commercially available Roche cobas 4800 CT/NG assay [14] to detect *Chlamydia trachomatis* or *Neisseria gonorrhoea* from a single swab or urine specimen (specimens are routinely tested for both bacteria).

Data collection

Laboratory data were obtained for tests performed in the 3 years from 1 July 2012 to 1 July 2015. The first positive chlamydia or gonorrhoea result for an individual occurring in the first two and a half years of data collection (1 July 2012 to 31 Dec 2014) was designated as the first 'index event' for that person, with follow-up to 1 July 2015 ensuring each person had a minimum of 6 months follow up (maximum 3 years). Exclusion criteria included: index events requested in secondary care (hospitals and specialists) with the exception of sexual health specialists; and tests performed for 0–9 year-olds (16 positives removed, all of which were neonatal eye infections). A small number of individuals with missing age and/or gender data were also excluded prior to analysis.

The dataset included laboratory number (assigned by the lab to unique individuals), National Health Index NHI (a unique patient identifier assigned to all New Zealanders at birth that enables health record linkage) [15], gender, date of birth, visit date, type of specimen, result, requestor name (Dr, nurse), requesting location (clinic). No patient names, addresses or contact details were obtained. Prioritized ethnicity and NZDeprivation06 (NZDep06) scores were obtained via NHI matching from nationally held datasets. Ethnicity refers to the ethnic group with which an individual self-identifies and is collected via self-report using the standardized New Zealand 2001 census question [16]. NZDep06 is a validated, census-derived, area-based index of socioeconomic deprivation, grouped into deciles 1 to 10, where 1 represents least deprived areas and 10 most deprived areas [17]. NHI and gender are not mandatory fields for laboratory requests so are not routinely provided by some requestors, and therefore ethnicity and NZDep could not be ascertained for some individuals.

Data processing and identification of cohort for analysis

SAS Enterprise Guide (v7.1) was used to clean and format data. Duplicate records were removed where multiple specimens were tested for one individual on the same day, or when retesting occurred within a few days of the index event due to inadequate specimen collection. Unique laboratory numbers were used to identify multiple tests for a given individual, and a single line of data created for each test-retest event. A test undertaken at least 6 weeks (42 days) after the index event was considered a 'retest' (outcome 1) and examined as to whether the retest was positive for chlamydia or gonorrhoea (outcome 2). Retesting soon after treatment is more likely to have been performed as 'test of cure' and carries with it a higher likelihood of false positives. Any repeat positives within 42 days of diagnosis were not therefore considered new infections in this analysis (assumes a median time to treatment of 6 days [18], plus 5 weeks).

Each person could contribute more than one index event test sequence to the dataset. If the retest following an index event was negative, that marked the end of the test-retest sequence; however any subsequent positive test (>42 days later) for that person became a new index event which was followed-up for retesting outcomes using the protocol above.

Statistical analyses

Proportions of the overall cohort testing positive for chlamydia and gonorrhoea infection were described with respect to gender, age and ethnicity. Kaplan-Meier curves were used to depict time from first index test to retest by gender (to a maximum of 2 years follow-up). All individuals included in this analysis had a minimum of 6 months follow-up, 80% had at least 12 months and 39% had at least 24 months follow-up.

Outcome measures were i) proportion of individuals retested for chlamydia and gonorrhoea 6 weeks to 6 months after a positive test (described by age, sex, ethnicity, NZDep); and ii) the proportion of retested individuals with positive results for chlamydia/gonorrhoea (described by age, sex, ethnicity, NZDep). Logistic regression models were used to examine associations between the outcomes and exposure variables (type of infection at index presentation, age, sex, ethnicity, NZDep). These models explicitly allowed for individuals to have multiple index events in the analysis by accounting for the non-independence of observations that arises when some individuals have more than one index event (using a generalized linear mixed model with a binomial link function and random intercepts to account for correlation between multiple index events from the same individual). Separate analyses were conducted for retesting between 6 weeks and 6 months of an index event (outcome one: denominator is index events), and for having a positive test on retesting within this timeframe (outcome two: denominator is all retests). Statistical analyses were conducted using Stata 12 (StataCorp, Tx).

Results

Description of the study cohort

Figure 1 depicts the process by which index events (positive tests) were selected for inclusion in outcome analyses. During the two-and-a-half-year period, a total of 94,426 tests were performed in primary care and sexual health clinics (18,217 for males and 76,209 for females) with 6817 testing positive overall (7.2% positivity). There were clear differences in rates of positivity by gender, age and ethnicity for the cohort tested. Males made up only 19.3% of those tested, but were more likely than females to test positive for chlamydia (11% versus 5.9%) and gonorrhoea (1.8% versus 0.4%). The majority of those testing positive were aged under 25 years (65%). In this age group (detail not included in Fig. 1), 16.1% of males and 9.5% of females were diagnosed with chlamydia, and 5.7% of males and 0.6% of females diagnosed with gonorrhoea. Individuals of Pacific ethnicities had the highest proportion of positive results (16.3%), followed by Maori (14.1%), European (5.2%) and Asian (5.1%). Following application of test-retest criteria (and removal of two cases with no age data), 6530 positive index events were included in the dataset for further analysis (2140 index tests for males, 4390 index tests for females).

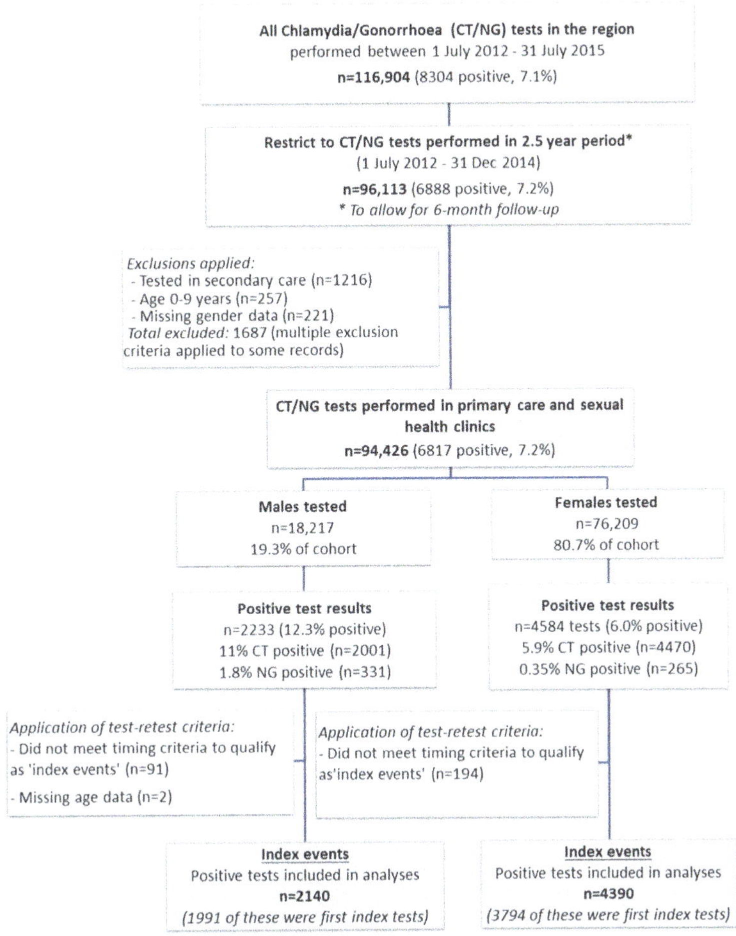

Fig. 1 Process by which index events (positive tests) were selected for inclusion in outcome analyses

Repeat testing

Table 1 presents the unadjusted data for 6530 index events for individuals who tested positive during the study period (n = 5785) and the number and percentage who were then a) retested between 6 weeks and 6 months of a chlamydia or gonorrhoea diagnosis, and b) diagnosed with a positive result on retest. During this period, 29.4% (1919/6530) of the cohort were retested for chlamydia and gonorrhoea within the recommended 6 month period, of whom 18% (347/1919) tested positive. Unadjusted retesting and repeat positivity rates varied by age, gender, ethnicity and index test location. Gender differences were observed in proportions retested within the recommended timeframe, with 35% of females retested (95% CI 33.6–36.4) but only 17.9% of males (95% CI 16.3–19.6). When retested, 21.1% of males had repeat positives (95% CI 17.2–25.6) compared to 17.3% of females (95% CI 15.5–19.3).

Time to retesting

Figure 2 presents Kaplan-Meier curves showing time from first index event to retesting for 5785 males and females (recommended retesting period is highlighted in grey). Within 6 weeks of the first index positive, 11.6% of females (440/3794) and 9.3% of males (186/1991) had been retested, of whom 22.0% (97/440) of females and 29.0% (54/186) of males retested positive. By 6 months, 44.5% of females and 26.2% of males had been retested (including tests within 6 weeks of index events). Gender differences persisted over time, with 58.2% of females and only 34% of males retested within 0–12 months; and 68.8% of females and 40.5% of males retested within 0–24 months.

Correlates of retesting and repeat positivity

Table 2 presents the odds ratios and confidence intervals from logistic regression analyses (generalized linear mixed models) examining factors independently associated with retesting and repeat positivity (separate analyses) between 6 weeks and 6 months of a positive chlamydia or gonorrhoea index event. Factors associated with significantly lower odds of retesting included male gender (OR 0.4, 95% CI 0.34–0.48, reference female),

Table 1 Characteristics of the cohort with index positive tests (n = 6530), proportions retested and positive on retesting

Patient characteristics[a]	Males					Females				
	Index Positive	Retested 6wks-6mths		Positive on retest		Index Positive	Retested 6wks-6mths		Positive on retest	
	n	*n*	(%)	*n*	(%)	*n*	*n*	(%)	*n*	(%)
Total	2140	383	(17.9)	81	(21.1)	4390	1536	(35.0)	266	(17.3)
Index infection										
Chlamydia	1825	330	(18.1)	67	(20.3)	4139	1454	(35.1)	245	(17.5)
Gonorrhoea	220	44	(20.0)	9	(20.5)	105	30	(28.6)	3	(10.0)
Both	95	9	(9.5)	5	(55.6)	146	52	(35.6)	18	(34.6)
Age-band										
10–14	0	-[b]	–	–	–	39	18	(46.2)	6	(33.3)
15–19	301	40	(13.3)	14	(35.0)	1277	524	(41.0)	129	(24.6)
20–24	842	157	(18.6)	39	(24.8)	1840	646	(35.1)	96	(14.9)
25–29	422	66	(15.6)	9	(13.6)	673	206	(30.6)	19	(9.2)
30–34	209	37	(17.7)	5	(13.5)	292	82	(28.1)	12	(14.6)
35–39	131	25	(19.1)	3	(12.0)	129	31	(24.0)	3	(9.7)
40–44	96	17	(17.7)	4	(23.5)	71	13	(18.3)	1	(7.7)
45–49	62	16	(25.8)	2	(12.5)	42	9	(21.4)	0	(0.0)
50–54	41	14	(34.1)	4	(28.6)	17	6	(35.3)	0	(0.0)
55–59	15	2	(13.3)	1	(50.0)	5	1	(20.0)	0	(0.0)
60+	21	9	(42.9)	0	(0.0)	5	0	(0.0)	–	–
Ethnicity										
European	951	201	(21.1)	36	(17.9)	1817	716	(39.4)	95	(13.3)
NZ Maori	440	62	(14.1)	21	(33.9)	1485	533	(35.9)	113	(21.2)
Pacific	245	34	(13.9)	9	(26.5)	618	163	(26.4)	37	(22.7)
Asian	105	31	(29.5)	3	(9.7)	221	80	(36.2)	15	(18.8)
MELAA/Other[c]	42	12	(28.6)	3	(25.0)	47	22	(46.8)	4	(18.2)
Not known	357	43	(12.0)	9	(20.9)	202	22	(10.9)	2	(9.1)
Socioeconomic deprivation (NZDep)										
Least deprived (1–3)	425	77	(18.1)	14	(18.2)	773	290	(37.5)	40	(13.8)
Moderately dep (4–7)	538	94	(17.5)	19	(20.2)	1362	522	(38.3)	83	(15.9)
Most deprived (8–10)	730	157	(21.5)	37	(23.6)	1981	689	(34.8)	140	(20.3)
Not known	447	55	(12.3)	11	(20.0)	274	35	(12.8)	3	(8.6)
Test location/clinic[d]										
General Practice	913	142	(15.6)	37	(26.1)	2069	606	(29.3)	109	(18.0)
Sexual Health	604	134	(22.2)	20	(14.9)	208	45	(21.6)	3	(6.7)
Student/Youth	323	59	(18.3)	17	(28.8)	999	434	(43.4)	80	(18.4)
Family Planning	300	48	(16.0)	7	(14.6)	1114	451	(40.5)	74	(16.4)

[a]The dataset includes 5785 unique individuals, some with multiple index tests
[b]The - sign indicates cells with no information (either no index tests in group, or no retests performed and reinfection frequency is zero by definition)
[c]MELAA is an ethnic grouping that includes Middle Eastern, Latin American and African
[d]Includes 112 individual locations/clinics

NZ Maori ethnicity (OR 0.72, 0.61–0.85, reference European) and Pacific ethnicity (OR 0.49, 0.39–0.62, reference European). Factors associated with significantly higher odds of repeat positivity when retested included male gender (OR 2.0, 1.41–2.81), younger age (for ages 15–19, OR 1.78, 1.32–2.41, reference 20–24), co-infection with both chlamydia and gonorrhoea at the index event (OR 2.39, 1.32–4.35, reference chlamydia only), and NZ Maori (OR 1.6, 1.18–2.17, reference European) and Pacific ethnicities (OR1.88, 1.22–2.9, reference European).

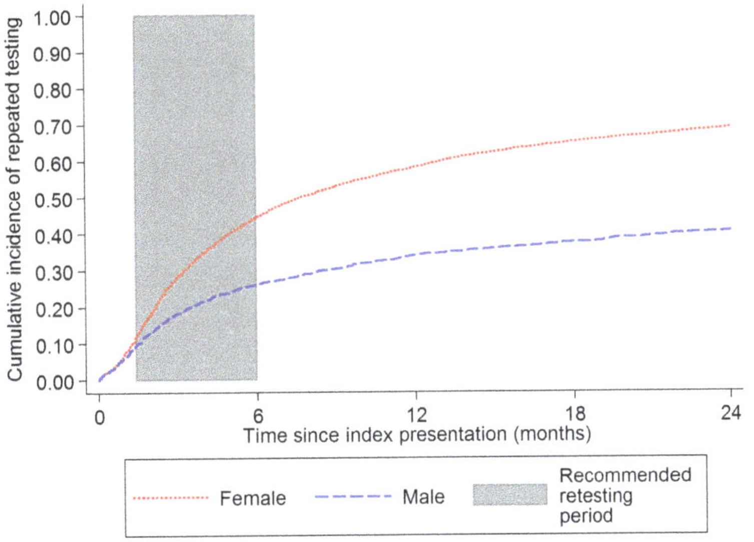

Fig. 2 Kaplan-Meier curves for time from first index event to subsequent test during two year follow-up

Discussion

This analysis suggests many clinicians are not following guideline recommendations to routinely test for reinfection at three to 6 months. Marked gender and ethnic disparities were observed both in retesting and reinfection rates. Males, Maori and Pacific ethnic groups were less likely to be retested within the recommended period, but when retested, these groups were among those most likely to return positive results. Overall rates of repeat positivity were high among those retested, with a quarter of females and a third of males aged 15–19 years testing positive, a finding likely to be indicative of low levels of partner treatment. Younger age groups (24 years and under) were more likely to be retested than those aged 25 years and older, in line with known risk profiles, but retesting rates were still low, particularly for young males. Co-infection with chlamydia and gonorrhoea was a risk factor for having a subsequent positive retest result, yet individuals in this group were tested no more frequently than those with a single-bacterial infection.

Whereas some studies reporting reinfection and retesting rates have focussed only specific patient populations (often limited to females) [4, 19, 20], a strength of our study was the robust sample comprising laboratory data for all males and females diagnosed with chlamydia or gonorrhoea in the region over a two-and-a-half-year period. Test locations included over 100 primary health care (general practice, youth health, student health and family planning) and sexual health clinics and all individuals had a minimum of 6 months follow-up. Limitations of the analysis included lack of behavioural and clinical data that would have helped in the interpretation of study findings (such as condom use, change of sexual partner, number and gender of recent partners, presence of symptoms, and treatment outcomes for index cases and their partners). While most of those with repeat positives will have represented new infections; a small proportion would have been persistent infection due to treatment failure or compliance issues (regardless, any repeat positive is important to pick up on retesting). Reasons for retesting were unknown, but would presumably include patient/clinician concerns about reinfection as well as opportunistic retesting as per guideline recommendations. We do not know what advice was given about reinfection or retesting, nor the extent to which individuals may have re-presented for care but not been offered retesting. Some cohort members will have moved during follow-up, and any retesting outside the study region will have been missed (hence underestimating retesting rates). Retesting may have been targeted towards those individuals identified as being at higher risk for reinfection, thus over-estimating the prevalence of reinfection in this cohort.

Only one other estimate of repeat testing rates has so far been published in New Zealand - approximately 32% of females and 16% of males were retested within 6 months of a positive chlamydia result in the Waikato region between 2008 and 2010 [18]. Our data were more recent and related to a different region but showed very similar levels of retesting. This suggests retesting may be falling well short of best practice guidelines throughout New Zealand – a finding that warrants urgent attention, particularly in light of our persistently high initial infection rates. Although proportions retested within 12 months in our study were good, retesting sooner – closer to

Table 2 Logistic regression analyses for factors associated with retesting for chlamydia/gonorrhoea and repeat positivity on retesting

Patient characteristics[a]	Retested at 6-weeks to 6-months (n = 6530)			Repeat positive on retesting (n = 1919)		
	Odds Ratio	(95% CI)	Factor p-value	Odds Ratio	(95% CI)	Factor p-value
Gender			<0.001			<0.001
Male	0.40	(0.34, 0.48)		2.00	(1.41, 2.82)	
Female	Reference			Reference		
Index infection						
Chlamydia	Reference		0.593	Reference		0.011
Gonorrhoea	1.00	(0.72, 1.39)		0.76	(0.38, 1.52)	
Both	0.83	(0.58, 1.19)		2.39	(1.32, 4.35)	
Age-band						
10–14	1.77	(0.80, 3.94)		2.60	(0.86, 7.85)	
15–19	1.23	(1.04, 1.46)		1.78	(1.32, 2.41)	
20–24	Reference		0.001	Reference		<0.001
25–29	0.83	(0.68, 1.01)		0.53	(0.33, 0.84)	
30–34	0.79	(0.60, 1.04)		0.71	(0.39, 1.27)	
35–39	0.69	(0.48, 1.01)		0.54	(0.22, 1.37)	
40+	0.91	(0.67, 1.25)		0.61	(0.30, 1.23)	
Ethnicity						
European	Reference		<0.001	Reference		0.018
NZ Maori	0.72	(0.61, 0.85)		1.60	(1.18, 2.17)	
Pacific	0.49	(0.39, 0.62)		1.88	(1.22, 2.90)	
Asian	1.12	(0.83, 1.52)		1.38	(0.77, 2.47)	
MELAA/Other[b]	1.62	(0.93, 2.84)		1.50	(0.59, 3.82)	
Not known	0.68	(0.40, 1.15)		2.33	(0.58, 9.43)	
Socioeconomic deprivation (NZDep)						
Least deprived (1–3)	Reference		<0.001	Reference		0.226
Moderately dep (4–7)	1.10	(0.90, 1.33)		1.11	(0.75, 1.63)	
Most deprived (8–10)	1.11	(0.92, 1.35)		1.35	(0.93, 1.96)	
Not known	0.43	(0.27, 0.69)		0.61	(0.17, 2.15)	

[a]The dataset includes 5785 unique individuals, some with multiple index tests
[b]MELAA is an ethnic grouping that includes Middle Eastern, Latin American and African

3 months - may be more likely to prevent the development of long-term reproductive health complications [21]. Our retesting rates were similar to rates reported in Australia, where 12% of heterosexual males and 18% of heterosexual females were retested in the 4 months following treatment for chlamydia in a study of sexual health services [22], and 14% of males and 29% of females were retested in a study based in general practice [23]. In the largest US study to date, laboratory data for over 3 million chlamydia tests showed that only 22% of males and 38% of non-pregnant females were retested within 12 months [24].

The high rate of repeat positivity observed in the current analysis was in line with reinfection rates reported previously [4, 20]. Estimated chlamydia reinfection rates among 16–24 year-old females recruited into a UK study were 22 per 100 person years for those treated in Family Planning clinics and 29.9 per 100 person years for those treated in general practice [20]. The incidence of reinfection among adolescent women attending primary care clinics in the US was 34 episodes per 100 woman-years of follow-up [4]. The high rates of repeat positivity observed here and in past studies reinforces the importance of timely access to retesting to detect and treat reinfection early.

Our analysis shows that greater effort needs to be put into ensuring equitable access to timely retesting (and initial testing) for males, Maori and Pacific groups in New Zealand. The lower rates of retesting for males in this study may reflect patterns of initial testing, where males made up only a fifth of the total cohort tested.

Males present to primary care less frequently than females [25], and diagnostic testing is more likely to be for symptomatic infection or on presentation as a contact of a known case. By contrast, females more often receive opportunistic screening, typically when presenting to primary care for contraception or cervical smears. Pacific people and Maori had substantially lower odds than Europeans to receive retesting (OR 0.5 and 0.7 respectively), yet amongst those retested the odds of reinfection were over 60% higher among Maori and 88% higher among Pacific (compared to European). Ethnic disparities in STI rates are well documented in New Zealand and are indicative (at least in part) of issues relating to inequitable access to appropriate healthcare [26]. Cost and other access-related issues may be prohibitive to return visits for some. Results from the 2012/13 New Zealand Health Survey showed that that Maori (and to a lesser extent Pacific) were more likely than European to report recent unmet need for healthcare due to cost [25].

The relatively low rates of retesting and high rates of repeat positivity in this study are suggestive of low levels of clinician awareness of this important aspect of patient care, and a lack of a systematic approach to partner notification and retesting. This suggestion is supported by the findings of a survey conducted in the same region in which 121 primary care clinicians (doctors and nurses among those with the highest annual STI diagnosis rates in the region) were asked about their approaches to partner notification and testing for reinfection [27]. Results showed that while partner notification was typically discussed at the time of treatment, a range of challenges were perceived to limit their ability to effectively undertake this discussion and follow-up on notification outcomes was rare. The survey also highlighted confusion among participants regarding the need for 'test of cure' versus a 'test of reinfection', with the majority indicating that active recall for repeat testing was uncommon [27]. Patient-factors including lack of knowledge about retesting and continued exposure to untreated partners are also likely to be important factors contributing to our study findings that need addressing.

Strategies to improve re-attendance rates among sexual health clinic attendees have demonstrated moderate levels of success. In two Australian studies, retesting rates increased by 9 and 22% when a text (SMS) message was sent to remind patients about a 3-month test of reinfection [28, 29]. A similar study in the Netherlands demonstrated a 21% increase in retesting [30]. The provision of a postal home sample-collection kit (in addition to an SMS) further improved retesting rates (an additional 22% retested compared to SMS alone) in another Australian study [31]. Missed opportunities for retesting in general practice have been reported, with patients re-presenting but not receiving retesting [23], which highlights the potential role of electronic chart prompts/flags to facilitate the offer of opportunistic testing when patients next present for care [1, 23]. Encouraging patients to put a reminder in their mobile phone, or offering drop-in clinics that allow asymptomatic patients to provide a self-sample, have also been suggested as strategies that may facilitate retesting [32].

Conclusions

This study highlights the need to raise awareness of retesting for chlamydia and gonorrhoea reinfection at 3 months post-treatment as an important aspect of best practice STI patient management. Provision of verbal advice and use of a proactive approach to retesting should be accompanied by reinfection risk reduction counselling that includes the importance of partner treatment, advice not to have sex for 7 days following completion of own and partners' treatment, consistent condom use and behavioural change if relevant. Prioritizing strategies to detect and prevent reinfection among those diagnosed will be critical if we are to reduce the burden and sequelae of bacterial STIs in our communities.

Acknowledgements

We thank Aotea Pathology (now Wellington Southern Community Laboratories) for extraction and provision of laboratory testing data for analysis.

Funding

This study was part of a wider project funded by a New Zealand Health Research Council (HRC) feasibility study grant (15/419).

Authors' contributions

SR led the research and development of study protocol, participated in interpretation of the findings and drafted the manuscript. SG participated in protocol development, preparation of data for analysis and revision of the manuscript. JS participated in protocol development, planned and performed the statistical analyses, participated in interpretation of the findings and revision of the manuscript. SP participated in protocol development, interpretation of the findings and revision of the manuscript. All authors read and approved the final manuscript.

Consent for publication

Not applicable

Competing interests

The authors declare that they have no competing interests.

Author details

[1]Department of Primary Health Care and General Practice, University of Otago, Wellington, PO Box 7343, Wellington South 6242, New Zealand. [2]Biostatistical Group, University of Otago, Wellington, P O Box 7343, Wellington South 6242, New Zealand.

References

1. California Department of Public Health (CDPH), Sexually Transmitted Diseases (STD) Control Branch: Best Practices for the Prevention and Early Detection of Repeat Chlamydial and Gonococcal Infections: Effective Partner Treatment and Patient Retesting Strategies for Implementation in California Health Care settings. 2011. https://archive.cdph.ca.gov/programs/std/Documents/Best-Practices-for-Prevention-and-Early-Detection-of-Repeat-CT-and-GC.pdf. Accessed 27 July 2017.
2. Centers for Disease Control and Prevention (CDC). CDC grand rounds: Chlamydia prevention: challenges and strategies for reducing disease burden and Sequelae. Morb Mortal Wkly Rep. 2011;60:370–3.
3. Heijne JC, Althaus CL, Herzog SA, Kretzschmar M, Low N. The role of reinfection and partner notification in the efficacy of Chlamydia screening programs. J Infect Dis. 2011;203:372–7.
4. Batteiger BE, Tu W, Ofner S, Van Der Pol B, Stothard DR, Orr DP, et al. Repeated Chlamydia trachomatis genital infections in adolescent women. J Infect Dis. 2010;201:42–51.
5. Centers for Disease Control and Prevention (CDC). Sexually transmitted diseases treatment guidelines. Morb Mortal Wkly Rep. 2015;64:3.
6. McClean H, Radcliffe K, Sullivan A, Ahmed-Jushuf I, British Association for Sexual Health and HIV (BASHH). BASHH statement on partner notification for sexually transmissible infections. 2012, http://www.bashh.org/documents/4445.pdf. Accessed 25 Aug 2016.
7. Nwokolo NC, Dragovic B, Patel S, Tong CYW, Barker G, Radcliffe K. 2015 UK national guideline for the management of infection with Chlamydia trachomatis. Int J STD AIDS. 2016;27(4):251–67.
8. Public Health Agency of Canada. Canadian guidelines on sexually transmitted infections. 2015. http://www.phac-aspc.gc.ca/std-mts/sti-its/cgsti-ldcits/index-eng.php. Accessed 21 Feb 2017.
9. New Zealand Sexual Health Society. Best practice guidelines: STI summary of guidelines. 2015. http://www.nzshs.org/guidelines.html. Accessed 17 Feb 2017.
10. Ministry of Health: Chlamydia management guidelines. 2008. https://bn6team-10.wikispaces.com/file/view/chlamydia-management-guidelines.pdf. Accessed 15 May 2017.
11. The Institute of Environmental Science and Research Ltd. Sexually transmitted infections in New Zealand: annual surveillance report 2014. Porirua; 2015. https://surv.esr.cri.nz/PDF_surveillance/STISurvRpt/2014/FINAL2014AnnualSTIReport.pdf. Accessed 27 July 2017.
12. Centers for Disease Control and Prevention (CDC). 2014 sexually transmitted diseases surveillance: Chlamydia. 2015. https://www.cdc.gov/std/stats14/chlamydia.htm. Accessed 15 May 2017.
13. Public Health England. Sexually transmitted infections (STIs): annual data tables. Table 9: selected STI diagnoses & rates in the UK by gender & age group, 2011–2015. 2015. https://www.gov.uk/government/uploads/system/uploads/attachment_data/file/572281/2015_Table_9_Selected_STI_diagnoses__rates_in_the_UK_by_gender__age_group__2011-2015.pdf. Accessed 27 July 2017.
14. Rockett R, Goire N, Limnios A, Turra M, Higgens G, Lambert SB, et al. Evaluation of the cobas 4800 CT/NG test for detecting Chlamydia trachomatis and Neisseria gonorrhoeae. Sex Transm Infect. 2010;86:470–3.
15. New Zealand Health Information Service. National Health Index. Wellington: Ministry of Health; 2010. http://www.health.govt.nz/our-work/health-identity/national-health-index. Accessed 12 Sept 2016
16. Statistics New Zealand. Ethnicity definition. Wellington; 2006. http://www.stats.govt.nz/methods/classifications-and-standards/classification-related-stats-standards/ethnicity/definition.aspx Accessed 15 Feb 2017
17. Salmond C, Crampton P, Aitkenson J. NZDep2006 index of deprivation. User's manual. Wellington: Department of Public Health, University of Otago, Wellington; 2007. p. 1–16. http://www.otago.ac.nz/wellington/otago020337.pdf. Accessed 10 Dec 2016
18. Morgan J, Woodhall S. Repeat chlamydia testing across a New Zealand district: 3 years of laboratory data. Sex Transm Infect. 2013;89:28–31.
19. Nielsen A, Marrone G, De Costa A. Chlamydia trachomatis among youth - testing behaviour and incidence of repeat testing in Stockholm County, Sweden 2010–2012. PLoS One. 2016;11(9):e0163597.
20. Scott Lamontagne D, Baster K, Emmett L, Nichols T, Randall S, McLean L, et al. Incidence and reinfection rates of genital chlamydial infection among women aged 16–24 years attending general practice, family planning and genitourinary medicine clinics in England: a prospective cohort study by the Chlamydia recall study advisory group. Sex Transm Infect. 2007;83(4):292–303.
21. Hosenfeld CB, Workowski KA, Berman S, Zaidi A, Dyson J, Mosure D, et al. Repeat infection with Chlamydia and gonorrhea among females: a systematic review of the literature. Sex Transm Dis. 2009;36(8):478–89.
22. Guy R, Wand H, Franklin N, Fairley CK, Chen MY, O'Connor CC, et al. Re-testing for chlamydia at sexual health services in Australia, 2004–08. Sex Health. 2011;8(2):242–7.
23. Bowring AL, Gouillou M, Guy R, Kong FYS, Hocking J, Pirotta M, et al. Missed opportunities—low levels of chlamydia retesting at Australian general practices, 2008–2009. Sex Transm Infect. 2012;88(5):330–4.
24. Hoover KW, Tao G, Nye MB, Body BA. Suboptimal adherence to repeat testing recommendations for men and women with positive Chlamydia tests in the United States, 2008–2010. Clin Infect Dis. 2013;56(1):51–7.
25. Ministry of Health: New Zealand Health Survey. Annual update of key findings 2012/13. Part 3: health service use, unmet need and oral health. Wellington; 2013. https://www.health.govt.nz/system/files/documents/publications/new-zealand-health-survey-annual-update-2012-13-dec13-v3.pdf. Accessed 27 July 2017.
26. Ellison-Loschmann L, Pearce N. Improving access to health care among New Zealand's Maori population. Am J Public Health. 2006;96(4):612–7.
27. Rose SB, Garrett SM, Pullon SRH. Partner notification – overcoming challenges when diagnosing Chlamydia and Gonorrhoea in primary care: a postal survey of doctors and nurses. J Prim Health Care. 2017;9(2):136–44.
28. Downing SG, Cashman C, McNamee H, Penney D, Russell DB, Hellard ME. Increasing chlamydia test of re-infection rates using SMS reminders and incentives. Sex Transm Infect. 2013;89(1):16–9.
29. Guy R, Wand H, Knight V, Kenigsberg A, Read P, McNulty AM. SMS reminders improve re-screening in women and heterosexual men with chlamydia infection at Sydney sexual health Centre: a before-and-after study. Sex Transm Infect. 2013;89(1):11–5.
30. Kampman C, Koedijk F, Driessen-Hulshof H, Hautvast J, van den Broek I. Retesting young STI clinic visitors with urogenital Chlamydia trachomatis infection in the Netherlands; response to a text message reminder and reinfection rates: a prospective study with historical controls. Sex Transm Infect. 2016;92(2):124–9.
31. Smith KS, Hocking JS, Chen MY, Fairley CK, McNulty AM, Read P, et al. Dual intervention to increase Chlamydia retesting: a randomized controlled trial in three populations. Am J Prev Med. 2015;49(1):1–11.
32. Nakatsukasa-Ono W, Howard H. Practical Strategies for Improving Chlamydia and Gonorrhea Retesting. Expert Commentary 2012, National Chlamydia Coalition (NCC) Research Translation Committee; 2012. p. 14. http://nnptc.org/resources/practical-strategies-for-improving-chlamydia-and-gonorrhea-retesting/. Accessed 18 Oct 2016

Antimicrobial resistance and *Neisseria gonorrhoeae* multiantigen sequence typing (NG-MAST) genotypes in N. *gonorrhoeae* during 2012–2014 in Karachi, Pakistan

Kauser Jabeen[1*], Pushpa Bhawan Mal[1], Erum Khan[1], Saeeda Chandio[1], Susanne Jacobsson[2] and Magnus Unemo[2]

Abstract

Background: Globally, increasing antimicrobial resistance (AMR) in *Neisseria gonorrhoea* has led to decreased treatment options for gonorrhoea. Continuous monitoring of resistance is crucial to determine evolving resistance trends in *Neisseria gonorrhoea* and to suggest treatment recommendations. Quality assured gonococcal AMR data from Pakistan are mainly lacking. This study was performed to determine prevalence and trends of gonococcal AMR and molecular epidemiology of local strains during 2012–2014 in Karachi, Pakistan.

Methods: Gonococcal isolates ($n = 100$) were obtained from urogenital specimens submitted to the Aga Khan University Laboratory, Karachi, Pakistan. Antimicrobial susceptibility was determined using Etest and molecular epidemiology was assessed by *N. gonorrhoeae* multiantigen sequence typing (NG-MAST). Quality control was performed using *N. gonorrhoeae* WHO reference strains C, F, G, K, L, M, N, O, and P, and ATCC 49226.

Results: Susceptibility to spectinomycin, ceftriaxone and cefixime was 100 % and to azithromycin was 99 %. All isolates had low ceftriaxone MICs, i.e., ≤0.032 mg/L. Resistance to ciprofloxacin, tetracycline and penicillin G were 86 %, 51 % and 43 %, respectively. NG-MAST analysis identified 74 different sequence types (STs).

Conclusions: A highly diversified gonococcal population, 74 NG-MAST STs (62 novel STs) with an increased resistance to penicillin G, ciprofloxacin and tetracycline circulated in Karachi, Pakistan. Fortunately, no resistance to ceftriaxone was detected. Accordingly, ceftriaxone can continuously be recommended as the treatment of choice. However it is recommended to increase the dose of ceftriaxone from 125 mg intramuscularly to 250 mg intramuscularly due to ceftriaxone MIC creep and emerging resistance reported in the region. Furthermore, due to the high level of resistance to ciprofloxacin (86 %) it is essential to exclude ciprofloxacin from the recommended first-line therapy. It is imperative to significantly broaden the gonococcal AMR monitoring with participation from other laboratories and cities in Pakistan.

Keywords: *Neisseria gonorrhoeae*, Gonorrhoea, Antimicrobial resistance, Antimicrobial resistance surveillance, Extended-spectrum cephalosporins (ESCs), Ceftriaxone, Treatment, *N. gonorrhoeae* multiantigen sequence typing (NG-MAST), Pakistan

* Correspondence: kausar.jabeen@aku.edu
[1]Department of Pathology and Laboratory Medicine, Aga Khan University, Stadium Road, Karachi, Pakistan
Full list of author information is available at the end of the article

Background

Global *Neisseria gonorrhoeae* incidence among adults is 78 million of the estimated 357 million cases of new sexually transmitted infections (STIs). Gonorrhoea is one of the most commonly reported STI with 111 cases per 100,000 population in the United States of America in 2014 [1–3]. Unfortunately, due to the lack of appropriate etiological diagnosis of gonorrhoea in many settings of Pakistan, no reliable figures regarding the incidence of gonococcal infections nationally exist.

N. gonorrhoeae was recently assigned as a "superbug" due to its ability to develop and retain *in vitro* and clinical resistance, i.e. resulting in treatment failures, to all antimicrobial agents available for treatment of gonorrhoea [2, 4–7]. The evolving resistance to ceftriaxone, the last treatment option for empirical therapy of gonorrhoeae has resulted in a fear of an era with extremely difficult to cure or possibly untreatable gonorrhoea [5–7]. Due to this emergent public health concern, the World Health Organization (WHO) in 2012 recommended a global action plan to halt the progression of *N. gonorrhoeae* antimicrobial resistance (AMR). This action plan strongly emphasizes the need of significantly enhanced surveillance of gonococcal AMR, using quality assured methods to monitor resistance trends, identify any emerging resistance and inform revisions of evidence-based treatment guidelines. The WHO has also suggested strong liaisons with other regional and national GASPs by re-launching the WHO Global Gonococcal Antimicrobial Surveillance Program (GASP) [7].

Despite these recommendations, surveillance of AMR in *N. gonorrhoeae* is difficult in settings where no national or regional GASP has been initiated. Inadequacy or complete absence of appropriate GASPs has been recently highlighted in Latin America, the Caribbean, Eastern Europe, Central Asia and Africa [2, 7–9]. This is certainly true also for the WHO Eastern Mediterranean Region (EMR). The WHO EMR includes the highly populated Pakistan with 182 million inhabitants, where no programme-based surveillance of gonococcal infections or AMR exists. In Pakistan, inadequate capacity to detect *N. gonorrhoeae* and perform quality assured AMR testing of *N. gonorrhoeae* in many laboratories are major factors that contribute to the absence of any national gonococcal AMR data. In small research studies, an increasing resistance to ciprofloxacin, penicillin and tetracycline in *N. gonorrhoeae* has been reported, but no resistance to extended-spectrum cephalosporins (ESCs) has yet been identified in Pakistan [10, 11]. However, in these studies very limited numbers of *N. gonorrhoeae* isolates were examined, and in general mainly qualitative disc diffusion methods have been used for AMR testing rather than the more reliable and quality assured quantitative methods, agar dilution and Etest, measuring the minimum inhibitory concentrations (MICs) of antimicrobials. In Pakistan, ceftriaxone 125 mg intramuscularly (IM) single dose (mostly used), cefixime 400 mg oral single dose or ciprofloxacin 500 mg oral single dose are currently the recommended first-line for empirical therapy of gonorrhoea. Alternative treatment option is azithromycin, 1 g oral single dose [12]. However, additional less effective antimicrobials such as penicillins and tetracyclines can also be used in both the private and public sector, and antimicrobials are freely available "over-the-counter" without prescriptions.

In addition to gonococcal AMR surveillance, understanding of the transmission of different gonococcal strains in the population is critical for effective control of gonorrhoea. *N. gonorrhoeae* multiantigen sequence typing (NG-MAST) [13] has been used globally to study prevalent strain genotypes, their transmission in sexual networks and core groups, and to describe distributions of AMR strains [14]. Although gonococcal prevalence surveys from Pakistan have reported rates ranging from 4.7 % to 20.2 % in high risk sex workers that suggest a high transmission in core groups, no molecular epidemiological data on high number of strains using NG-MAST is available [15]. A recent study evaluating AMR and genetic characteristics of gonococcal strains from Pakistan, India and Bhutan reported a highly diversified strain population [16]. However, this study included a low number ($n = 18$) of gonococcal isolates from Pakistan and recommended the need for expanded and ongoing surveillance with large number of gonococcal isolates in Pakistan.

The present study evaluated the prevalence and trends of *N. gonorrhoeae* AMR and described the genotypic distribution, using NG-MAST, of *N. gonorrhoeae* isolates cultured in 2012–2014 in Karachi, Pakistan.

Methods

Biological samples

The present research was conducted at the Aga Khan University (AKU) laboratories based in Karachi, Pakistan. The AKU laboratories comprise the largest laboratory network in Pakistan with satellite units in major cities and towns. The AKU Laboratory in Karachi was included as a sentinel site in the WHO GASP in 2012. Since then the laboratory regularly participates in the external quality assessment schemes of the WHO GASP with excellent result. In the current research, 100 mainly consecutive *N. gonorrhoeae* isolates cultured from urethral swabs ($n = 85$), high vaginal and cervical swabs ($n = 14$) and conjunctival swab ($n = 1$) as part of routine clinical care from January 2012 to February 2014 were included. *N. gonorrhoeae* isolates were identified by colony morphology, Gram staining, oxidase test, sugar utilization and Remel RapidNH® Panel (BioMerieux, France). These *N. gonorrhoeae* isolates have also been used in a study evaluating two different disc diffusion methods for susceptibility testing of *N. gonorrhoeae* (BMC Microbiology, accepted). All isolates were preserved in sterile 10 % glycerol phosphate broth at −70 °C and subsequently shipped with professional courier service (World Courier) on dry ice to Örebro University Hospital, Örebro, Sweden for the NG-MAST analysis. All cultures were performed according to standard protocol as part of the routine diagnostics and did not include patients' identification. The study was approved by the Ethical Review Committee of Aga Khan University (Exemption #4052-Pat-ERC-16), and did not require informed consent as samples were taken as part of routine clinical care.

Antimicrobial susceptibility testing

Antimicrobial susceptibility testing was done at the Microbiology laboratory of the Aga Khan University, Karachi, Pakistan. The MICs (mg/L) of ceftriaxone, cefixime, penicillin G, spectinomycin, ciprofloxacin, azithromycin and tetracycline were determined by the Etest (BioMerieux AB, Solna, Sweden) on GC agar base (Difco GC agar base medium, Becton, Dickinson, Sparks, MD, USA) with 1 % BBL IsoVitalex Enrichment (Becton, Dickinson, Sparks, MD, USA), according to the instructions from the manufacturer. MICs were interpreted using breakpoints for resistance, intermediate susceptibility and susceptibility according to the Clinical and Laboratory Standards Institute (CLSI) [17]. For azithromycin, breakpoints are not available as per CLSI, accordingly, the MIC breakpoints from the European Committee on Antimicrobial Susceptibility Testing (EUCAST; www.eucast.org) were applied. For quality controls, as recommended by the CLSI the *N. gonorrhoeae* reference strain ATCC 49226 was included in each testing. In addition, the *N. gonorrhoeae* WHO *N. gonorrhoeae* reference strains C, F, G, K, L, M, N, O, and P [18] were used as quality controls. β-lactamase production was identified by a chromogenic cephalosporin method using nitrocefin reagent (Oxoid, Hampshire, UK).

Molecular epidemiological typing (NG-MAST)

Genomic DNA was isolated from cultured gonococcal isolates using the NorDiag Bullet robot (NorDiag ASA Company, Oslo, Norway) with BUGS'n BEADS STI-fast kit (NorDiag ASA Company, Oslo, Norway), according to the manufacturer's instructions. NG-MAST [13] was performed as previously described [19]. NG-MAST allele numbers of the more variable segments of *porB* and *tbpB*, and sequence types (STs) were evaluated using the NG-MAST website (www.ng-mast.net). NG-MAST genogroups, comprising the main ST plus genetically associated STs, were assigned as reported in past studies. Briefly, a genogroup was defined as all STs which shared one allele and exhibited >99 % homogeneity in the other allele (≤5 bp difference for *porB* and ≤4 bp for *tbpB*) [20].

Result

Patient characteristics

N. gonorrhoeae isolates were grown from 86 (86 %) males and 14 (14 %) females. The mean age for the males was 30 years (median age: 29 years; range: 1.3 to 55 years) and for the females 29 years (median age: 29 years; range: 5 to 47 years).

Antimicrobial susceptibility of *N. gonorrhoeae* isolates in 2012–2014 ($n = 100$) in Karachi, Pakistan

Summary of result of antimicrobial susceptibilities are given in Table 1.

During 2012–2014, all (100 %) isolates were susceptible to ceftriaxone, cefixime and spectinomycin, and 99 % susceptible to azithromycin, that is, only one isolate was resistant to azithromycin (MIC = 4 mg/L). Furthermore, all isolates had MICs < 0.016 mg/L and MICs ≤0.032 mg/L of cefixime and ceftriaxone, respectively. However, the pattern of resistance the levels of resistance to ciprofloxacin, tetracycline and penicillin G were high that is, 86 %, 51 % and 43 %, respectively (Table 1). The resistance to ciprofloxacin (75–100 %), tetracycline (42–50 %) and penicillin G (25–42 %) during 2012–2014 remained high. Nevertheless, the resistance to penicillin G decreased from 42 % to 25 %, which was due to the decrease of β-lactamase producing isolates in 2014 (Table 2).

Neisseria gonorrhoeae multiantigen sequence typing (NG-MAST)

In total, 94 (94 %) isolates could be successfully typed with NG-MAST. Remaining six (6 %) isolates were not revived due to contamination. Seventy-four different STs were identified and 62 STs (83.8 %) of these had not been previously described. The most prevalent STs were ST338 ($n = 3$ isolates), ST3328 ($n = 3$), ST10876 ($n = 3$), and ST10886 ($n = 3$). Twelve STs were represented by two isolates and 58 STs were represented by single isolates. In total, 36 *porB* alleles and 32 *tbpB* alleles were found. The most common *porB* alleles and *tbpB* alleles were *porB1173* (12 isolates), *porB90* ($n = 11$), *porB251* ($n = 11$), *tbpB136* ($n = 12$) and *tbpB121* ($n = 10$). ST338, ST3328 and ST10878 could be grouped in to the genogroup G338 ($n = 8$).

In Additional file 1: Table S1, the AMR of isolates assigned as the more prevalent NG-MAST STs is described. Out of the 74 identified STs, 33 (44 %) STs included *N. gonorrhoeae* isolates ($n = 36$) showing resistance to penicillin G, 43 (57 %) STs having resistance to tetracycline ($n = 44$), and 61 (81 %) STs displaying resistance to ciprofloxacin ($n = 73$). The only azithromycin resistant isolate (MIC = 4 mg/L) was assigned as ST8580.

Table 1 Antimicrobial susceptibility of *Neisseria gonorrhoeae* isolates ($n = 100$) in Karachi, Pakistan, 2012–2014

Antimicrobial	MIC range (mg/L)	MIC_{50} (mg/L)	MIC_{90} (mg/L)	S (%)	I (%)	R (%)
Ceftriaxone	0.002–0.032	0.008	0.016	100	0	0
Cefixime	<0.016	<0.016	<0.016	100	0	0
Spectinomycin	0.25–16	4	8	100	0	0
Azithromycin	0.016–4	0.094	0.25	99	-	1
Penicillin G	0.004–32	0.5	12	8	49	43
Tetracycline	0.12–96	3	24	12	37	51
Ciprofloxacin	0.25–32	4	14	0	14	86

MIC Minimum inhibitory concentration of an antibiotic necessary to inhibit the growth of a target organism, MIC_{90} Minimum inhibitory concentration of an antibiotic at which 90 % of the isolates were inhibited, MIC_{50} Minimum inhibitory concentration of an antibiotic at which 50 % of the isolates were inhibited, *S* Susceptibility; *I* Intermediate susceptibility, *R* Resistance

Discussion

This study showed that the susceptibility to ceftriaxone (100 %), cefixime (100 %), spectinomycin (100 %) and azithromycin (99 %) has remained high in Karachi, Pakistan. Accordingly, the results of the current study support using ceftriaxone as empiric treatment of choice in Pakistan for gonorrhoea, which has been recommended since year 2010 [12]. However, due to the increasing MICs of ceftriaxone and the emerging ceftriaxone resistance internationally the dose in Pakistan is recommended to be increased from 125 mg IM to at least 250 mg IM. Furthermore, because of increased resistance to ciprofloxacin (86 %) in Karachi it is important to exclude ciprofloxacin from the recommended first-line therapies. The reasons for the retained high susceptibility to ceftriaxone in Pakistan are unknown. This showed that gonococcal strain with decreased susceptibility to ESCs has neither been imported or if imported has not been successful to retain and establish local spread. However, it might also reflect that the ESCs resistance selection pressure has been low in gonococcal infections because ceftriaxone for therapy has only been recommended since 2010 (and instead ciprofloxacin was frequently used). In cases of ceftriaxone resistance, unavailability of ceftriaxone or severe β-lactam allergy, spectinomycin can be used as the second-line treatment. Azithromycin 2 g, should be added to the spectinomycin regimen in case of pharyngeal gonorrhoea, in accordance to European gonorrhea treatment guideline [21]. In current study, only one (1 %) azithromycin resistant isolate (ST8580) was found. Consequently, azithromycin remains effective against *N. gonorrhoeae* in Pakistan. However, due to the risk of selecting resistance (including high-level resistance) to azithromycin in *N. gonorrhoeae* [5], as well as in etiological agents of other sexually transmitted infections, this antimicrobial should mainly not be used in gonorrhoea monotherapy and, if it has to be used (e.g., due to severe β-lactam allergy or resistance or unavailability of ceftriaxone and spectinomycin), azithromycin 2 g single oral dose should be used. Instead, it is recommended in the US [22] and European [21] gonorrhoea treatment guidelines that azithromycin should be added to ceftriaxone in the recommended first-line regimen. These dual antimicrobial therapies can be recommended in settings where ceftriaxone resistance has been verified or has not been excluded. Combined antimicrobial therapy will not only successfully eliminate gonorrhoea but also *Chlamydia trachomatis* infections and many *M. genitalium* infections. High levels of resistance to ciprofloxacin (86 %), tetracycline (51 %) and penicillin G (43 %) were identified in Karachi, Pakistan. Because of increased resistance to these antibiotics locally and also in most other countries worldwide, none of them ought to be suggested for empirical therapy of choice of gonorrhea in Pakistan or internationally [2, 5, 8–11]. Worryingly, in Pakistan penicillins, tetracyclines, fluoroquinolones, and macrolides are still commonly used as treatment options for gonorrhoea and these antibiotics are easily accessible "over-the-counter". Due to this practice, it is crucial to substantially enhance the continuous monitoring of gonococcal AMR with a focus on emergence of resistance to ceftriaxone, spectinomycin and azithromycin, using MIC determination and also monitor treatment failures and gonococcal molecular epidemiological characteristics in Pakistan. It is therefore recommended to evaluate AMR annually with representation from more cities or

Table 2 Percentage (%) of antimicrobial resistance and β-lactamase production in *Neisseria gonorrhoeae* isolates ($n = 100$) obtained in Karachi, Pakistan, separated in 2012, 2013 and 2014

Antimicrobial	2012 ($n = 48$)	2013 ($n = 40$)	2014 ($n = 12$)
Ceftriaxone	0	0	0
Cefixime	0	0	0
Spectinomycin	0	0	0
Azithromycin	2	0	0
Penicillin G	42	42	25
Tetracycline	50	45	42
Ciprofloxacin	75	88	100
β-lactamase production	42	40	25

regions to generate national data. It is also imperative to associate AMR to epidemiological data for development of effective control and prevention strategies. Consequently, financial assurance or support, both national and international, is crucial to emphasize continuous monitoring. The political commitment of the country leadership to curtail AMR in Pakistan and other countries in the WHO EMR will also be required.

NG-MAST has been used as a standard technique to evaluate clonal spread of gonococcal strains within high risk populations and to relate therapeutic failure with dissemination of particular strain types [14]. In the present study, 74 different NG-MAST STs among 94 isolates were identified. The high number of STs represented by only one isolate ($n = 58$) and STs that have not been previously described (62 novel STs) make the results hard to value. These results may be associated with the large catchment area, poor diagnostic capabilities in laboratories, lack sexual contacts tracing, and evolution of STs in Pakistan. Nevertheless, some NG-MAST ST clusters identified, e.g. G338 ($n = 8$), were associated with resistance to all three of the previously used antimicrobials ciprofloxacin, penicillin G and tetracycline. The successful ST1407 clone or genetically closely related STs belonging to genogroup 1407 associated with cefixime and ceftriaxone treatment failure internationally [5, 6], were not found in the present study.

The present study was performed on small number of strains which were collected as per physicians request and the researchers had no main control over patient selection. Therefore the results could not be generalized to the entire population. Additionally clinical data was not available from the patients to evaluate risk factors and treatment response. Despite these limitations, the results of this study are exceedingly important and will provide a baseline for future studies.

Conclusions

A highly diversified gonococcal population, 74 NG-MAST STs ($n = 62$ novel STs) identified, with a high resistance to ciprofloxacin, penicillin G and tetracycline circulated in Karachi, Pakistan. Fortunately, no resistance to ceftriaxone was detected and ceftriaxone can continuously be recommended as the drug of choice. However it is recommended to increase the dose of ceftriaxone from 125 mg intramuscularly to 250 mg intramuscularly due to ceftriaxone MIC creep and emerging resistance reported in the region. Furthermore, due to the high resistance to ciprofloxacin (86 %) in Karachi it is essential to exclude ciprofloxacin from the recommended first-line therapies. It is important to emphasize the continuous monitoring of gonococcal AMR and investigate therapeutic failure in patients from other regions of Pakistan.

Abbreviations

AKU, Aga Khan University; AMR, antimicrobial resistance; CLSI, Clinical and Laboratory Standards Institute; ESCs, extended-spectrum cephalosporins; EUCAST, European Committee on Antimicrobial Susceptibility Testing; GASP, gonococcal antimicrobial surveillance programme; MIC, minimum inhibitory concentration; NG-MAST, *N. gonorrhoeae* multiantigen sequence typing; WHO EMR, WHO Eastern Mediterranean Region; WHO, World Health Organization

Acknowledgements

The laboratory work was supported by the Örebro County Council Research Committee and the Foundation for Medical Research at Örebro University Hospital, Sweden.

Funding

The laboratory work was funded by the Örebro County Council Research Committee and the Foundation for Medical Research at Örebro University Hospital, Sweden.

Authors' contributions

KJ, SJ and MU designed, initiated and coordinated the study. KJ, PB, EK, SC, SJ and MU coordinated and performed all the laboratory analyses. KJ and MU analysed and interpreted all the data, and wrote a first draft of the paper. All authors read, commented and approved the final manuscript.

Competing interests

The authors declare that they have no competing interests.

Consent for publication

Not applicable.

Author details

[1]Department of Pathology and Laboratory Medicine, Aga Khan University, Stadium Road, Karachi, Pakistan. [2]WHO Collaborating Centre for Gonorrhoea and Other STIs, National Reference Laboratory for Pathogenic Neisseria, Department of Laboratory Medicine, Microbiology, Faculty of Medicine and Health, Örebro University, Örebro, Sweden.

References

1. Newman L, Rowley J, Vander Hoorn S, Wijesooriya NS, Unemo M, Low N, et al. Global estimates of the prevalence and incidence of four curable sexually transmitted infections in 2012 based on systematic review and global reporting. PLoS One. 2015;10:e0143304.
2. World Health Organization (WHO). Department of Reproductive Health and Research: Global action plan to control the spread and impact of antimicrobial resistance in *Neisseria gonorrhoeae*. Geneva: WHO; 2012. p. 1–36.
3. Centers for Disease Control and Prevention. Sexually Transmitted Disease Surveillance, 2014. Gonorrhea statistics. Available at: http://www.cdc.gov/std/gonorrhea/stats.htm
4. Chen SC, Yin YP, Dai XQ, Unemo M, Chen XS. First nationwide study regarding ceftriaxone resistance and molecular epidemiology of *Neisseria gonorrhoeae* in China. J Antimicrob Chemother. 2016;71:92–9.
5. Unemo M, Shafer WM. Antimicrobial resistance in *Neisseria gonorrhoeae* in the 21st Century: past, evolution, and future. Clin Microbiol Rev. 2014;27:587–613.
6. Unemo M, Nicholas RA. Emergence of multidrug-resistant, extensively drug-resistant and untreatable gonorrhea. Future Microbiol. 2012;7:1401–22.
7. Ndowa F, Lusti-Narasimhan M, Unemo M. The serious threat of multidrug-resistant and untreatable gonorrhoea: the pressing need for global action to control the spread of antimicrobial resistance, and mitigate the impact on sexual and reproductive health. Sex Transm Infect. 2012;88:317–8.
8. Unemo M, Ison CA, Cole M, Spiteri G, Van de Laar M, Khotenashvili L. Gonorrhoea and gonococcal antimicrobial resistance surveillance networks in the WHO European Region, including the independent countries of the former Soviet Union. Sex Transm Infect. 2013;89 Suppl 4:iv42–6.

9. Ndowa FJ, Francis JM, Machiha A, Faye-Kette H, Fonkoua MC. Gonococcal antimicrobial resistance: perspectives from the African region. Sex Transm Infect. 2013;89 Suppl 4:iv11–5.
10. Zafar A, Jabeen K. Antimicrobial resistance in *Neisseria gonorrhoeae* and limited treatment options. J Pak Med Assoc. 2007;57:333–4.
11. Nizamuddin S, Jabeen K, Zafar A. Evaluation of predominant *Neisseria gonorrhoeae* strain types and its correlation with fluoroquinolone resistance in Pakistan. J Pak Med Assoc. 2011;61(5):446-9.
12. Medical Microbiology & Infectious Disease society of Pakistan. http://www.mmidsp.com/wp-content/uploads/2012/06/Guidelines-for-Antimicrobial-Use-2.pdf
13. Martin IM, Ison CA, Aanensen DM, Fenton KA, Spratt BG. Rapid sequence-based identification of gonococcal transmission clusters in a large metropolitan area. J Infect Dis. 2004;189:1497–505.
14. Unemo M, Dillon JA. Review and international recommendation of methods for typing *Neisseria gonorrhoeae* isolates and their implications for improved knowledge of gonococcal epidemiology, treatment, and biology. Clin Microbiol Rev. 2011;24:447–58.
15. Sexually Transmitted Infections and HIV Among People With High Risk Behaviours: Results of Behavioural and Biological Surveys in Rawalpindi and Abbottabad, Pakistan. London School of Hygiene & Tropical Medicine. 2008.
16. Sethi S, Golparian D, Bala M, Dorji D, Ibrahim M, Jabeen K, et al. Antimicrobial susceptibility and genetic characteristics of *Neisseria gonorrhoeae* isolates from India, Pakistan and Bhutan in 2007–2011. BMC Infect Dis. 2013;13:35.
17. Clinical and Laboratory Standards Institute. Performance standards for antimicrobial susceptibility testing; 24th informational supplement. CLSI document M100-S24. Wayne: Clinical and Laboratory Standards Institute; 2014.
18. Unemo M, Fasth O, Fredlund H, Limnios A, Tapsall J. Phenotypic and genetic characterization of the 2008 WHO *Neisseria gonorrhoeae* reference strain panel intended for global quality assurance and quality control of gonococcal antimicrobial resistance surveillance for public health purposes. J Antimicrob Chemother. 2009;63:1142–51.
19. Unemo M, Sjöstrand A, Akhras M, Gharizadeh B, Lindbäck E, Pourmand N, et al. Molecular characterization of *Neisseria gonorrhoeae* identifies transmission and resistance of one ciprofloxacin-resistant strain. APMIS. 2007;115:231–41.
20. Chisholm SA, Unemo M, Quaye N, Johansson E, Cole MJ, Ison CA, Van de Laar MJ. Molecular epidemiological typing within the European Gonococcal Antimicrobial Resistance Surveillance Programme reveals predominance of a multidrug-resistant clone. Euro Surveill. 2013;18:20358.
21. Bignell C, Unemo M, on behalf of the European STI Guidelines Editorial Board. European guideline on the diagnosis and treatment of gonorrhoea in adults. Int J STD AIDS. 2013;24:85–92.
22. Workowski KA, Bolan GA. Sexually transmitted diseases treatment guidelines, 2015. MMWR Recomm Rep. 2015;64(RR-03):1–137.

17

Effect of previous test results, age group and reason for testing on (re-)infection with Chlamydia trachomatis in Germany

Alexandra Sarah Lang[1*], Matthias an der Heiden[1], Klaus Jansen[1], Andrea Sailer[1], Viviane Bremer[1], Sandra Dudareva[1,2], Chlamydia trachomatis laboratory sentinel team

Abstract

Background: Infection with *Chlamydia trachomatis* (Ct) is the most commonly reported sexually transmitted infection in Europe. In Germany, Ct screening is offered free of charge to pregnant women since 1995 and to women < 25 years of age since 2008. For symptomatic individuals, testing is covered by statutory health insurance. Study results have shown that repeat Ct infection occurs in 10–20% of previously infected women and men. Our aim was to describe persons tested for Ct and to investigate the determinants of (repeat) Ct infection in women and men in Germany.

Methods: We analysed Ct test results from men and women tested between 2008 and 2014 in laboratories participating in the German *Chlamydia trachomatis Laboratory Sentinel surveillance*. Reinfection was defined as at least 2 positive laboratory tests within more than 30 days. We performed logistic regression stratified by sex and, for women, reason for testing to determine the effect of previous test results and age group on subsequent test results.

Results: In total, 2,574,635 Ct tests could be attributed to 1,815,494 women and 123,033 men. 5% of women and 14% of men tested positive at least once. 15–19- and 20–24-year-old women tested positive at least once respectively in 6.8 and 6.0%, while men respectively in 16.6 and 21.2%. Altogether, 23.1% of tested women and 11.9% of tested men were tested repeatedly between 2008 and 2014. Among those who previously tested positive, reinfection occurred in 2.0% of women and 6.6% of men. Likelihood to be tested Ct positive was higher in women and men with a positive Ct test in the past compared to previously tested Ct negative, odds ratios 4.7 and 2.6 ($p < 0.01$) respectively. Odds ratios ranged by age group and test reason.

Conclusion: A history of Ct infection increased the likelihood of infection with Ct in women and men taking into account the result of the previous test. Health education, safer sex and treatment of partners are necessary for women and men who have tested positive to prevent reinfection and complications and to interrupt the chain of transmission. To identify potential reinfection repeat testing after treatment should be performed.

Keywords: Chlamydia trachomatis, Sexually transmitted infections, STI, Reinfection, Screening, Infertility, Sentinel

* Correspondence: LangAl@rki.de
[1]Department for Infectious Disease Epidemiology, Robert Koch Institute, Berlin, Germany
Full list of author information is available at the end of the article

Background

Infection with *Chlamydia trachomatis* (Ct) is the most commonly reported sexually transmitted infection (STI) in Europe [1]. According to data of the European Center for Disease prevention and control (ECDC), young people are particularly affected, with two-thirds (67%) of the 384,555 reported cases in 2013 diagnosed amongst 15 to 24-year-olds [2]. This is however strongly influenced by testing practices in reporting countries [2]. In contrast to other STIs, Ct infection is very common in the general population with prevalence ranging from 3.0 to 5.3% among women 18–26-years old and 2.4–7.3% among men 18–26 years old [3]. Population-based estimations for Germany showed prevalence of 4.4% for sexually active 17-year-olds, 4.5% for 18- to 19-year-old women and 4.9% for 25- to 29-year-old men [4]. Overall, women aged 20 to 24 years are the group most frequently diagnosed with Ct [5, 6]. The most consistent risk factors associated with Ct infection in other studies are young age and a high number of sexual partners [5, 7–9].

Ct causes infection in the lower genital tract. Untreated infected women may suffer from ascending infection, which can lead to complications such as chronic pain, inflammation and occlusion of the fallopian tubes, which may result in infertility and ectopic pregnancy [10, 11]. Ct increases the susceptibility and transmission of HIV-infection [12]. The infection is asymptomatic in up to 50% of women and 80% of men or may only display mild symptoms. Therefore, Ct infection often remains unnoticed and undiagnosed, and thus untreated [13].

Because of the considerable burden of Ct infection and its sequelae, particularly in young women, many countries have implemented Ct-related public health activities to enhance detection and to prevent negative consequences by treating infected individuals as soon as possible. Approximately half of the European countries offer opportunistic testing as a measure for Ct control. Only a few countries have a systematic approach with standard guidance for treatment and repeated testing [14]; however, there are guidelines on the management of Ct infection available for Europe [15]. Germany published a guideline in 2016 to enable optimal diagnostics and therapy of Ct [16]. In Germany, opportunistic screening has been offered free of charge for statutory insured pregnant women since 1995 and once annually for statutory insured sexually active women under 25 years of age since 2008. Currently, tests for men are refunded by statutory health insurance if carried out for diagnostic purposes, i.e. suspect infection based on symptoms or anamnesis. There is no screening program for men in Germany. There are no regulations for the contract tracing in Germany and usually it is performed. With the aim of gathering representative data on Ct tests, the Robert Koch-Institute (RKI) established a voluntary nationwide, laboratory-based Ct surveillance system, the 'Ct laboratory sentinel', in 2010 that accompanied the implementation of the Ct screening programme for women under 25 years old. Information on routine Ct-testing in combination with test results, reason for testing and patient-related information were collected from 24 microbiological laboratories in Germany offering Ct-diagnostics. The Ct laboratory sentinel covers 34% of all Ct tests performed in Germany. Study results based on the sentinel data found an overall positive result rate of 3.9% amongst women and 11.0% amongst men of all age groups [17]. Reinfection with Ct is possible and increases the likelihood of complications and future acquisition and transmission of the disease [18]. Based on international studies it was estimated that 13.9% of women and 11.3% of men have repeatedly been infected with Ct [19, 20] .

The association of previous infections, age and test reason on reinfection have not yet been analysed yet in Germany. The main aims of this study were to gather evidence on whether current infection was more frequent in women and men who had tested positive previously compared to those who had tested negative previously and, furthermore, to identify whether the age group and, for women, the reason for testing, along with previous test results, influences the result of a subsequent test. Our findings will contribute to identify special risk groups for Ct who are in need of health education and to generate evidence for targeted Ct testing programmes.

Methods

The study population was composed of women and men who were tested for Ct in Germany between January 1, 2008 and December 31, 2014 and whose assays were tested in one of the laboratories participating in the Ct Laboratory Sentinel that provided traceable patient-IDs for a minimum of 3 years. The patient-IDs consisted of an encrypted 32-digit hash code. If patients were tested more than once within the same laboratory, data from several samples could be assigned by this unique identifier to one patient [16].

The following variables were used for analysis: patient-ID, assay-ID, laboratory code, testing date, age, sex, test result and test reason.

If information on sex or age was missing for some of the assays with the same patient-ID, the missing values were replaced by the information on sex and birth date available from the other assays. If sex was missing in all assays with the same patient-ID, these assays were excluded from analysis.

Multiple assays with the same patient-ID that were examined on the same day or within 7 consecutive days were considered as only one test. In this case, the test result was recorded as positive if at least one assay tested positive and recorded as negative if all assays were negative. The decision to summarize multiple assays was based on information regarding the time difference between the date when the sample was taken (available for 26% of all assays in the sample) and the date of testing. Assays taken the same day by the physician were tested within 7 days. Thus, multiple assays (such as vaginal and rectal swabs) belonging to the same test-event might have been tested in the laboratory on different days.

Assays with missing information on the test result were excluded from analysis. Assays with missing information on age group or reason for testing were kept in the analysis.

The nucleic acid amplification test (NAAT) that is predominantly used in Germany for Ct testing is very sensitive and can still be detected 3 weeks after therapy even though the pathogen is no longer vital [21, 22]. Thus, we included only those tests with a time interval of at least 30 days from the preceding test in the analysis. Reinfection was consequently defined as at least 2 positive laboratory tests within a time interval of more than 30 days, following the definition of Brunham et al. [23] and the European Guideline for the management of Ct which recommends a test of cure 4 weeks after completion of therapy [15].

We described the number and proportions of performed Ct tests, the number of tested persons and the number of tests per person by sex, age group, reason for testing and test result. Among repeat testers we calculated median time between Ct tests by initial and subsequent test result. "Initial test result" is defined as the first Ct test that we have captured in the sentinel, however, this might not be the first test of the individual.

We tested the association between the variables *previous test result* and *age group* and the outcome variable *test result* by using logistic regression. Because of the large sample size a *p*-value less than alpha = 0.01 was considered significant in all calculations. We included only tests from women and men at least 15 years old. Separate models were calculated for men and women, and for women, the analysis was additionally stratified according to the reason for testing. The persons tested only once in the surveillance period contribute to the calculation of the proportion tested positive. To include these persons into regression analysis, we defined the variable *previous test result* as "unknown" as this group is mixture of those previously never tested and those tested positive or negative. The stratified univariable analysis was compared to the results of a multivariable logistic regression model. We tested improved goodness of fit by using likelihood ratio tests (LRTs), and we calculated odds ratios (OR), probabilities (Pr), and the according 99% confidence intervals. Including the interaction in a model with two variables means that every combination of age group and previous test result was estimated separately. Since the result is a single odds it can directly be transformed into a probability ($P = O/(O + 1)$). We chose to present the probabilities, since for most people this is the more familiar measure. This implied that the probability of a positive test result had to be estimated separately in all strata. The data were extracted from an SQL dataset and analysed using STATA 14.

Results

Study population

General characteristics of Ct testing in Germany

During 2008–2014, 3,877,589 Ct tests were reported. Of those, 2,574,635 tests were analysed, including 2,429,942 in women and 144,693 in men (Fig. 1). These tests could be attributed to 1,815,494 women and 123,033 men. The median age at the first Ct test was 26 years in women (IQR: 22–32) and 33 years (IQR: 25–43) in men. Note that this might not be the first test of the individual. In women, most tests (45.0%) were performed because of screening in pregnancy, followed by screening under 25 years (27.9%) and diagnostic testing (27.2%). The median age at the time of the first positive test was 22 years for women (IQR: 19–25) and 28 years for men (IQR: 23–36). Number of Ct tests and proportion of positive Ct tests by reason of testing and age group among women and men is given in Table 1.

Altogether, 23.1% ($n = 420,220$) of tested women and 11.9% ($n = 14,680$) of tested men were tested more than once during the 7-year-surveillance period. Most of those were tested twice (69.5% of women and 73.6% of men). While 20.1 and 10.4% of women and 16.4 and 10.0% of men were tested 3 and 4 or more times, respectively.

Amongst women and men tested more than once 13.6% ($n = 57,133$) and 34.6% ($n = 5073$) respectively had at least one positive Ct test. In women and men, the median time until the date of the subsequent test was shorter if the previous test was positive (Table 2).

Overall, in 0.5% ($n = 8369$) of women and in 0.8% ($n = 963$) of men in all the tested men and women reinfection was detected. Amongst repeatedly tested women and men, reinfection was detected in 2.0 and 6.6%, respectively. The median time from the first to the second positive test (reinfection) was 4.2 months in women (IQR: 2.1–13.0) and 6.7 months in men (IQR: 2.3–16.6).

Uni- and multivariable analysis

In the univariable logistic regression, the variables *age group* and *previous test result* were significantly associated with a positive result in a subsequent test (for detailed results of univariable analysis for women see Additional file 1: Table S1). A multivariable logistic regression model including the variables *age group* and *previous test result*

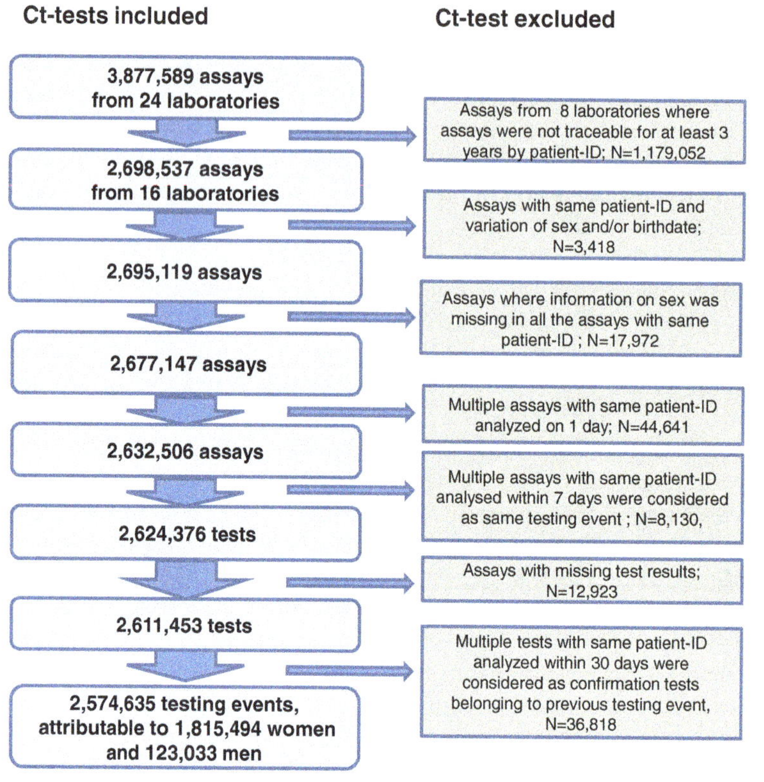

Fig. 1 Flowchart of sample selection

Table 1 Number of Ct tests and proportion of positive Ct tests by reason of testing and age group among women and men, 2008–2014, *n* = 2,574,635

	Women		Men	
	Number (Proportion in %)	Proportion Ct positive in %	Number (Proportion in %)	Proportion Ct positive in %
Tests				
Total	2,429,942 (100)	4.0	144,693 (100)	12.4
Reason for testing (tests)				
Screening under 25 years	571,054 (23.5)	5.0	n. a.	n. a.
Screening in pregnancy	920,133 (37.9)	2.5	n. a.	n. a.
Diagnostic testing	555,853 (22.9)	4.6	144,693 (100)	12.4
Unknown	382,902 (15.8)	5.1	n. a.	n. a.
Age group (tests)				
0–15 years	13,106 (0.5)	3.4	1048 (0.7)	3.0
15–19 years	342,892 (14.1)	6.8	6634 (4.6)	16.6
20–24 years	736,040 (30.3)	6.0	24,545 (17.0)	21.2
25–29 years	494,432 (20.4)	3.3	24,924 (17.2)	17.1
30–34 years	445,559 (18.3)	1.6	21,165 (14.6)	12.1
35–39 years	238,306 (9.8)	1.2	17,211 (11.9)	9.3
40+ years	157,824 (6.5)	1.3	46,868 (32.6)	5.7
Unknown	1783 (0.1)	5.1	2298 (1.6)	7.7

Table 2 Median time interval until subsequent test in women and men stratified by previous test result, 2008–2014, $n = 1{,}074{,}430$

Time interval until subsequent test	Women Median time in months (IQR)	Men Median time in months (IQR)
Negative test	15.5 (IQR: 9.4–25.6)	7.4 (IQR: 3.1–15.2)
Positive test	3.0 (IQR: 1.7–8.9)	2.8 (IQR: 1.5–8.1).

showed that their interaction had a significant effect (Likelihood-Ratio-Test: $p < 0.01$). In regard to the probability of a positive test result, a similar result was reported in women for each test reason. Women and men of all age groups who had previously tested positive showed a higher probability of testing positive compared to their peers who had previously tested negative. The estimated probabilities for women and men are shown in Table 3 and Figs. 2, 3 and 4. A different presentation of the results for women and men in odds ratios can be found in Additional file 2: Figure S1 and Additional file 3: Figure S2.

In women who were tested in the frame of screening programmes (Table 3, Fig. 2), the probability to test positive generally decreased with increasing age. The proportion of previously positive pregnant women testing positive again was highest amongst the 15–19 and 20–24-year-olds. However, the difference in regard to the previous test result was most pronounced in pregnant women in older age groups. Previously positive tested women aged 35–39 years were 21.1 times and women aged 40+ 20.5 times more likely to test positive compared to their previously negative tested peers.

Amongst diagnostic tests the probability to test positive was highest in the age groups 15–19 and 20–24 years in women who had previously tested positive. Overall, the probability to test positive decreased with increasing age, regardless of the previous test result. We observed a slight increase in the probability of a positive test result in the group of previously positive 35- to 39-year-olds. The difference between women who had previously tested positive and their previously negative tested peers was most pronounced in the age groups 35–39 and 40+ years (OR: 7.1 and 5.4, respectively).

The probability to test positive in men (Table 3, Fig. 4) was highest amongst 15–19 and 20- to 24-year-olds who had previously tested positive. The probability to test positive decreased with increasing age; however, amongst men who had previously tested positive, we observed a slight increase in the age group 40+. The difference between previously positive and previously negative tested men was most distinct in the age groups 35–39 and 40+ years (OR: 2.6 and 2.8, respectively).

Table 3 Probability (Pr) of positive test result by previous test result and age group among women according to reason for testing and men, 2008–2014

Previous test result	Age group, years	Pr to test positive in % (99%-CI)			
		Women			Men
		Screening under 25 years	Screening in pregnancy	Diagnostic testing	All tests
Negative	15–19	4.3 (4.1–4.6)	6.5 (6.0–8.1)	5.3 (4.8–5.8)	9.2 (5.9–14.1)
	20–24	3.4 (3.2–3.5)	3.0 (2.9–3.4)	4.6 (4.3–4.9)	10.7 (9.0–12.6)
	25–29	–	1.1 (1.0–1.3)	3.1 (2.9–3.4)	9.5 (8.0–11.2)
	30–34	–	0.4 (0.4–0.5)	1.6 (1.4–1.9)	7.8 (6.5–9.3)
	35–39	–	0.3 (0.2–0.4)	1.2 (1.0–1.5)	6.4 (5.2–7.9)
	40+	–	0.3 (0.1–0.6)	1.1 (0.9–1.3)	5.5 (4.8–6.3)
Positive	15–19	12.6 (11.3–14.0)	28.4 (34.3–45.7)	16.8 (15.7–18.1)	18.6 (12.7–26.4)
	20–24	9.8 (9.1–10.4)	18.5 (20.6–24.9)	12.7 (12.0–13.4)	19.2 (16.7–22.0)
	25–29	–	10.4 (10.0–13.3	10.1 (9.2–11.0)	16.6 (14.3–19.3)
	30–34	–	7.9 (6.8–10.8)	7.1 (6.0–8.4)	16.4 (13.8–19.5)
	35–39	–	6.4 (4.3–10.7)	8.8 (6.9–11.0)	15.4 (12.3–19.1)
	40+	–	5.9 (2.3–17.2)	5.9 (4.3–8.1)	16.9 (14.7–19.4)
Unknown	15–19	4.9 (4.7–5.0)	9.7 (10.2–11.3)	8.1 (7.7–8.4)	16.9 (15.7–18.2)
	20–24	5.7 (5.6–5.8)	5.8 (6.0–6.4)	8.3 (8.0–8.6)	22.3 (21.6–23.1)
	25–29	–	2.2 (2.1–2.3)	5.1 (5.0–5.3)	18.0 (17.3–18.7)
	30–34	–	1.1 (1.0–1.1)	2.9 (2.7–3.0)	12.4 (11.8–13.1)
	35–39	–	0.7 (0.6–0.8)	1.9 (1.8–2.1)	9.4 (8.8–10.1)
	40+	–	0.6 (0.5–0.8)	1.6 (1.5–1.7)	6.1 (5.8–6.4)

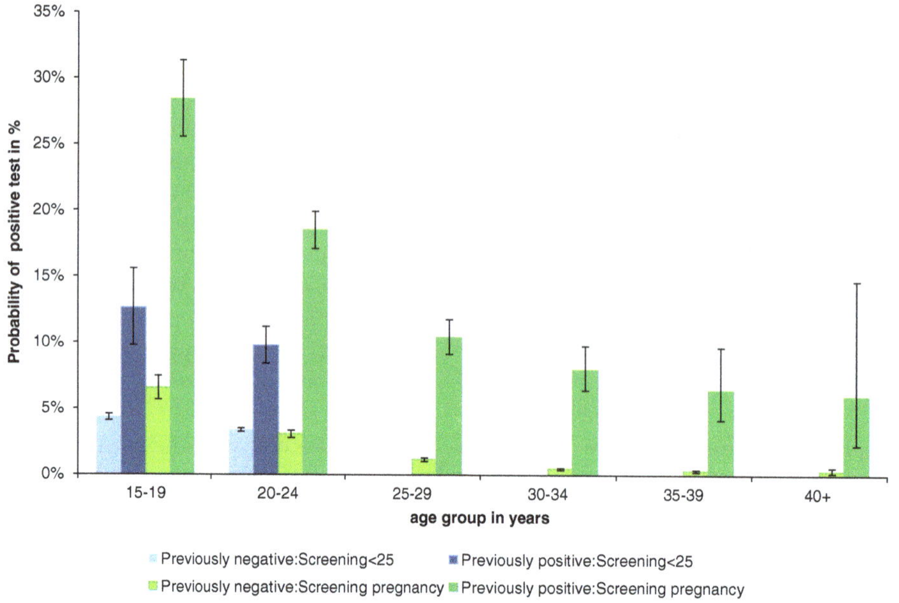

Fig. 2 Probability and 99%-CI of positive test results according to age group and previous test results in women tested in the frame of screening programmes by age group, 2008–2014

Discussion

To our best knowledge, this was the first German study using a comparably large dataset of routine Ct tests to examine the likelihood of infection while taking into account the result of the previous test.

The likelihood of being diagnosed with Ct differed based on the reason for testing and age in women. In particular, young pregnant women who had a history of Ct infection were at a high risk to test positive. As in Germany the mean age of women at the time of the birth of their first child was 29.3 years in 2015 [26], it is possible that many pregnancies in the age group 15–19 years were unwanted and screening for Ct has been carried out in the context of an abortion and can be related to behaviour with higher risk to acquire a STI as discussed before [17].

The proportion of positive tests was considerably higher in men compared to women.

This can be explained by the fact that men are usually tested because of symptoms or anamnestic reasons. Furthermore, past analysis of the Ct laboratory sentinel showed

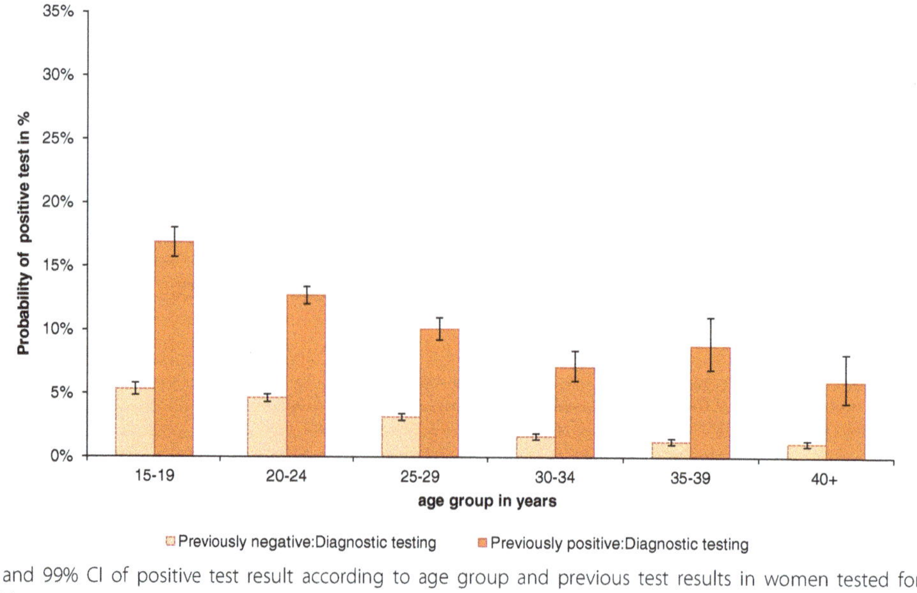

Fig. 3 Probability and 99% CI of positive test result according to age group and previous test results in women tested for diagnostic reasons, 2008–2014

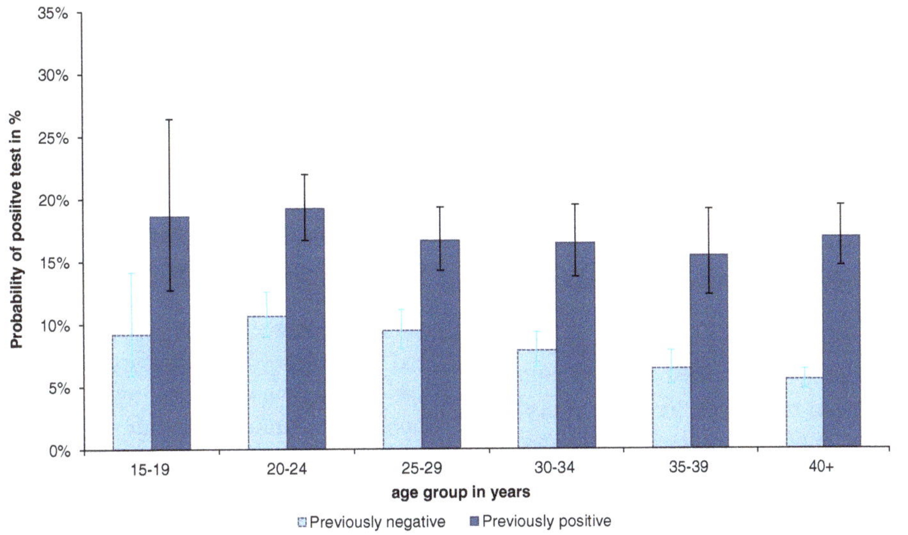

Fig. 4 Probability and 99% CI of positive test result according to age group and previous test results in men, 2008–2014

that a substantial proportion of tested material is rectal swabs [27] . Based on previous national and international studies, it is known that the proportion of positive tests is higher among MSM than heterosexual men [13, 29]. This aspect might have influenced the data we observe.

Less than one fourth of all tested women and men were tested repeatedly during the study period. Because screening for women < 25 years of age should be performed annually, and women can also be tested because of screening in pregnancy and for diagnostic reasons, we expected higher proportion of repeatedly tested women. The small proportion of repeatedly tested women suggests that screening programmes might not be sufficiently implemented in Germany yet. To tackle insufficient coverage of the existing screening programs, the Federal Agency for Health Education (BZgA) designed an information campaign and information materials on chlamydia screening for physicians and attendees of medical praxes, in addition to an ongoing poster campaign on STIs and corresponding symptoms [28].

In all age groups and regardless of the reason for testing, women and men with prior Ct infection had a high probability to be tested positive for Ct (women: Pr: 5.9–28.4%, men: Pr: 15.4–19.2%). The probability of reinfection varied substantially among women by age and test reason with highest probabilities in young women, especially if tested within screening in pregnancy. Studies have shown that early first intercourse was associated with subsequent sexual risk behavior [9, 24] which also leads to a higher probability of acquiring an STI. We observed less age-related variation for reinfection among men, though younger men had a higher probability for reinfection. We believe that this might be related to a mixed population of men in our data set. The group that repeatedly tested positive might be more at risk of infection, for example HIV positive MSM. Bacterial STI are more common in HIV positive MSM [13, 30]. However, we lack data in current study to analyse this in more detail. Additionally, the detection rate of STI, especially asymptomatic infections, among men frequently accessing testing might be higher.

Currently, evidence remains insufficient to recommend routine Ct-screening for all sexually active young men in Germany, partially because men rarely develop sequelae [31]. Nonetheless, the benefit of a screening programme for high-risk populations of men has been supported, for example Gift et al. found that Ct-screening programme targeting high-risk men was cost-saving compared to programme expanding screening of lower-risk women [32].

Interestingly, previously positive tested women and men in the older age groups showed the highest odds ratios to test positive; women especially when screened in pregnancy. This finding could indicate that these women and men aged 30 years and older with repeat infection, may represent a small group with ongoing sexual risk behavior that is thus more likely to contract repeat infection than their previously negative tested peers. Nevertheless, the absolute risk differences (in percent points) between previously positive and previously negative tested women and men by age group are much higher in the young age groups. The increased probability of infection for women and men with a history of Ct infection has been found by several other studies. In a study population of adolescent girls, Batteiger et al. found that incident Ct infections occurred in 78.1% of participants with infections at baseline compared to 51.7% of participants without infection at baseline [33]. The results of Dunne et al. showed a 1.2-fold risk for men with previous Ct infection amongst men screened for Ct infection [34], whereas Rietmejer et al. found a 2.4-fold increased risk of reinfection for women and men with Ct infection at baseline amongst female and male patients of an STI clinic [25]. However, because of wide variations amongst the definitions of reinfection, the study designs and the composition of study populations, it is difficult to compare these numbers directly to our results.

Untreated infections of current partners and unprotected sex with new partners contribute to repeated infections [17, 35]. Although treatment with antibiotics is highly effective [33], a small proportion of alleged reinfection might be ongoing infections after treatment failure or insufficient adherence to treatment. Several studies have shown that persons with prior Ct infection were at a high risk of reinfection [9, 20, 25, 33, 34]. However, a link between previously diagnosed and treated Ct infections and the development of immunity against Ct has also been discussed [23].

The testing interval was considerably shorter if a previous Ct test was positive. A median time to repeat testing after a positive test result of approximately 3 months might indicate compliance to European guideline that recommends repeat testing in women and men < 25 years of age within 3 to 6 months after a positive Ct test result [15]. Additionally, test of cure is recommended for pregnant women, if symptoms persist, if non-compliance is suspected or if second- and third-line treatments have been used [15]. However, the median time to the reinfection depends largely on the testing patterns and cannot directly be related to the natural history of infection.

The relatively small proportion of persons with reinfection we found in our whole sample was likely a consequence of the small proportion of repeatedly tested persons in our sample. While among those tested repeatedly during the study period, the reinfection was observed in 2% of women and 6.5% of men. The median time to reinfection was 4.2 month in women and 6.7 months in men. Similar to our results, studies from the United States and Australia have found a median time to reinfection of 5.2 months amongst 19-year-old women [29] and of 4.6 months amongst women aged 16 to 25 years [9]. The treatment failure can still be observed 7–8 weeks after antibiotic treatment. Therefore, it is important to be able to distinguishing between actual reinfection with Ct and treatment failure [36]. As we have no information on treatment and detailed follow up data, we cannot distinguish between treatment failure and reinfection. Therefore, our approach to define a reinfection as each infection that occurs after a 30 days period is sensitive and potentially misclassifies those with treatment failure. In a sensitivity analysis, where we defined a reinfection as a subsequent positive test occurring after 42 days, we observed a reinfection in 1.9% (instead of 2.0%) of repeatedly tested women and in 6.4% (instead of 6.6%) of repeatedly tested men. With this approach, it is probable that some of the true reinfections are misclassified treatment failures.

Limitations

First, because several samples of a person only received the same patient-ID if tested in the same laboratory, the true number and proportion of reinfection in the study population may have been underestimated. If samples of one person were sent to different laboratories, e.g., because someone changed physician or the physician changed the diagnosing laboratory, these persons were either lost to follow-up or their tests were sampled in the Ct laboratory sentinel again, but with a new patient-ID. However, we expect that the proportion of previously tested persons having received a new patient-ID represents only a small fraction of the analysed tests.

Another limitation is that the *Ct laboratory sentinel* dataset offers no information on whether a person who tested positive received therapy and whether the treatment was successful. Thus, ongoing Ct-infections due to non-compliance or treatment failure could have been falsely classified as reinfection in this study. Furthermore, there is no information on behavioural factors that may influence the likelihood to be tested positive.

Finally, the Ct Laboratory Sentinel data might lack representativeness for the target population in Germany, even though the sentinel generally reached a good coverage in the period 2008–2014 and it was possible to collect a large number of samples representing one third of all performed Ct tests in Germany [17]. Still, the participation of laboratories was voluntary and it is unclear whether participating laboratories differed systematically from the non-participating laboratories, e. g. in terms of tested population. Data from the laboratories with continuous follow-up for at least 3 years used in current analysis did not substantially differ from rest of the participating laboratories regarding distribution of sex, age and proportion tested positive.

Conclusions

We describe how history of Ct infection increased the likelihood of infection with Ct in women and men, taking into account age and reason for testing (in women). This helps to identify groups in need of health education and generates evidence for a more targeted testing strategy.

The high proportion of positive tests and of reinfection found amongst men supports risk-based screening of sexually active young men. However, future studies must determine all potential risk factors and identify the categories of transmission in men to identify for which group Ct screening is most beneficial.

We recommend that women and men who have been diagnosed positive with Ct should be consulted on prevention, symptoms and possible consequences of Ct infection to avoid reinfection.

To identify potential reinfection – and persisting infection – repeat testing after treatment should be performed. To increase the number of those getting tested, preventive measures for young women and men like awareness campaigns on Ct infection and testing opportunities as well as sex education in schools should be implemented. Till now, preventional campaigns for Ct in Germany do not address a higher risk for infection of persons who were tested positive before specifically. On basis of our data, we recommend to adjust the respective materials to emphasize this. Awareness about Ct infection, increased risk of reinfection for person tested Ct positive before, and adaequate screening should also be raised amongst physicians and gynaecologists to enhance the coverage of the screening programmes. Further studies are necessary to examine whether these measures show the desired effect.

Abbreviations

CDC: Centers for Disease Control and Prevention; Ct: Chlamydia trachomatis; ECDC: European Center for Disease Control and Prevention; LRT: Likelihood ratio test; MSM: Men having sex with men; NAAT: Nucleic acid amplification test; OR: Odds ratio; Pr: Probability; STI: Sexually transmitted infection

Acknowledgements

Chlamydia trachomatis laboratory sentinel team:
Michael Baier, Eberhard Straube (Institut für Medizinische Mikrobiologie, Universitätsklinikum Jena)
Armin Baillot (Niedersächsisches Landesgesundheitsamt, Hannover)
Patricia Bartsch (MVZ Dr. Eberhard & Partner, Dortmund)
Thomas Brüning (LADR GmbH MVZ Nord-West Schüttorf)
Josef Cremer (Medizinisch-Diagnostisches Labor Kempten, Kempten)
Helga Dallügge-Tamm (amedes MVZ wagnerstibbe, Hannover)
Arndt Gröning (amedes MVZ wagnerstibbe, Hannover)
Stephan Eicke (Labor Dr. Eicke, Berlin)
Dagmar Emrich (MVZ Labor 28 GmbH, Berlin)
Florian Mielack, Martina Woitkowiak (MVZ Labor 28 GmbH, Berlin)
Gundula Fritsche (Labor MVZ Westmecklenburg, Schwerin)
Rosi Gjavotchanoff (Labor Alfredstraße, Essen)
Peter Gohl (Bioscientia Institut für Medizinische Diagnostik GmbH, Ingelheim)
Matthias Götzrath, Axel Meye (Medizinisches Labor Ostsachsen MVZ GbR, Dresden)
Ingrid Ehrhard, Beate Köpke (Landesuntersuchungsanstalt Sachsen, Dresden)
Birgit Henrich (Institut für Medizinische Mikrobiologie und Krankenhaushygiene, Universitätsklinikum Düsseldorf)
Caroline Kastilan (MVZ Labor Diagnostik Karlsruhe GmbH, Karlsruhe)
Susanne Lehmann (Diagnosticum, Plauen)
Anneliese Märzacker (Labor Schottdorf MVZ GmbH, Augsburg)
Stefan Odenbreit, Claudio Perocco (Labor Schottdorf MVZ GmbH, Augsburg)
Bernhard Miller (Labor PD Dr. Volkmann und Kollegen GbR, Karlsruhe)
Gerrit Mohrmann (Labor Lademannbogen MVZ GmbH, Hamburg)
Christian Pache (MVZ Labor Passau)
Thomas Miedl (MVZ Labor Passau)
Roland Pfüller (MDI Laboratorien GmbH, Berlin)
Carsten Tiemann (Labor Krone, Bad Salzuflen)
Frank Hilwalserbäumer (Labor Krone, Bad Salzuflen)
Hilmar Wisplinghoff (Labor Dr. Wisplinghoff, Köln; Institut für Mikrobiologie, Universität Witten/Herdecke; Institut für Medizinische Mikrobiologie, Universität zu Köln)
Thomas Müller, Christian Aepinus (synlab MVZ Weiden GmbH, Weiden)
Manuela Wudy (synlab MVZ Weiden GmbH, Weiden)
Further acknowledgements:
Harald Fauther (LADR GmbH MVZ Nord-West Schüttorf),
Ekkehard Hennebach (Landesuntersuchungsanstalt Sachsen, Dresden),
Frank Hilwalserbäumer (Labor Krone, Bad Salzuflen),
Thomas Kröger (MVZ Dr. Eberhard & Partner, Dortmund),
Thomas Miedl (MVZ Labor Passau),
Florian Mielack, Martina Woitkowiak (MVZ Labor 28 GmbH, Berlin),
Stefan Odenbreit, Claudio Perocco (Labor Schottdorf MVZ GmbH, Augsburg),
Udo Schallenberg (Labor Dr. Wisplinghoff, Köln),
Steffen Schmudlach (Labor MVZ Westmecklenburg, Schwerin),
Manuela Wudy (synlab MVZ Weiden GmbH, Weiden),
Ekkehard Hennebach, Dr. Eva Krause, Kristina Kunath, Markus Naake, Sarah Störr, Susanne Schäfer, Susanne Ullrich (Landesuntersuchungsanstalt Sachsen, Dresden);
Hermann Claus, Eberhard Pape, Alexandra Hofmann, Ole Wichmann (Robert Koch Institute, Berlin)
National association of statutory health insurance for the kind distribution of data

Funding

The project was designed by Robert Koch Institute and funded by German Federal Ministry of Health. German Federal Ministry of Health was not involved in data collection, analysis and writing of the manuscript.

Authors' contributions

AL, SD and VB developed the concept of the analysis of repeated testers in the Chlamydia trachomatis laboratory sentinel study. AL, MadH and SD developed data analysis plan. AL performed the data analysis. SD and MadH supervised the data analysis. AS supported the data management. AL, SD, KJ, VB, AS and MadH critically discussed study results and data interpretation. AL drafted the paper. SD, KJ, VB, AS and MadH revised the paper. All authors read and approved the final manuscript.

Consent for publication

Not applicable.

Competing interests

KJ is member of the editorial board member at BMC Infectious Diseases. However, there are no competing interests of all authors.

Author details

[1]Department for Infectious Disease Epidemiology, Robert Koch Institute, Berlin, Germany. [2]Charité Universitätsmedizin Berlin Berlin, Germany.

References

1. WHO: Report on global sexually transmitted infection surveillance 2013. 2014.
2. ECDC. Sexually transmitted infections in Europe – 2013. In: Surveillance report. Stockholm: European Center for Disease Control and Prevention; 2015.
3. Redmond SM, Alexander-Kisslig K, Woodhall SC, van den Broek IV, van Bergen J, Ward H, Uuskula A, Herrmann B, Andersen B, Gotz HM, et al. Genital chlamydia prevalence in Europe and non-European high income countries: systematic review and meta-analysis. PLoS One. 2015;10(1):e0115753.

4. Desai S, Meyer T, Thamm M, Hamouda O, Bremer V. Prevalence of chlamydia trachomatis among young German adolescents, 2005-06. Sex Health. 2011;8(1):120–2.
5. Haar K, Bremer V, Houareau C, Meyer T, Desai S, Thamm M, Hamouda O. Risk factors for Chlamydia trachomatis infection in adolescents: results from a representative population-based survey in Germany, 2003–2006. Euro Surveill. 2013;18:1–10.
6. Bremer V, Hofmann A, Hamouda O. Epidemiologie der Chlamydia-trachomatis-Infektionen. Hautarzt. 2007;58:13–23.
7. ECDC. Chlamydia control in Europe: literature review. In: ECDC, editor. Technical report. European Center for Disease Control and Prevention: Stockholm; 2014.
8. Torrone E, Papp J, Weinstock H. Prevalence of Chlamydia trachomatis genital infection among persons aged 14-39 years--United States, 2007-2012. MMWR Morbidity and mortality weekly report. 2014;63(38):834–38.
9. Walker J, Tabrizi SN, Fairley CK, Chen MY, Bradshaw CS, Twin J, Taylor N, Donovan B, Kaldor JM, McNamee K, et al. Chlamydia trachomatis incidence and re-infection among young women–behavioural and microbiological characteristics. PLoS One. 2012;7(5):e37778.
10. Svenstrup HF, Fedder J, Kristoffersen SE, Trolle B, Birkelund S, Christiansen G. Mycoplasma genitalium, Chlamydia trachomatis, and tubal factor infertility–a prospective study. Fertil Steril. 2008;90(3):513–20.
11. Malik A, Jain S, Rizvi M, Shukla I, Hakim S. Chlamydia trachomatis infection in women with secondary infertility. Fertil Steril. 2009;91(1):91–5.
12. Bernstein KT, Marcus J, Nieri G, Philip S, Klausner J. Rectal Gonorrhea and Chlamydia reinfection is associated with increased risk of HIV seroconversion. J Aquir Immune Defic Syndr. 2009;00(0):1–7.
13. Dudareva-Vizule S, Haar K, Sailer A, Wisplinghoff H, Wisplinghoff F, Marcus U, group Ps. Prevalence of pharyngeal and rectal Chlamydia trachomatis and Neisseria gonorrhoeae infections among men who have sex with men in Germany. Sex Transm Infect. 2014;90(1):46–51.
14. van den Broek IV, Sfetcu O, van der Sande MA, Andersen B, Herrmann B, Ward H, Gotz HM, Uuskula A, Woodhall SC, Redmond SM, et al. Changes in chlamydia control activities in Europe between 2007 and 2012: a cross-national survey. Eur J Pub Health. 2016;26(3):382–8.
15. Lanjouw E, Ouburg S, de Vries HJ, Stary A, Radcliffe K, Unemo M. 2015 European guideline on the management of Chlamydia trachomatis infections. Int J STD AIDS. 2016;27(5):333–48.
16. STI-Gesellschaft D: S2k-Leitlinie: Infektionen mit Chlamydia trachomatis. 2016.
17. Dudareva-Vizule S, Haar K, Sailer A, Jansen K, Hamouda O, Wisplinghoff H, Tiemann C, Pape E, Bremer V, Chlamydia trachomatis laboratory sentinel t: Establishment of a voluntary electronic Chlamydia trachomatis laboratory surveillance system in Germany, 2008 to 2014. Euro Surveill. 2017;22(6):1–10.
18. Hillis SD, Owens LM, Marchbanks PA, Amsterdam LF, Mac Kenzie WR. Recurrent chlamydial infections increase the risks of hospitalization for ectopic pregnancy and pelvic inflammatory disease. Am J Obstet Gynecol. 1997;176(1 Pt 1):103–7.
19. Hosenfeld CB, Workowski KA, Berman S, Zaidi A, Dyson J, Mosure D, Bolan G, Bauer HM. Repeat infection with Chlamydia and gonorrhea among females: a systematic review of the literature. Sex Transm Dis. 2009;36(8):478–89.
20. Fung M, Scott KC, Kent CK, Klausner JD. Chlamydial and gonococcal reinfection among men: a systematic review of data to evaluate the need for retesting. Sex Transm Infect. 2007;83(4):304–9.
21. Dukers-Muijrers NH, Morre SA, Speksnijder A, van der Sande MA, Hoebe CJ. Chlamydia trachomatis test-of-cure cannot be based on a single highly sensitive laboratory test taken at least 3 weeks after treatment. PLoS One. 2012;7(3):e34108.
22. Papp JR, Schachter J, Gaydos CA, Pol BVD. Recommendations for the laboratory-based detection of Chlamydia trachomatis and Neisseria gonorrhoeae — 2014. MMWR Recomm Rep. 2014;63:1–19.
23. Brunham R. The unexpected impact of a chlamydia trachomatis infection control program on susceptibility to reinfection. J Infect Dis. 2005;192:1836–44.
24. Heywood W, Patrick K, Smith AM, Pitts MK. Associations between early first sexual intercourse and later sexual and reproductive outcomes: a systematic review of population-based data. Arch Sex Behav. 2015;44(3):531–69.
25. Rietmejier CA: Incidence and repeat infection rates of chlamydia trachomatis among male and female patients in an STD clinic: implications for screening and rescreening. 2001.
26. Eurostat: Frauen in der EU sind bei der Geburt ihres ersten Kindes durchschnittlich fast 29 Jahre alt. ; 2015.
27. Dudareva-Vizule S, Haar K, Sailer A, Jansen K, Hamouda O, Pape E, Bremer V, team* Ctls. Establishment of a voluntary electronic Chlamydia trachomatis laboratory surveillance system in Germany, 2008-2014. Eurosurveillance:2017.
28. Liebesleben – Es ist deins. Schütze es. http://www.liebesleben.de/. Access 20 June 2017.
29. Niccolai LM, Hochberg AL, Ethier KA, Lewis JB, Ickovics JR. Burden of recurrent Chlamydia trachomatis infections in young women. Arch Pediatr Adolesc. 2007;161:246.
30. The EMIS Network. EMIS 2010: the European men-who-have-sex-with-men internet survey. Findings from 38 countries. Stockholm: European Centre for Disease Prevention and Control; 2013.
31. Mund M, Sander G, Potthoff P, Schicht H, Matthias K. Introduction of Chlamydia trachomatis screening for young women in Germany. J Dtsch Dermatol Ges. 2008;6(12):1032–7.
32. Gift TL, Blake DR, Gaydos CA, Marrazzo JM. The cost-effectiveness of screening men for Chlamydia trachomatis: a review of the literature. Sex Transm Dis. 2008;35(11 Suppl):S51–60.
33. Batteiger BE, Tu W, Ofner S, Van Der Pol B, Stothard DR, Orr DP, Katz BP, Fortenberry JD. Repeated Chlamydia trachomatis genital infections in adolescent women. J Infect Dis. 2010;201(1):42–51.
34. Dunne EF, Chapin JB, Rietmeijer CA, Kent CK, Ellen JM, Gaydos CA, Willard NJ, Kohn R, Lloyd L, Thomas S, et al. Rate and predictors of repeat Chlamydia trachomatis infection among men. Sex Transm Dis. 2008;35(11 Suppl):S40–4.
35. LaMontagne DS, Fenton KA, Randall S, Anderson S, Carter P. Establishing the National Chlamydia Screening Programme in England: results from the first full year of screening. Sex Transm Infect. 2004;80(5):335–41.
36. Hocking JS, Vodstrcil LA, Huston WM, Timms P, Chen MY, Worthington K, McIver R, Tabrizi SN. Australian Chlamydia treatment study i: a cohort study of Chlamydia trachomatis treatment failure in women: a study protocol. BMC Infect Dis. 2013;13:379.

18

Macrolide-resistant *Mycoplasma genitalium* infections in Cuban patients: an underestimated health problem

Brian Arturo Mondeja[1], Javier Couri[1,2], Nadia Maria Rodríguez[1], Orestes Blanco[1], Carmen Fernández[1] and Jørgen Skov Jensen[3*]

Abstract

Background: The increasing prevalence of macrolide resistant *Mycoplasma genitalium* is a major concern worldwide. In Cuba, several cases of clinical treatment failure with 1 g single dose and extended azithromycin regimen have been detected and the aim of the present investigation was to retrospectively determine the prevalence of macrolide-resistance mediating mutations (MRMM) in *M. genitalium*-positive samples conserved at the Cuban National Reference Laboratory of Mycoplasma Research between 2009 and 2016.

Methods: A total of 280 positive DNA extracts were analysed by a 5′ nuclease assay for detection of *M. genitalium* MRMM. Ten urogenital specimens from patients with azithromycin treatment failure and MRMM were inoculated in Vero cell to obtain the isolates for subsequent determination of antimicrobial susceptibility.

Results: The overall prevalence of MRMM was 32%. No MRMM was detected in samples collected between 2009 and 2013 but since 2014 a dramatic increase to 90% (95% CI, 76–96%) in 2016 was seen. Three new *M. genitalium* isolates were isolated in Vero cell cultures and confirmed phenotypic resistance to macrolides in a cell-culture assisted susceptibility test. Preliminary observations suggest that combination therapy with levofloxacin and doxycycline may represent an affordable option for treatment of macrolide resistant *M. genitalium* infections.

Conclusions: This investigation showed the rapid emergence and high prevalence of MRMM in *M. genitalium*-infected patients in Cuba and confirmed the phenotypic resistance in isolates carrying MRMM. We suggest that Cuban guidelines for sexually transmitted infections are modified to include testing for *M. genitalium* and detection of MRMM in patients with failure of syndromic treatment, to ensure that in these cases, the treatment will be guided by etiologic diagnosis.

Keywords: *Mycoplasma genitalium*, Antimicrobial susceptibility, Macrolide resistance, Sexually transmitted infections

Background

Mycoplasma genitalium is an emerging sexually transmitted pathogen and the increase of macrolide resistance is considered a health problem globally [1]. In this bacterium, macrolide resistance is mediated mainly by point mutations in the A2058 and A2059 (*Escherichia coli* numbering) positions in region V of the 23S ribosomal RNA. These mutations are associated with azithromycin treatment failure and high minimal inhibitory concentration (MIC) for macrolides as documented in several *M. genitalium* strains [2, 3].

The prevalence of strains with macrolide resistance mediating mutations (MRMM) is highly variable and unknown in many regions. In Europe, Australia and Asia, it is generally above 30% and in extreme cases, as in Greenland, 100% of *M. genitalium* strains carry MRMM [4–8]. In Cuba, macrolides are used as the first line treatment for urogenital syndromes caused by sexually transmitted infections (STI), including *M. genitalium* and chlamydia infections. Since 2007, *M. genitalium* diagnosis has been performed at the Pedro Kourí Tropical Medicine Institute (IPK), and several cases of treatment failure with 1 g single dose and extended azithromycin regimens have

* Correspondence: jsj@ssi.dk
[3]Statens Serum Institut, Research Unit for Reproductive Tract Microbiology, Artillerivej 5, DK-2300 Copenhagen S, Denmark
Full list of author information is available at the end of the article

been detected in the IPK - STI clinic within recent years. In 2015, a new macrolide resistant *M. genitalium* strain (B19, A2059G mutation) was isolated from one of these patients using Vero cell co-culture [9], and antimicrobial susceptibility patterns were determined using a cell-assisted procedure [10]. However, no data about the prevalence of MRMM carrying *M. genitalium* strains in Cuba are available, but clinical experience of macrolide treatment failures and the isolation of at least one MRMM strain suggest the possible circulation of MRMM carrying *M. genitalium* strains in Cuban patients after 2015, which has direct implications for the effectiveness of syndromic management of STI.

The aim of the present investigation was to retrospectively determine MRMM prevalence in *M. genitalium*--positive samples conserved at the Cuban National Reference Laboratory of Mycoplasma Research on IPK between 2009 and 2016.

Materials and methods

Study design

A retrospective study was conducted at the Cuban National Reference Laboratory of Mycoplasma Research – IPK, for the direct detection of MRMM in *M. genitalium* positive clinical samples archived since 2009. This study was approved by The Pedro Kourí Tropical Medicine Institute Ethical Board (approval CEI-IPK 57–16) and written informed consent to participate and publish was obtained from all patients.

M. genitalium positives specimens

For the study, a total of 280 *M. genitalium* positive DNA extracts from Cuban patients with urogenital syndromes, spontaneous abortion and infertility were analysed. These were representing all samples submitted to IPK for *M. genitalium* diagnosis since 2009 and up to December 2016. DNA was extracted by the Chelex 100 method and conserved at – 80 °C [11]. Until December of 2014, *M. genitalium* diagnosis was performed by a 16S rRNA singleplex-PCR with internal control [12] and confirmation by a qPCR based in the amplification of *mgpB* gene [11]). Since January of 2015, *M. genitalium* diagnosis was performed by the same *mgpB* gene qPCR mentioned above and the confirmation was with a *mgpA* gene – qPCR [13]. For each patient, only the first positive specimen was included in the study.

Detection of MRMM

DNA specimens were analyzed by a modification of the 5′ nuclease genotyping assay for *M. genitalium* MRMM testing, described by Kristiansen et al. [14]. In brief, a qPCR mix was prepared in a final volume of 25 µL containing 500 nM of the 23S rRNA gene primers described by Jensen et al. [15], 200 nM of wild-type probe: Cy5-GGA CGG AAA GAC CCC GTG AAG CTT T-BHQ2, 100 nM of each MRMM probes MRMM-A2058G: FAM-GAC GGG AAG ACC CCG TGA AGC TTT-BHQ1 and MRMM-A2059G: FAM- GAC GGA GAG ACC CCG TGA AGC TTT-BHQ1 [14], and 1.5 U of Top*Taq*-polymerase (Qiagen,Hilden, Germany). As positive controls for MRMM, DNA from *M. genitalium* strains M6271 (A2058G), M6489 (A2059G) and M6302 (A2058C) were used, and as wild-type *M. genitalium* strains the Danish strains M2300, M2321 and M2341 were used [3].

Samples were amplified and analysed in a Rotor-Gene Q 5-plex instrument (Qiagen) using the same amplification program as described by Kristiansen et al. [14]. Results were analysed using the Rotor-Gene Q Software Version 2.1.0.9 (Qiagen) by the Scatter Analysis module with the reading combination of the green and red fluorescence channel.

Isolation and determination of antimicrobial susceptibility of MRMM strains from clinical specimens

Ten urogenital specimens from patients with azithromycin treatment failure and with an *M. genitalium* load > 10,000 genome equivalents (geq) per mL, were inoculated in Vero cell as previously described [16] in an attempt to obtain new isolates. The specimens comprised seven male urethral swabs (three male homosexual couples and one heterosexual man) and three endocervical swabs (one of them from the female partner of the male patient providing the sample yielding the B19 strain previously described [10]). In order to document lack of cross-contamination between cell cultures, an *mgpB* based DNA typing method [17] was applied to primary samples and isolated strains.

Antimicrobial susceptibility testing was performed by a cell-assisted procedure as previously described, but with an incubation time of 28 days [10]. MICs to azithromycin, erythromycin, doxycycline, tetracycline, ciprofloxacin, ofloxacin, moxifloxacin and levofloxacin was defined as the lowest concentration of antimicrobial capable of inhibiting 99% of the *M. genitalium* growth in the test well compared with the *M. genitalium* growth in the control wells [18]. MRMM identification of the isolates was done by the nuclease genotyping assay described above, using genomic DNA of the isolate and of the corresponding clinical specimen.

Treatment of patients with macrolide resistant *M. genitalium* infection

Between July 2015 and December 2017, all 46 *M. genitalium* positive patients with treatment failure after azithromycin (500 mg day 1 followed by 250 mg days 2–5) and attending the STD clinic of the IPK Hospital have been treated with doxycycline 100 mg 2 times daily plus levofloxacin 500 mg 2 times daily for 14 days. This regimen has been used due to the limited availability of moxifloxacin in Cuba. Microbiological cure was evaluated 30 days after treatment using the same PCR methodology as used for the primary diagnosis.

Statistical analysis

The statistical comparisons between the frequency of resistant *M. genitalium* in each year of the study and for the proportion of MRMM between men and women was compared with Fisher's exact test with p for trend (two-sided p values). Differences with $p < 0.05$ were considered statistically significant (StatsDirect version 3.1.14 (StatsDirect Ltd., Cheshire, UK)).

Results

Distribution of *M. genitalium* positive patients

Of the 280 *M. genitalium* positive patients, 100 (35.7%) were men and 180 (64.3%) were women (Fig. 1).

Prevalence of MRMM in the clinical specimens

Of the 280 samples analysed, 202 (72%) were amplifiable by the MRMM qPCR. Of these 202, 138 (68%; 95% CI 57–81%) were identified as wild-type genotype (macrolide susceptible) and 64 (32%; 95% CI 24–40%) were identified as carrier of mutant genotypes. MRMM was not detected in any of the 65 successfully amplified samples collected between 2009 and 2013 0% (95% CI: 0–6%). In contrast, MRMM was detected in 64 of 137 clinical samples 47% (95% CI: 39–55%) collected since 2014 with a dramatic increase to 90% (95% CI: 76–96%) in 2016 ($p < 0.0001$, $p < 0.0001$ for trend) (Fig. 2).

No differences between the MRMM prevalence in men and women were detected ($p = 0.88$).

Genotype distribution among MRMM positive samples

Out of a total of 64 MRMM positive samples, 52 samples (81%) were identified as A2058G/A2059G and 12 (19%) as A2058C/T. The latter genotype was more commonly found in female than in male specimens.

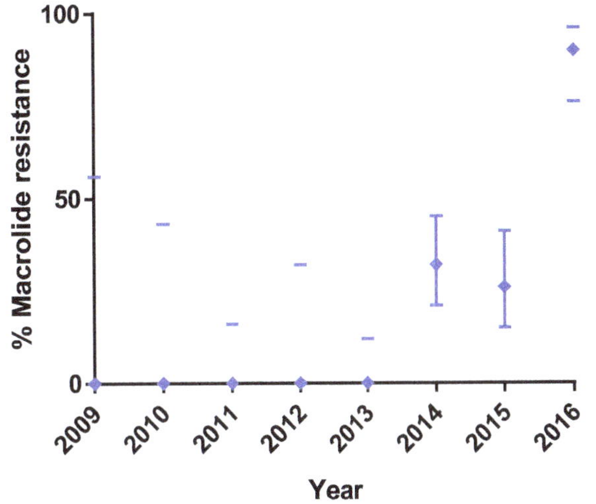

Fig. 2 Prevalence of MRMM genotype in percent of clinical specimens per year of study. Error-bars show 95% confidence intervals

Antimicrobial susceptibility pattern of MRMM strains from clinical specimens

Of the ten *M. genitalium* positive specimens, only three were capable of growing in the Vero cell culture and yielded new isolates. The B25 and B26 strains were isolated from a male couple and showed the same *mgpB* type (not previously described and denominated Cuba3; Acc# MH407699). The B30 strain was isolated from the female partner of the male patient yielding the B19 isolate previously reported [10]. The B30 strain showed an identical *mgpB* type to that of the B19 strain (genotype 4). For all three isolates, the same *mgpB* type was detected from isolate and the corresponding clinical specimen.

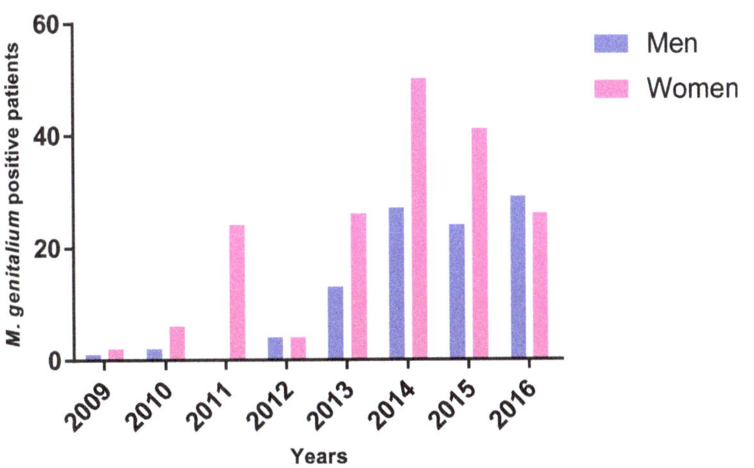

Fig. 1 Gender distribution and number of *M. genitalium* positive patients per year of study

The three new clinical *M. genitalium* isolates were resistant to macrolides with a MIC value of > 8 mg/L. MIC values for tetracyclines were 0.5–2 mg/L and for quinolones, a MIC of 0.125 mg/L was found for moxifloxacin (Table 1).

All the isolates and the corresponding clinical specimen were identified as MRMM A2058G/A2059G by the 5' nuclease assay and as A2059G by sequencing (Table 1) clearly confirming the good concordance between detection of MRMM by the molecular assay and the demonstration of a phenotypic resistance in vitro in the cell-assisted assay as well as in vivo documented by macrolide treatment failure.

Treatment of patients with macrolide resistant *M. genitalium* infection

All 46 cases with azithromycin treatment failure were found to carry *M. genitalium* with MRMM. Dual therapy with doxycycline and levofloxacin for 14 days eradicated *M. genitalium* from all patients as documented by PCR 30 days after treatment.

Discussion

The emergence of MRMM in *M. genitalium* in several countries is a worrying reality. For several years, this sexually transmitted pathogen has been underestimated as responsible for STI syndromes in men and women. In the Unites States Center for Diseases Control STI treatment guidelines the infection got attention with a separate chapter for the first time in 2015 [19]. In 2016 the European guideline on *Mycoplasma genitalium* infections was published as the first international guideline addressing diagnosis and treatment [20]. This was the first step to harmonize the international recognition and treatment of *M. genitalium* as an STI.

Since 2004, *M. genitalium* infections have been studied at IPK, and diagnosis was established in 2009 as part of an aetiological surveillance of STIs in Cuba. For many years, empiric treatment with macrolides and tetracyclines was used for the control of mycoplasma and chlamydia infections. In 2001, Cuba implemented syndromic management of STI, and the 1 g single dose azithromycin treatment became the recommended treatment for non-gonococcal urogenital infections in men and women. At this time, few studies were available that evaluated the treatment efficacy of macrolides and the emergence of resistance was an unknown problem. The latter, has become recognised as a worldwide problem after 2008 [2].

In the present investigation, we have determined the presence of MRMM in *M. genitalium* in Cuban clinical specimens archived since 2009, nine years after the initiation of azithromycin syndromic treatment of urogenital syndromes, and until 2016. From our data, it appears that *M. genitalium* with MRMM was very rare in Cuba before 2014. However, the number of analysed *M. genitalium* positive samples between 2009 and 2013 was relatively low, so it is difficult to make definite conclusions. Nevertheless, the explosion in the prevalence of *M. genitalium* with MRMM reaching 90% in 2016 is extremely worrying and threatening the current recommended syndromic management. In Cuba, more than 4000 cases of urogenital syndromes (lower abdominal pain, vaginal discharge and urethral syndrome) are reported to the Ministry of Public Health every year. However, it is not common that *M. genitalium* tests are ordered, even when macrolide treatment has failed. This finding is very similar in other countries and is partly due to lack of awareness among clinicians, but also due to lack of testing availability in many settings.

The genotyping assay used for MRMM detection was able to characterise more than 70% of the *M. genitalium* positive specimens, compared with 94.5% reported in the original paper by Kristiansen et al. [14]. However, when we analysed samples from 2016, 15 of the 17 non-amplified specimens were successfully re-amplified by the *mgpB* qPCR. These samples showed an *M. genitalium* load < 1000 geq/mL which may explain the failure of amplification in the genotyping assay. Other factors such as destruction of DNA, even when conserved at -80 °C, could be playing a role in the success of the genotyping assay, as has been shown for another *M. genitalium* molecular test [21]. Unfortunately, it was not possible to provide information about the exact positions of the MRMM as the method applied did not provide this level of discrimination. Most of the samples were used up for culture attempts and additional PCRs for MRMM was not possible. In Cuba, Sanger sequencing is difficult and expensive and consequently, a qPCR for the detection of MRMM directly from the clinical samples

Table 1 Minimal Inhibitory Concentrations (MICs) for the three MRMM carrying Cuban *M. genitalium* isolates as determined by a modified cell-culture-based method

M. genitalium isolates		MIC VALUES (mg/L)							
	MRMM	Azithromycin	Erythromycin	Ciprofloxacin	Ofloxacin	Levofloxacin	Moxifloxacin	Tetracycline	Doxycycline
B25	A2059G	> 8	> 8	4	1	2	0.125	1	0.5
B26	A2059G	> 8	> 8	4	1	0.5	0.125	1	0.5
B30	A2059G	> 8	> 8	8	1	1	0.125	2	0.5

was introduced. Furthermore, as the type of mutation is not relevant for the clinical management, and as an increasing amount of surveillance data is produced by PCR based testing, even in more resourced settings, we do not consider this to be a major limitation of the study.

The three new Cuban *M. genitalium* strains isolated from samples with MRMM have an antimicrobial resistance profile with susceptibility to tetracyclines and moxifloxacin according to CLSI guidelines for *M. pneumoniae* [22]. The patient from whom the B25 strain was isolated is a Cuban man living in Switzerland, where he was infected, diagnosed and treated for *M. genitalium*. His Cuban male partner never lived outside of Cuba and was infected after unprotected sex during a visit of patient B25. Thus, introduction of the MRMM *M. genitalium* strain from Europe is the most plausible explanation, and confirmation of the same *mgpB* type (Cuba3) in clinical samples and MRMM strains, support this. Fortunately, both the B25 and B26 strains were susceptible to doxycycline and the patients were cured after combined treatment with doxycycline and levofloxacin for 14 days. The B30 female patient was a woman having had sex with foreign men and she was the sexual contact reported by the B19 male patient described in our previous study [10] at the time of *M. genitalium* diagnosis. The same *mgpB* type (type 4) was found in the clinical specimens and isolated strains B19 and B30, reaffirming the sexual transmission between the partners. However, it is impossible to determine if the MRMM strain was imported or not. Both patients were cured with levofloxacin plus doxycycline.

All three new isolates showed phenotypic resistance to macrolides. In these cases, a total concordance between the 5'nuclease genotyping assay, the macrolide resistance pattern determined by the Vero cell culture assay, and clinical and microbiological failure of azithromycin treatment was documented. This fact reaffirm the utility of the genotyping assay to predict azithromycin treatment failure in patients infected with *M. genitalium* when MRMM are detected. Unfortunately, no isolates with MRMM were obtained from the seven other clinical specimens inoculated in Vero cells.

In this investigation, the overall macrolide resistance rate was 32% but with all of the resistant strains detected within the last three years of the study. The A2058G/A2059G was the most frequently detected MRMM genotype detected in *M. genitalium* positives specimens as in most other studies. Comparable rates of macrolide resistance have been reported recently from Denmark [4], United Kingdom [6], and Australia [8], where the prevalence of macrolide resistance–associated mutations was 40, 41 and 43%, respectively. These studies also found similar distributions of the most common A2058G and A2059G mutations but did not see the same dramatic increase in the prevalence of MRMM strains. The A2058C/T was detected in 19% of Cuban MRMM specimens. Unfortunately, neither of the isolated strains had this mutation pattern but no influence on the MICs values for macrolides have been recorded in other investigations for the different mutation-types [2, 3].

Based on the findings reported here, a new molecular diagnostic strategy for *M. genitalium* at IPK has been established since January 2017. In this strategy, we use the *mgp*B qPCR as screening test and positive specimens are immediately confirmed by the 5'nuclease genotyping assay and by the *mgpA* qPCR for *mgpB* positive samples with less than 1000 geq/mL. This approach is in accordance with the European guideline on *M. genitalium* infections [20] where determination of MRMM is recommended for all *M. genitalium* positive samples.

The prevalence of MRMM carrying *M. genitalium* strains has been high after 2014 in Cuba. Since 2015, all *M. genitalium* positive patients with MRMM seen at the STD clinic at the IPK Hospital have demonstrated treatment failure after azithromycin. In these 46 cases, MRMM *M. genitalium* was successfully eradicated with a 14-days second-line combined therapy of levofloxacin plus doxycycline (Orestes Blanco, unpublished). This regimen has been used due to the limited availability of moxifloxacin in Cuba and may be applicable elsewhere. The choice of this combination regimen was based on the synergistic in vitro activity of doxycycline and moxifloxacin in fluoroquinolone susceptible *M. genitalium* strains [23]. Experimental work documenting the synergy between levofloxacin and doxycycline is currently underway. The high efficacy was somewhat unexpected as doxycycline monotherapy has a microbiological cure rate of approximately 30% and that of levofloxacin monotherapy is rarely exceeding 50% [24].

No data about MRMM prevalence in other Latin-American countries are available, but it will probably be found at a similar rate in countries with similar macrolide treatment strategy for STIs as Cuba.

Conclusions

The results obtained in this investigation showed for the first time the rapid emergence and high prevalence of MRMM carrying *M. genitalium* strains in Cuban patients. No data about macrolide failure in syndromic STI management outside IPK are available, but macrolide resistance in *M. genitalium*-infected Cuban patients could be an underestimated health problem. We suggest that Cuban guidelines for STI treatment are modified to include testing for *M. genitalium* and detection of macrolide resistance–mediating mutations at least in patients failing syndromic treatment to ensure that in these cases the treatment will be guided by the aetiological diagnosis.

Abbreviations
IPK: Pedro Kourí Tropical Medicine Institute; MRMM: Macrolide resistance mediating mutations; qPCR: Quantitative Polymerase Chain Reaction; STI: Sexually transmitted infections

Acknowledgements
Lic. Ruxana Sardiñas provided excellent technical assistance with *M. genitalium* PCR diagnosis.

Consent to publication
Written informed consent to participate and publish was obtained from all patients.

Funding
No specific funding was received for this study. The work was supported in part by the Pedro Kourí Tropical Medicine Institute, Cuba, with the collaboration and economical support of Statens Serum Institut, Denmark. No funding bodies had any role in study design, data collection and analysis, decision to publish, or preparation of the manuscript.

Authors' contributions
Conceptualization: BAM JSJ. Data curation: BAM JC OB JSJ. Formal analysis: BAM JSJ. Funding acquisition: BAM NMR JSJ. Investigation: BAM JC OB CF JSJ. Methodology: BAM NMR CF JSJ. Project administration: BAM NMR. Resources: JSJ OB NMR. Supervision: JSJ NMR CF. Validation: NMR. Visualization: BAM NMR JSJ. Writing – original draft: BAM JSJ. Writing – review& editing: BAM NMR JC OB CF JSJ.All authors read and approved the final manuscript.

Competing interests
BM, JC, NM, OB, and CF report no conflict of interest. JSJ has received speaker's fee from Hologic and serves a scientific advisory board of Roche Molecular Systems. SSI has received remuneration for contract work from SpeeDx, Hologic, NYTor, Diagenode, Nabriva, GSK, and Angelini.The authors declare that they have no competing interest.

Author details
[1]Pedro Kourí Tropical Medicine Institute, La Habana, Cuba. [2]Faculty of Biology, University of Havana, La Habana, Cuba. [3]Statens Serum Institut, Research Unit for Reproductive Tract Microbiology, Artillerivej 5, DK-2300 Copenhagen S, Denmark.

References
1. Unemo M, Jensen JS. Antimicrobial-resistant sexually transmitted infections: gonorrhoea and *Mycoplasma genitalium*. Nat Rev Urol. 2017;14:139–52.
2. Jensen JS, Bradshaw CS, Tabrizi SN, Fairley CK, Hamasuna R. Azithromycin treatment failure in *Mycoplasma genitalium*-positive patients with nongonococcal urethritis is associated with induced macrolide resistance. Clin Infect Dis. 2008;47:1546–53.
3. Jensen JS, Fernandes P, Unemo M. In vitro activity of the new fluoroketolide solithromycin (CEM-101) against macrolide-resistant and - susceptible *Mycoplasma genitalium* strains. Antimicrob Agents Chemother. 2014;58:3151–6.
4. Salado-Rasmussen K, Jensen JS. *Mycoplasma genitalium* testing pattern and macrolide resistance: a Danish nationwide retrospective survey. Clin Infect Dis. 2014;59:24–30.
5. Gesink DC, Mulvad G, Montgomery-Andersen R, Poppel U, Montgomery-Andersen S, Binzer A, et al. *Mycoplasma genitalium* presence resistance and epidemiology in Greenland. *Int J Circumpolar Health*. 2012;71:1–8.
6. Pond MJ, Nori AV, Witney AA, Lopeman RC, Butcher PD, Sadiq ST. High prevalence of antibiotic-resistant *Mycoplasma genitalium* in nongonococcal urethritis: the need for routine testing and the inadequacy of current treatment options. Clin Infect Dis. 2014;58:631–7.
7. Nijhuis RH, Severs TT, Van der Vegt DS, Van Zwet AA, Kusters JG. High levels of macrolide resistance-associated mutations in *Mycoplasma genitalium* warrant antibiotic susceptibility-guided treatment. J Antimicrob Chemother. 2015;70:2515–8.
8. Tagg KA, Jeoffreys NJ, Couldwell DL, Donald JA, Gilbert GL. Fluoroquinolone and macrolide resistance-associated mutations in *Mycoplasma genitalium*. J Clin Microbiol. 2013;51:2245–9.
9. Jensen JS, Hansen HT, Lind K. Isolation of *Mycoplasma genitalium* strains from the male urethra. J Clin Microbiol. 1996;34:286–91.
10. Mondeja BA, Rodriguez NM, Barroto B, Blanco O, Jensen JS. Antimicrobial susceptibility patterns of recent Cuban *Mycoplasma genitalium* isolates determined by a modified cell-culture-based method. PLoS One. 2016;11:e0162924.
11. Jensen JS, Björnelius E, Dohn B, Lidbrink P. Use of TaqMan 5′ nuclease real-time PCR for quantitative detection of *Mycoplasma genitalium* DNA in males with and without urethritis who were attendees at a sexually transmitted disease clinic. J Clin Microbiol. 2004;42:683–92.
12. Jensen JS, Borre MB, Dohn B. Detection of *Mycoplasma genitalium* by PCR amplification of the 16S rRNA gene. J Clin Microbiol. 2003;41:261–6.
13. McGowin CL, Annan RS, Quayle AJ, Greene SJ, Ma L, Mancuso MM, et al. Persistent *Mycoplasma genitalium* infection of human endocervical epithelial cells elicits chronic inflammatory cytokine secretion. Infect Immun. 2012;80:3842–9.
14. Kristiansen GQ, Lisby JG, Schonning K. A 5′ nuclease genotyping assay for identification of macrolide-resistant *Mycoplasma genitalium* in clinical specimens. J Clin Microbiol. 2016;54:1593–7.
15. Jensen JS. Protocol for the detection of *Mycoplasma genitalium* by PCR from clinical specimens and subsequent detection of macrolide resistance-mediating mutations in region V of the 23S rRNA gene. In: CR MK, Henrich B, editors. Diagnosis of Sexually Transmitted Diseases; Methods and Protocols. 903rd ed. New York: Humana Press, Springer; 2012. p. 129–39.
16. Mondeja BA, Jensen JS, Rodriguez I, Morier LF, Kouri V, Rodriguez NM, et al. Isolation of mycoplasma genitalium from patients with urogenital infections: first report from the Latin-American region. New Microbes New Infect. 2013;1:22–6.
17. Hjorth SV, Björnelius E, Lidbrink P, Falk L, Dohn B, Berthelsen L, et al. Sequence-based typing of *Mycoplasma genitalium* reveals sexual transmission. J Clin Microbiol. 2006;44:2078–83.
18. Hamasuna R, Osada Y, Jensen JS. Antibiotic susceptibility testing of *Mycoplasma genitalium* by TaqMan 5′ nuclease real-time PCR. Antimicrob Agents Chemother. 2005;49:4993–8.
19. Workowski KA, Bolan GA. Sexually transmitted diseases treatment guidelines, 2015. *MMWR Recomm Rep*. 2015;64:1–137.
20. Jensen JS, Cusini M, Gomberg M, Moi H. 2016 European guideline on *Mycoplasma genitalium* infections. J Eur Acad Dermatol Venereol. 2016;30:1650–6.
21. Carlsen KH, Jensen JS. *Mycoplasma genitalium* PCR: does freezing of specimens affect sensitivity? J Clin Microbiol. 2010;48:3624–7.
22. CLSI (Eds):Methods for antimicrobial susceptibility testing for human mycoplasmas; Approved guideline. In *CLSI document* 2011, M43-A.
23. Bradshaw CS, Jensen JS, Waites KB. New horizons in *Mycoplasma genitalium* treatment. J Infect Dis. 2017;216:S412–9.
24. Jensen JS, Bradshaw C. Management of *Mycoplasma genitalium* infections - can we hit a moving target? BMC Infect Dis. 2015;15:343.

19

Syphilis reinfection is associated with an attenuated immune profile in the same individual

Chris Kenyon[1,2*], Kara Krista Osbak[1], Tania Crucitti[3] and Luc Kestens[4,5]

Abstract

Background: Ascertaining if the clinical and immunological response to repeat syphilis differs from that in initial syphilis may assist in designing optimal syphilis screening strategies and vaccine design.

Methods: We prospectively recruited 120 patients with a new diagnosis of (baseline) syphilis. During a 24-month follow-up period, 11 of these patients had a further diagnosis of (repeat) syphilis. We conducted a paired comparison of their plasma cyto-chemokines at baseline and repeat syphilis.

Results: Comparing to their baseline infection, paired analyses of the 11 individuals with repeat infections during follow-up revealed that these reinfections had lower concentrations of Interferon (IFN)α (0.8 [Interquartile range (IQR) 0.8–0.8 vs. 12.2 [IQR 1.6–24.2], $P = 0.004$) and Chemokine (C-C motif) ligand (CCL) 4 (0.9 [IQR 0.9–12.2 vs. 17.5 [IQR 4.9–32.8], $P = 0.022$].

Conclusion: In this small study of 11 individuals, repeat syphilis was found to present with an attenuated immune response. The relevance of these findings to the design of optimal syphilis screening programs is discussed.

Keywords: Syphilis, Immunology, Repeat, Screening, Cytokine

Background

A striking feature of the current epidemics of syphilis in high-income countries is the increasing proportion of cases of syphilis that are repeat episodes of syphilis [1–3]. These infections occur predominantly in men who have sex with men (MSM) with high rates of partner change [1, 4]. There is growing recognition that part of the difficulty with controlling these epidemics is the fact that repeat syphilis is less likely to present with symptoms [4–8]. As a result, persons with repeat syphilis may have delayed diagnoses and be more likely to transmit syphilis [1, 6]. At our medical centre in Antwerp, Belgium, reinfections now constitute approximately half of all syphilis infections [1]. In a study that followed up 120 patients with a new diagnosis of syphilis over a 12-month period we previously confirmed that repeat syphilis was not only less likely to be symptomatic than initial syphilis but also had an altered immune profile [4]. These differences included variations in the magnitude and decay curves of rapid plasma reagin (RPR) as well as repeaters being less likely to have elevated plasma interleukin (IL)-10. These differences in plasma IL-10 persisted at 6-month follow-up such that those with initial but not those with repeat syphilis had higher levels of IL-10 than the control group. While following up this cohort for a 24-month period a total of 11 individuals had a further repeat episode of syphilis. This manuscript compares the immune responses of these 11 repeat episodes with the paired baseline episodes.

* Correspondence: ckenyon@itg.be
[1]HIV/STI Unit, Institute of Tropical Medicine, Antwerp, Belgium
[2]Division of Infectious Diseases and HIV Medicine, University of Cape Town, Anzio Road, Observatory, Cape Town 7700, South Africa
Full list of author information is available at the end of the article

Methods

The Institutional Review Board of the Institute of Tropical Medicine and the Ethics Committee of the University Hospital Antwerp approved this study (13/44/426). All study participants provided written informed consent. Between May 2014 and June 2015 all patients attending the Institute of Tropical Medicine, Antwerp's STI or HIV clinics and over the age of 17 years in whom a new diagnosis of syphilis was made were prospectively recruited into the study (ClinicalTrials.gov Registration Number: NCT02059525). The diagnosis and staging of syphilis was according to the Centers for Disease Control and Prevention classification [9]. Repeat syphilis, which included syphilis repeat infections and reactivations, was defined as an episode in a person who had a ≥ 4 increase in RPR titre after a previous diagnosis of syphilis who exhibited an appropriate response to therapy, defined as a ≥ 4-fold decrease in RPR titre. All patients were assessed according to a standardized protocol that collected detailed information about sexual behavior, clinical features and laboratory tests. Patients were followed up at 3, 6, 9, 12, 18, 24 months and at any other time if they developed symptoms or signs of syphilis. Patient clinical and laboratory characteristics were recorded at each consultation. Blood was drawn into plain and EDTA-coated tubes (Sarstedt Monovette, Nümbrecht, Germany) and centrifuged at 2000 *g* for 10 min at ambient temperature. Serum and plasma was stored at − 20 °C (plain) and − 80 °C (plasma), respectively. Samples were processed and frozen within 3 h of acquisition.

Interferon (IFN)α, IFNγ, IL-1β, IL-12p40, IL-12p70, Interferon gamma inducible protein (IP)-10, Monocyte chemoattractant protein (MCP)-1, Macrophage inflammatory protein (MIP)-1α// Chemokine (C-C motif) ligand (CCL)3, CCL4 (MIP-1β), IL-4, IL-5, IL-6, IL-7, IL-8, IL-10 and IL-17A from the baseline, 6 month follow-up and repeat episodes of syphilis were measured in a single experiment using a magnetic bead Luminex multiplex assay (EMD Millipore, Billerica, MA, United States (US)) according to the manufacturer's instructions. Samples below the limit of quantification were assigned the value of half the lowest limit detected for each cytokine (for further study details including quality assessment data please see [4]). Macro Vue RPR card test (Becton, Dickinson and Company, Sparks, MD, US) and *Treponema pallidum* agglutination chemiluminescent immunoassay (Ortho-Clinical Diagnostics, Rochester, NY, US) performed on the Vitros 5600 Integrated System (Ortho-Clinical Diagnostics) were performed at each study visit.

T. pallidum PCR

An in-house real time PCR targeting *polA* was used to detect *T. pallidum* DNA in serum. DNA was extracted from 400 μL serum using the custom-plasma program of the Abbott m2000sp automated extraction platform (Abbott, Maidenhead, UK), according to the manufacturer's specifications. The extracted DNA was eluated in 100 μL eluate solution. The 25 μL PCR mixture contained Platinum® Quantitative PCR SuperMix-Uracil DNA Glycosylase (Invitrogen by life technologies, Thermo Fisher Scientific) 0.9 μM forward primer TP-1, 0.9 μM reverse primer TP-2,0.14 μM probe TP-3 (Integrated DNA technologies, Leuven, Belgium) [10] and 10 μL DNA extract. The amplifications were performed using the Rotor Gene 6000 (Qiagen, Venlo, the Netherlands) and included 45 cycles of 20 s at 95 °C followed by 45 s at 60 °C per cycle.

Statistical analysis

Values are summarized as medians and interquartile ranges (IQR). Wilcoxon's signed rank test was used to evaluate intraindividual changes from baseline to repeat syphilis. Spearman's correlation was used to assess if there was an association between the number of prior episodes of syphilis and plasma cytokine and chemokine concentrations at the time of syphilis diagnosis (baseline and repeat infections combined, $N = 22$). All analyses were performed in Stata 13 (StataCorp LP, College Station, TX, USA). Due to the small sample size we did not conduct multivariable analyses.

Results

The cohort was followed up for 24 months. During this time period 11 individuals (all men, MSM and 10 HIV-infected) were diagnosed with a syphilis reinfection a median 456 (IQR 364–503) days after their baseline infection (Table 1). The median CD4+ T-cell count of the 10 HIV-infected individuals was 554/μL (IQR 489–677) at the baseline visit. All HIV-infected individuals were on antiretroviral therapy with undetectable HIV viral loads. Serum PCR for *Treponema pallidum* was negative for all 11 individuals at baseline and for 6/6 at the time of reinfection. All 11 were treated with stage appropriate intramuscular benzyl penicillin G (BPG) therapy at baseline and reinfection syphilis.

Syphilis stage at reinfection

Two of these reinfections were primary, two secondary and seven early latent syphilis (Table 1).

Only one individual presented with confirmed initial syphilis

For 10 of these individuals, this represented at least their third episode of syphilis (Table 1). The 11th individual was the only one to present with an initial episode of syphilis. His first episode of syphilis was characterized by a diffuse maculopapular rash and a RPR titre of 1/32. He had tested TPA and RPR negative 6 months prior. He received 2.4MU BPG via intramuscular injection and his RPR titre declined to 1/4 at 3 months. At nine months following condomless sex, he presented with a less pronounced maculopapular

Table 1 Selected clinical and laboratory findings of 11 individuals with an episode of syphilis reinfection during study follow-up

		Baseline Episode of Syphilis						Nadir RPR	Repeat Episode of Syphilis		
Study nr	HIV Status	CD4 (T cells/ul)	HIV Viral Load	No. Previous Syphilis Infections[a]	Days since last syphilis	RPR titre baseline	Syphilis Stage	Nadir RPR pre- reinfection	RPR Repeat	Syphilis Stage	Days between baseline and repeat syphilis
1	Infected	563	< 20	3	1371	256	Secondary	64	256	Early Latent	391
2	Infected	546	< 20	4	692	128	Early Latent	16	256	Early Latent	532
3	Infected	677	< 20	1	360	64	Early Latent	8	128	Early Latent	456
4	Infected	456	< 20	1	347	256	Secondary	16	64	Early Latent	492
5	Infected	598	< 20	2	568	8	Early Latent	2	16	Primary	424
6	Uninfected	NA	NA	1	319	64	Secondary	2	8	Early Latent	725
7	Infected	489	< 20	6	684	128	Late Latent	16	64	Primary	496
8	Infected	1284	< 20	1	180	128	Secondary	8	32	Early Latent	308
9	Infected	689	< 20	1	797	128	Late Latent	32	256	Secondary	364
10	Infected	503	< 20	1	565	128	Secondary	4	256	Early Latent	503
11	Infected	483	< 20	0	NA	32	Secondary	0	32	Secondary	171

[a] Number of episodes of syphilis prior to current study
NA Not applicable

rash and an RPR titre rise to 1/32. Of the 11 individuals, his baseline syphilis contained the highest or second highest levels of IL-10, IFNα, CCL4 and IP-10 (Participant 11, Fig. 1). At the time of his reinfection his cytokine levels did not attain the levels of his initial infection (Fig. 1).

Paired comparisons of cytokines

Comparing to their baseline infections, paired analyses of the 11 individuals with reinfections during follow-up revealed that these reinfections had lower concentrations of IFNα (0.8 [IQR 0.8–0.8] vs. 12.2 [IQR 1.6–24.2], $P = 0.004$) and CCL4 (0.9 [IQR 0.9–12.2 vs. 17.5 [IQR 4.9–32.8], $P = 0.022$];

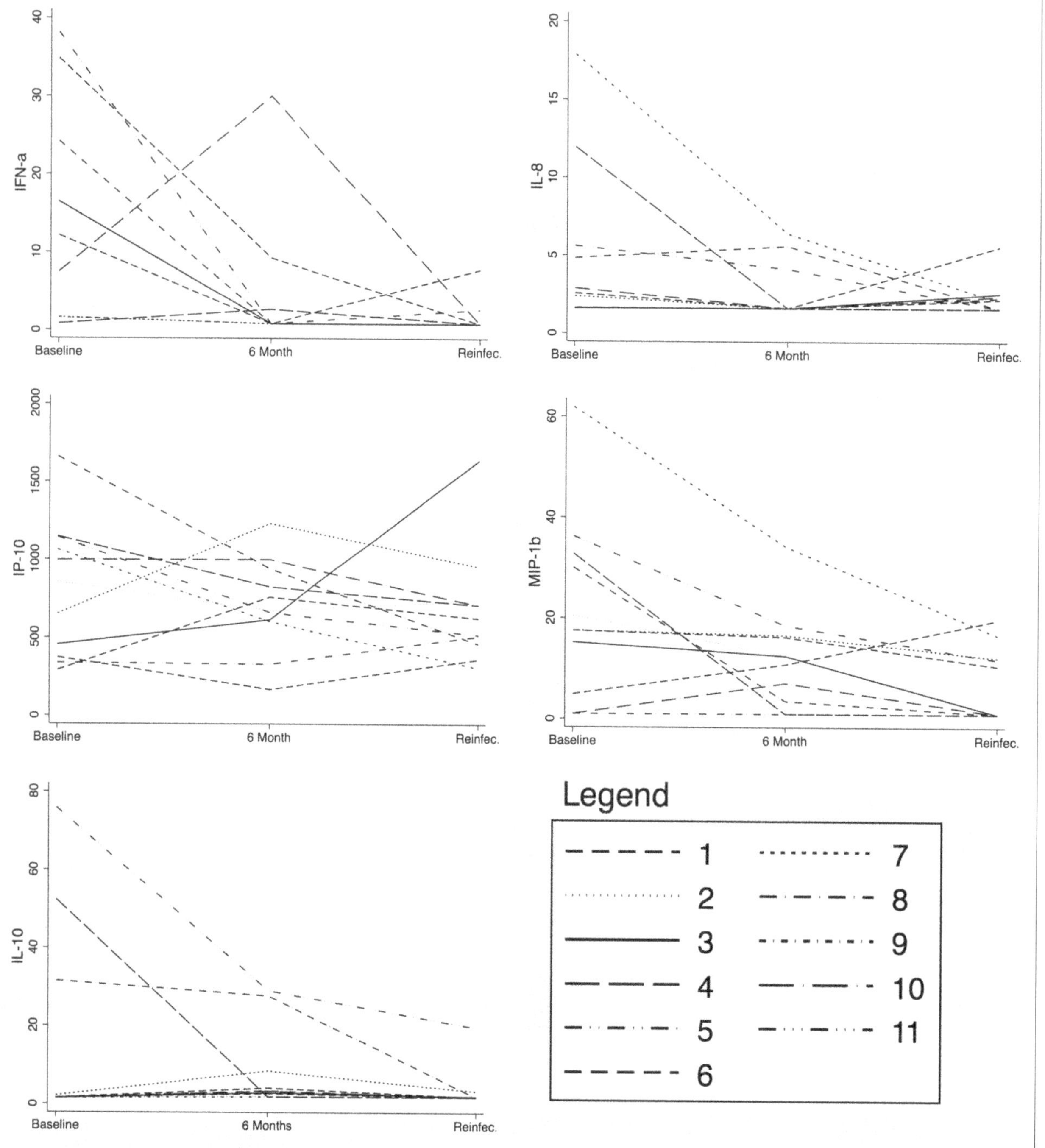

Fig. 1 Selected chemo- and cytokine profiles (in pg/ml) in 11 participants with reinfections during study follow up. Participant number 11 was the only individual whose baseline infection was an initial infection

Table 2). These associations remained after excluding the individual whose baseline infection was his first (initial) episode of syphilis. In general, there was a decline in cyto- and chemokines between baseline and 6-month visit with little or no increase at the time of reinfection (Fig. 1).

Correlation between number of prior episodes of syphilis and individual cyto/chemokines

There was a weak negative association between IFNα and the number of episodes of syphilis (Rho = – 0.42; *P* = 0.050; Table 3).

Discussion

A diagnosis of syphilis in humans and animal models is typically characterized by elevations in both plasma pro-inflammatory (TNFα, IFNγ, CCL4, IP-10) and anti-inflammatory cytokines (IL-10) [11–18]. This immunological profile however varies according to a number of parameters including stage of syphilis [4, 17–20], HIV-infection status [20] and the number of previous episodes of syphilis [4, 21, 22]. Our study is the first that we are aware of that has been able to assess the immune profile of the same individuals at the time of reinfection.

Our study is weakened by the small number included and the fact that only one of the 11 baseline episodes of syphilis was a confirmed initial episode of syphilis. Larger studies would be required to be able to conduct multivariable analyses to control for the role of confounders such as stage of syphilis, number of episodes of syphilis, time between episodes of syphilis and HIV status. With a sample size of only 11 we deemed the risk of type II errors too large to warrant conducting multivariable analyses. As a result we cannot exclude the possibility that our results are due to confounding. Nonetheless our results are commensurate with the thesis that repeat syphilis presents with an attenuated immune response. The individual with an initial syphilis at study inclusion had a more pronounced elevation in IL-10, IFNα, CCL4 and IP-10 than the individuals with repeat syphilis. His second episode of syphilis was also clinically less dramatic and characterized by little or no elevation in plasma cytokines (compared to his 6-month levels). Furthermore, shortly after completing the 24-month follow-up period (and therefore not included in this study) this individual had a third episode of syphilis which was asymptomatic.

In the paired comparisons, plasma IFNα and CCL4 were lower at the time of the reinfection. The fact that repeat episodes had lower IFNα and CCL4 even after excluding the only individual whose baseline syphilis represented an initial infection suggests that each additional episode of syphilis results in a more attenuated immune response than the previous episode. As noted above, this finding is weakened by the fact that in 10 out of 11 individuals the baseline episode of syphilis was not the individual's first episode of syphilis. What we are comparing is earlier with later episodes of syphilis in the same individual. Our

Table 2 Plasma cytokine and chemokine concentrations in baseline, 6-month follow-up and repeat episodes of syphilis (pg/ml)

	Baseline infection	6 month	Repeat infection	*P*-Value[a]
IFNα	12.1 (1.6–24.2)	0.8 (0.8–2.6)	0.8 (0.8–0.8)	0.004
IFNγ	1.5 (1.5–8.9)	1.7 (1.5–10.3)	1.54 (1.5–10.6)	0.714
IL1β	1.5 (1.5–1.5)	1.57 (1.5–1.5)	1.57 (1.5–1.5)	.
IL12p40	1.0 (1.0–1.0)	1.0 (1.0–1.0)	1.0 (1.0–1.0)	.
IL12p70	1.6 (1.6–1.6)	1.6 (1.6–1.6)	1.6 (1.6–1.6)	.
IP-10	855.4 (372.7–1143.6)	672.9 (602.6–941.6)	626.3 (462.0–740.4)	0.424
MCP-1	242.1 (212.8–303.1)	278.37(259.2–312.2)	260.7 (225.8–294.0)	0.533
CCL3	1.6 (1.6–4.9)	1.6 (1.6–1.6)	1.6 (1.6–1.6)	0.127
CCL4	17.5 (4.9–32.8)	12.4 (3.5–16.6)	0.9 (0.9–12.1)	0.022
IL-4	1.6 (1.6–1.6)	1.6 (1.6–1.6)	1.6 (1.6–1.6)	.
IL-5	1.6 (1.6–1.6)	1.6 (1.6–1.6)	1.6 (1.6–1.6)	.
IL-6	1.3 (1.3–1.3)	1.3 (1.3–1.3)	1.3 (1.3–1.3)	.
IL-7	1.1 (1.1–1.6)	1.1 (1.1–1.1)	1.1 (1.1–1.1)	.
IL-8	2.5 (1.6–5.6)	1.6 (1.6–4.1)	2.1 (1.6–2.4)	0.265
IL-10	1.5 (1.5–31.5)	3.3 (1.9–8.4)	1.8 (1.8–1.9)	0.787
IL-17A	1.5 (1.5–1.5)	1.5 (1.5–1.5)	1.5 (1.5–1.5)	0.489
RPR titre	128 (64–128)	8 (2–16)	32 (16–128)	0.07

All values are median and interquartile range

[a] P-value is for paired comparison of reinfections with baseline infections (Wilcoxon's signed rank test)

Table 3 Spearman's correlations between plasma cytokine and chemokine concentrations at the time of syphilis diagnosis and number of prior diagnoses of syphilis (baseline and repeat infections combined, $N = 22$)

	Spearman's correlation	*P*-Value
IFNα	−0.42	0.050
IFNγ	−0.07	0.761
IL1β	–	–
IL12p40	–	–
IL12p70	0.17	0.42
IP-10	−0.22	0.327
MCP-1	0.141	0.531
CCL3	−0.09	0.697
CCL4	−0.27	0.222
IL-4	–	–
IL-5	–	–
IL-6	0.17	0.428
IL-7	0.14	0.532
IL-8	−0.31	0.156
IL-10	−0.04	0.84
IL-17A	−0.28	0.202

findings of lower plasma IFNα and CCL4 in later episodes of syphilis is commensurate with immunological and clinical findings from other studies. Previous studies have, for example, found that each subsequent diagnosis of syphilis is associated with a step-wise increase in peak RPR at the time of diagnosis, a faster decay in RPR but then a higher nadir RPR result following the episode of syphilis [4, 21, 22]. One of these studies found that the RPR result did not serorevert in any individuals with four or more episodes of syphilis [4]. A recent study has found a stepwise increase in the probability that syphilis presents asymptomatically with increasing numbers of episodes of syphilis [3]. These findings suggest that individuals with multiple episodes of syphilis may develop a degree of immunity to infection by *T. pallidum* [1] and that each episode of syphilis has an additive effect in the development of immunity. Further studies are required to assess if the attenuated immune response is correlated with a lower bacterial load and hence infectivity. This would be relevant for studies modeling syphilis spread and might provide clues of use for *Treponema pallidum* vaccine design.

In a similar vein, our study builds on the findings of other contemporary studies which suggest a need to rethink the syphilis staging system used in settings such as ours where repeat syphilis constitutes an increasing proportion of all syphilis infections [1]. In a study of individuals with four or more episodes of syphilis from our center, for example, we found a step-wise increase in the proportion diagnosed with latent (asymptomatic) syphilis with increasing numbers of episodes of syphilis [3]. Similarly, in this study we found that 7 of the 11 episodes of repeat syphilis were latent syphilis. This classification was based on the fact that these 7 episodes were asymptomatic. The traditional staging system of syphilis typically depicts syphilis as progressing from primary to secondary and then early and late latent syphilis [23]. A large proportion of our patients with repeat syphilis do not develop symptoms of syphilis and thus classified as latent syphilis. This is likely due to the attenuated immune response to repeat syphilis and not reflective of a longer duration of infection as would be the case in initial episodes of latent syphilis. Future studies could explore this issue further by assessing if there are clinical, immunological, pathogen and pathological differences between individuals with early and late latent syphilis diagnosed during a first compared to a fourth (or higher) episode of syphilis. Consideration could be given to classifying latent syphilis in individuals with multiple previous episodes of syphilis as latent-repeat syphilis [1].

Unfortunately we were unable to sequence *T. pallidum* DNA from any of the episodes of syphilis included. We were thus unable to establish genotypically if the repeat syphilis was due to reinfection or reactivation as has been done in other studies [24, 25]. Given the high rates of partner change, low rates of condom usage and high syphilis incidence in this cohort [4] it is however likely that most if not all the repeat episodes are due to reinfections. We cannot, however, exclude the possibility that the episodes of repeat syphilis are due to reactivation rather than reinfection. Relapse syphilis may be characterized by a different immunological response to reinfection syphilis and this may influence our results. This misclassification bias would however be expected to bias the results towards the null-hypothesis.

Conclusions

This study makes a small contribution to the growing evidence that the clinical and immunological presentation of repeat syphilis is more attenuated than initial syphilis. This is of considerable clinical and public health consequence. It is important that both clinicians and patients are aware of this as it provides extra motivation for periodic serological screening in persons who have had a diagnosis of syphilis. These individuals are not only at a considerably higher risk of syphilis than the general population, their subsequent syphilis is also more likely to be asymptomatic and serological screening may be the only way to diagnose this syphilis episode in a timeous fashion.

Abbreviations

CCL: Chemokine ligand; IFN: Interferon; IL: Interleukin; IQR: Interquartile range; MIP: Macrophage inflammatory protein; MSM: Men who have sex with men; PCR: Polymerase chain reaction; RPR: Rapid plasma reagin; TNF: Tumour necrosis factor; USA: United States of America

Acknowledgements
We would like to thank Said Abdellati and Vicky Cuylaerts for performing the cytokine assays.

Funding
This work was supported by the grants from the Flemish Government, Department of Economy, Science and Innovation, SOFI-B Grant to CK (Project ID 757003), http://www.fwo.be. The funders played no role in the design of the study or the collection, analysis or interpretation of the data.

Authors' contributions
CK, KO, TC and LK conceived the study. CK conducted the data analyses and wrote the first draft. CK, KO, TC and LK all contributed to the final version of the manuscript. All authors read and approved the final manuscript'

Consent for publication
Not applicable.

Competing interests
The authors declare that they have no competing interests.

Author details
[1]HIV/STI Unit, Institute of Tropical Medicine, Antwerp, Belgium. [2]Division of Infectious Diseases and HIV Medicine, University of Cape Town, Anzio Road, Observatory, Cape Town 7700, South Africa. [3]HIV/STI Reference Laboratory, Institute of Tropical Medicine, Antwerp, Belgium. [4]Immunology Unit, Institute of Tropical Medicine, Antwerp, Belgium. [5]Department of Biomedical Sciences, University of Antwerp, Antwerp, Belgium.

References

1. Kenyon C, Lynen L, Florence E, Caluwaerts S, Vandenbruaene M, Apers L, Soentjens P, Van Esbroeck M, Bottieau E. Syphilis reinfections pose problems for syphilis diagnosis in Antwerp, Belgium - 1992 to 2012. Euro Surveill. 2014;19(45):20958.
2. Botham SJ, Ressler K-A, Maywood P, Hope KG, Bourne CP, Conaty SJ, Ferson MJ, Mayne DJ. Men who have sex with men, infectious syphilis and HIV coinfection in inner Sydney: results of enhanced surveillance. Sex Health. 2013;10(4):291–8.
3. Kenyon C, Osbak KK, Apers L. Repeat syphilis is more likely to be asymptomatic in HIV-infected individuals: a retrospective cohort analysis with important implications for screening. Open Forum Infect Dis. 2018; 5(6):ofy096.
4. Kenyon C, Tsoumanis A, Osbak K, Van Esbroeck M, Crucitti T, Kestens L. Repeat syphilis has a different immune response compared to initial syphilis: an analysis of biomarker kinetics in two cohorts. Sex Transm Infect. 2017; Epub ahead of print.
5. Courjon J, Hubiche T, Dupin N, Grange PA, Del Giudice P. Clinical aspects of syphilis reinfection in HIV-infected patients. Dermatology. 2015;230(4):302–7.
6. Brewer TH, Peterman TA, Newman DR, Schmitt K. Reinfections during the Florida syphilis epidemic, 2000-2008. Sex Transm Dis. 2011;38(1):12–7.
7. Kerani R, Lukehart S, Stenger M, Marra C, Pedersen R, Golden M. Is early latent syphilis more likely in patients with a prior syphilis infection? British Society for Sexual Health and HIV. London: Presentation at 18th international society for STD research; 2009. 28 June-1 July
8. Magnuson HJ, Thomas EW, Olansky S, Kaplan BI, De Mello L, Cutler JC. Inoculation syphilis in human volunteers. Medicine (Baltimore). 1956;35(1):33–82.
9. Workowski KA, Berman SM, Centers for disease C, prevention. Sexually transmitted diseases treatment guidelines, 2010. Atlanta: Department of Health and Human Services, Centers for Disease Control and Prevention; 2010.
10. Chen CY, Chi KH, George RW, Cox DL, Srivastava A, Rui Silva M, Carneiro F, Lauwers GY, Ballard RC. Diagnosis of gastric syphilis by direct immunofluorescence staining and real-time PCR testing. J Clin Microbiol. 2006;44(9):3452–6.
11. Bernardeschi C, Grange PA, Janier M, Gressier L, Dion PL, Benhaddou N, Bianchi A, Lassau F, Avril MF, Batteux F, et al. Treponema pallidum induces systemic TH17 and TH1 cytokine responses. Eur J Dermatol. 2012;22(6):797–8.
12. Wicher V, Scarozza AM, Ramsingh AI, Wicher K. Cytokine gene expression in skin of susceptible Guinea-pig infected with Treponema pallidum. Immunology. 1998;95(2):242–7.
13. Salazar JC, Cruz AR, Pope CD, Valderrama L, Trujillo R, Saravia NG, Radolf JD. Treponema pallidum elicits innate and adaptive cellular immune responses in skin and blood during secondary syphilis: a flow-cytometric analysis. J Infect Dis. 2007;195(6):879–87.
14. Kojima N, Bristow CC, Maecker H, Rosenberg-Hasson Y, Leon SR, Vargas SK, Konda KA, Caceres CF, Klausner JD. Similarities in the markers of inflammation between men with syphilis and women with increased risk of HIV acquisition. Clin Infect Dis. 2016;62(2):265–6.
15. Cruz AR, Ramirez LG, Zuluaga AV, Pillay A, Abreu C, Valencia CA, La Vake C, Cervantes JL, Dunham-Ems S, Cartun R, et al. Immune evasion and recognition of the syphilis spirochete in blood and skin of secondary syphilis patients: two immunologically distinct compartments. PLoS Negl Trop Dis. 2012;6(7):e1717.
16. Knudsen A, Benfield T, Kofoed K. Cytokine expression during syphilis infection in HIV-1-infected individuals. Sex Transm Dis. 2009;36(5):300–4.
17. Podwinska J, Lusiak M, Zaba R, Bowszyc J. The pattern and level of cytokines secreted by Th1 and Th2 lymphocytes of syphilitic patients correlate to the progression of the disease. FEMS Immunol Med Microbiol. 2000;28(1):1–14.
18. Pastuszczak M, Gozdzialska A, Jakiela B, Obtulowicz A, Jaskiewicz J, Wojas-Pelc A. Robust pro-inflammatory immune response is associated with serological cure in patients with syphilis: an observational study. Sex Transm Infect. 2017; 93(1):11–14.
19. Fitzgerald TJ. The Th1/Th2-like switch in syphilitic infection: is it detrimental? Infect Immun. 1992;60(9):3475–9.
20. Kenyon C, Osbak KK, Crucitti T, Kestens L. The immunological response to syphilis differs by HIV status; a prospective observational cohort study. BMC Infect Dis. 2017;17(1):111.
21. Brown ST, Zaidi A, Larsen SA, Reynolds GH. Serological response to syphilis treatment. A new analysis of old data. JAMA. 1985;253(9):1296–9.
22. Romanowski B, Sutherland R, Fick GH, Mooney D, Love EJ. Serologic response to treatment of infectious syphilis. Ann Intern Med. 1991;114(12):1005–9.
23. Tramont E, In S, Mandell GL, Bennett JE, Dolin R. Principles and Practice of Infectious Diseases. 8th ed. Atlanta: Churchill Livingstone Inc; 2015.
24. Myint M, Bashiri H, Harrington RD, Marra CM. Relapse of secondary syphilis after benzathine penicillin G: molecular analysis. Sex Transm Dis. 2004;31(3):196–9.
25. Florindo C, Reigado V, Gomes JP, Azevedo J, Santo I, Borrego MJ. Molecular typing of treponema pallidum clinical strains from Lisbon, Portugal. J Clin Microbiol. 2008;46(11):3802–3.

20

Prevalence of chlamydia trachomatis infection among reproductive age women in sub Saharan Africa

Siraj Hussen[1*], Demelash Wachamo[2], Zemenu Yohannes[3] and Endale Tadesse[1]

Abstract

Background: *Chlamydia trachomatis* is the most common curable sexual transmitted bacterial infection in the world, including Sub-Saharan Africa. There is nil systematic review and meta-analysis on *Chlamydia trachomatis* infection in Sub-Saharan Africa among reproductive age women. Therefore, this study was carried out to determine the pooled prevalence of *chlamydia trachomatis* infection in Sub-Saharan Africa among reproductive age women.

Methods: A comprehensive literature search was conducted from biomedical data bases: Medline, PubMed, EMBASE, Google scholar, HINARI and Cochrane Library using a special index search terms (medical subject headings (MeSH), title and abstract. The Cochrane Q test and I^2 statistics was used to test heterogeneity and publication bias was assessed using Begg's and Egger's tests. Results were presented in tables, figures and funnel plot. Data were pooled in a meta-analysis using a random effects model.

Results: Twenty-four studies were included in this meta–analysis. There was a high level of heterogeneity among studies. The pooled prevalence of *Chlamydia trachomatis* infection in Sub-Saharan Africa among reproductive age women *was* 7.8% (95% CI: 5.6–10.6).

Conclusion: This review showed that *Chlamydia trachomatis* infection is high in Sub-Saharan Africa among reproductive age group women. This evidence suggests that governmental and non-governmental organization shall give attention for primary prevention of this infection. Likewise, in resource limited countries policy makers, stakeholders and health care providers' due attention for *Chlamydia trachomatis* specific and rapid diagnostic test, treatment in any medical out and in patient clinics for reproductive age women.

Keywords: Systematic review, Meta-analysis, *Chlamydia trachomatis*, Reproductive age women, Sub-Saharan Africa

Background

Chlamydia trachomatis is the major public health concern across the globe,and the main cause of sexual transmitted infections throughout the world, especially Sub-Saharan Africa [1]. The World Health Organization (WHO) estimated that 50 million women were newly infected with *Chlamydia trachomatis* worldwide, of which 34 million were in Sub-Saharan Africa and South/Southeast Asia.It is the most implicated organism that causes infertility and pelvic inflammatory disease [2–5].

Chlamydia trachomatis is the most common curable sexual transmitted bacterial infection in the world, with an estimated 4–5 million new cases each year [6]. WHO estimated that, the incidence of *Chlamydia trachomatis* is high in sub-Saharan Africa, which is more than 10 million new infection annually [2].

Chlamydial infection in women is commonly asymptomatic. Undetected and untreated *Chlamydial* infection can ascend upper genitalia that may cause pelvic inflammatory disease (PID), infertility, ectopic pregnancy and chronic pelvic pain [7, 8]. *Chlamydial* infection in

* Correspondence: sirajhu123@gmail.com
[1]Department of Medical Laboratory Science, College of Medicine and Health Sciences, Hawassa University, Hawassa, Ethiopia
Full list of author information is available at the end of the article

women show that different clinical manifestations and associated disease like: cervicitis,endometritis, salpingitis, pelvic inflammatory disease, infertility, preterm rupture of membranes, perihepatitis, while most of women do not get medical care, because more than three forth of women are commonly asymptomatic [9].Untreated Chlamydial infection cause up to 40% of pelvic inflammatory disease cases, one in four of these will result in infertility [10].

Untreated genital infection in sub-Saharan Africa can cause up to 85% of infertility among women who seek infertility treatment and care. Undetected and untreated Chlamydial infections during pregnancy can increase risk of cervicitis, endometritis, salpingitis, pelvic inflammatory disease, infertility, perihepatitis, premature rupture of the membranes, low birth weight,chorio amnionitis, neonatal sepsis and conjunctivitis in new born [11, 12]. Whereas, the risk of developing PID after lower genital tract chlamydial infection varies considerably, up to 30%, and the risk of developing tubal infertility after PID is 10–20% [7].

Chlamydial infection can occur at any anatomical site of sexual contact including endocervix, urethra, rectum, and oropharynx, which causes pelvic inflammatory disease, infertility, ectopic pregnancy and chronic pelvic pain for women [13].

Throughout our search and knowledge, there is no systematic review and meta-analysis regarding *Chlamydia trachomatis* infection among reproductive age women in Sub-Saharan Africa. This study is used as an input for clinician, public health experts and stake holders for possible interventions.

Methods

Study design and search strategy

A systematic review and meta-analysis was done using published articles on prevalence of *Chlamydia trachomatis* in Sub-Saharan Africa. A comprehensive literature search was conducted from biomedical data bases: Medline, PubMed, EMBASE, Google scholar, HINARI and Cochrane Library using a special index search terms (medical subject headings (MeSH) "prevalence of *Chlamydia trachomatis AND* Sub-Saharan Africa, *Chlamydia trachomatis* AND reproductive age group, *Chlamydia trachomatis* OR Neisseria gonorrhea, *Chlamydia trachomatis* OR sexual transmitted infection", title and abstract. The limit of language was English and the limit of study group was human. Searching of articles were carried out from March to October 01, 2017.

Study selection and data extraction

Cross-sectional studies published in English language from 1997 to 2017 were included. Articles that assessed prevalence of *Chlamydia trachomatis* infection among reproductive age group who attended ANC, family planning clinic, STI clinic, Gynecology clinic and in general population were used. Age restriction was imposed. Reproductive age group women were defined as those of age 15–49 years.

The critical appraisal was done before the extraction of data. Data extraction was carried out using the Downs and Black checklist [14]. All essential information was extracted from the final selected studies. It contains study year, population characteristics, sample size, prevalence, age, and Chlamydia *trachomatis* screening technique. Four authors independently reviewed the studies and inconsistencies were resolved through discussion and consensus.

Quality assessment

The quality of selected articles were assessed using 12 point scoring system based on Downs and Black check lists. These are: (clarity of objective, reported response rate which scored ≥80%, clear data collection methods and procedures, study design clearly described, sample representativeness of the entire population, the main finding of the study clearly described, suitable sampling methods, reliable measurement of outcome variable, use of appropriate statistical analysis method, and quality assurance methods). Mean quality score was used to assess the quality of included studies in the meta-analysis. Studies which scored above the mean of the quality score were grouped into the high-quality score, and those below the mean were grouped as low-quality score and not include in the meta-analysis [14].

Statistical analysis

Data entry and analysis were done using Comprehensive Meta-Analysis (version 3.1).The pooled prevalence of *Chlamydia trachomatis* with 95%CI was obtained using the random effects model, due to the possibility of heterogeneity among the studies.

Sub-group analysis

Sub-group analysis was conducted based on type of study population; (Community based, FCSWS Health facility based), Geographical zone; (East Africa, Middle Africa, Southern Africa and West Africa), laboratory diagnostic methods (ICT and PCR) and Year of study; (1997–2001, 2002–2006, 2007–2011, and 2012–2016).

Heterogeneity and publication bias

The heterogeneity of studies were assessed using Cochran's Q test and I^2 test statistics. A Cochran's Q test $P < 0.10$ is indicated that heterogeneity between the studies [15]. The level of I^2 test statistics of 25, 50 and 75% are used low, medium and high heterogeneity, respectively [16]. Publication bias was assessed by Egger's and Begg's test, and *p*-value less than 0.05 is statistically significance, and there is publication bias [17].

Results

Identified studies

A total of 93 records were retrieved through electronic database searching. Records were screened using their titles, abstracts and through full article review. Accordingly, a total of 63 articles were excluded using their title and abstract review. Thirty articles were assessed for eligibility and six article was excluded by exclusion criteria in the study. Finally, 24 articles were included in this meta-analysis (Fig. 1). The Cohran's Q (905.3) and I^2 statistics (I^2 = 97.459%; $p < 0.0001$) revealed that high heterogeneity among studies. However, neither Egger's test ($p = 0.231$) nor Begg's test ($p = 0.085$) gave evidence of publication bias, which indicate to use random effects model.

Study characteristics

The total study population size screened for *Chlamydia trachomatis* and involved in this systematic review and meta-analysis were 17,119.Among these, 9606 were screened at community based studies [18–23], about 2638 were FCSWS [19, 20, 24–28] and 4875 were at health facility based studies [28–38]. The sample size of study population varied from 100 [24] to 4886 [19], and were conducted between the year 1997–2001 [19, 22, 30], 2002–2006 [25], 2007–2011 [21, 26, 31] and 2012–2016 [23, 27, 34–36]. Geographically,the population screened for *Chlamydia trachomatis* four regions of Sub-Saharan Africa: East Africa [19, 22, 27, 32–35, 37],West Africa [18, 20–24, 26, 28–30], Southern Africa [22, 31, 39], and middle Africa [25, 38] (Table 1).

Meta-analysis

The analysis of 24 studies, according to the Der Simonian-Laird random-effects model. The pooled prevalence of *C. trachomatis* among Sub-Saharan African reproductive age women was 7.8% (95% CI: 5.6–10.6) (Fig. 2). In particular, the pooled prevalence among subgroup was 9.7% (95% CI: 5.8–16.0) in FCSWs, 7.0% (95% CI; 3.2–14.7) in community based studies, and 7.6% (95% CI; 4.7–12.3) in health facility studies. Regarding year of study, 3.8% (95% CI; 2.1–6.7) from 1997 to 2001, 8.4% (95% CI; 1.8–31.1) from 2002 to 2006, 8.8% (95% CI; 3.7–19.5) from 2007 to 2011 and11.0% (95% CI; 7.3–16.4) from 2012 to 2016, while among diagnostic method 12.8% (95% CI; 7.6–20.6) screened by ICT, and 5.8% (95% CI; 3.8–8.6) screened by PCR (Table 2). Further, subgroup analysis was done among geographical location, 8.9% (95% CI; 4.5–16.6) in East Africa, 7.2% (95% CI; 1.8–24.6) Middle Africa, 5.9% (95% CI; 1.9–16.8) Southern Africa, and 7.4% (95% CI; 4.1–13.1) in West Africa (Fig. 3).

Discussion

Chlamydia trachomatis is an important public health problem across the globe, including Sub-Saharan Africa. Most developed countries have implemented specific chlamydial infection control programs that vary from case management to opportunistic screening of high risk groups and annual screening program for sexually active women age < 25 years to tackle the problem. These countries decreased chlamydial infection and its complication, while in developing countries the management is still syndromic approach, and its infection and complications are still huge burden in Sub-Saharan Africa [40], because of its asymptomatic nature of the infection in

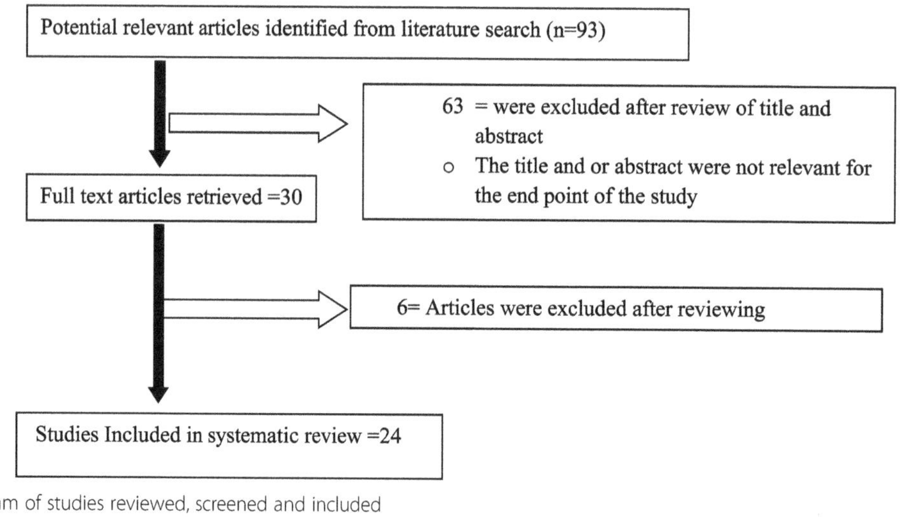

Fig. 1 Flow diagram of studies reviewed, screened and included

Table 1 *Chlamydia trachomatis infection* among reproductive age women in different study populations in different regions of Sub Saharan Africa from 1997 to 2016 [18–34]

Authors, publication year [Ref]	Country	Study population	Sample size	Prvalence(%)	Specimen	Age group	Diagnostic methods
Yirenya et al., 2014 [18]	Ghana	Community	191	6.3	Endocervical swabs	15–49	PCR
Obasi et al., 2001 [19]	Tanzania	Community	4686	2.4	Urine	15–19	PCR
Wariso et al., 2012 [20]	Nigeria	Student	400	11	Urine	16–30	PCR
Ikeme et al., 2011 [21]	Nigeria	Community	286	29.4	Blood	20–34	ICT
Buve et al., 2001 [22]	Benin	Community	962	1.3	Urine	15–49	*PCR*
Buve et al., 2001 [22]	Cameron	Community	1016	9.4	Urine	15–49	*PCR*
Buve et al., 2001 [22]	Kenya	Community	821	4.5	Urine	15–49	*PCR*
Buve et al., 2001 [22]	Zambia	Community	890	2.9	Urine	15–49	PCR
Arize et al., 2014 [23]	Nigeria	Students	354	30.2	Endocervical swabs	15–30	ICT
Abubakari et al.,2016 [24]	Ghana	FCSWs	100	19	Endocervical swabs	18–35	ICT
Vandepitte et al.,2007 [25]	Congo	FCSWs	502	8.4	Vaginal swabs	15–49	PCR
Opoku & Sarkodie,2014 [26]	Ghana	FCSWs	1070	4.8	vaginal swabs	18–35	*ICT*
Francis et al., 2014 [27]	Tanzania	FCSWs	966	12	Blood (Serum)	18–44	PCR
Apea-Kubi,2014 [28]	Ghana	OB and Gyn	465	3	Endocervical swabs	15–49	PCR
Gomes et al., 2001 [29]	Guinea-Bissau	STI and FP	200	4	Endocervical swabs	15–49	PCR
Luján et al., 2008 [30]	Mozambique	ANC	1119	4.1	urine	15–49	PCR
Kohli et al., 2013 [31]	Kenya	OPD	300	6	Vaginal swabs	18–45	ICT
Adesiji et al., 2015 [32]	Nigeria	FP and Gyn	140	0.7	Endocervical swabs	15–49	ICT
Tadesse et al., 2016 [33]	Hawassa	FP and Gyn	322	18.9	Endocervical swabs	15–49	ICT
Musa et al., 2016 [34]	Uganda	Gyn	324	26.5	Endocervical swabs	15–49	ICT
Mainaet al., 2016 [35]	Kenya	FP	261	13	Endocervical swabs	18–49	PCR
Peters et al., 2014 [36]	South Africa	ANC	603	16	Vaginal swabs	18–49	PCR
Mayaud *et al.*, 2016 [37]	Tanzania	ANC	660	5.9	Endocervical swabs	15–49	ICT
Blankhart*et al.*, 1999 [38]	C.A Rep.	ANC	481	6.2	Endocervical swab	15–49	PCR

ANC antenatal care, *OB* obstetrics, *FCSHS* Female commercial sex workers, *FP* Family planning, *Gyn* gynecology, Community based study (all reproductive age women who live in the study area), *ICT* Immuno chromatographic test and *PCR* Polymerase chain reaction

most patients left unnoticed and remain untreated for longer period of time, there by transmitting the infection to their sexual partner(s). Annual screening of *Chlamydia trachomatis* in low income countries in all sexually active women aged < 25 years isn't applied, whereas after complications the cost of diagnosis and treatment is high, which is compared to annual screening [7, 11]. In resource limited countries, reports of *Chlamydia trachomatis* represents only 'tip of ice berg', most of women have asymptomatic stage [11].

Based on the available data, the present study attempted to synthesize prevalence of *chlamydia trachomatis* in Sub-Saharan Africa among reproductive age women. In most studies the prevalence of *chlamydia trachomatis* is widely different from time to time, region to region, study population, study setting and type of laboratory diagnosis method.

This systematic review and meta-analysis showed that *Chlamydia trachomatis* among reproductive age group women in Sub-Saharan Africa was 7.8%, among diagnostic method 5.8% screened by PCR and 12.8% screened by ICT. This finding is inconsistent with WHO 2008 estimated in Africa is 2.6% [11], in 2005 is 4% [2] and global estimated is 4.2% [6].This finding is in line with systematic review in women attending antenatal care estimated prevalence of 6.9%, and the highest prevalence is predominantly at younger age < 25 years for chlamydial infection [41, 42].

In this study, the prevalence in east Africa was 8.9%. This finding is in agreement with the 6.9% reported in a systematic review and meta-analysis in East/Southern Africa, and 6.1% (95% CI: 4.0–8.3) in West/Central Africa. But, lower than a single counties reviewed studies like 4.9–14% in China, 0.1–35.9% in India, 5.7–16.2% in Thailand, 19.3% in Mongolia, and 41–44% in Bangladesh [1]. The difference might be, in this study, most of studies takes place in health facilities and around urban area, whereas studies in Asia is nationwide and screening

Model	Group by Diagnostic	Study name	Events/Total	Statistics for each study		Statistics for each	
			Total	Event rate	Lower limit	Upper limit	Relative weight
	ICT	Ikeme et al., 2011[21]	84 / 286	0.294	0.244	0.349	12.09
	ICT	Arize et al., 2014 [23]	107 / 354	0.302	0.256	0.352	12.15
	ICT	Abubakari et al.,2016 [24]	19 / 100	0.190	0.125	0.279	11.32
	ICT	Opoku and Sarkodie , 2010 [26]	51 / 1070	0.048	0.037	0.063	12.03
	ICT	Kohli et al., 2013 [31]	18 / 300	0.060	0.038	0.093	11.40
	ICT	Adesiji et al., 2015 [32]	1 / 140	0.007	0.001	0.049	4.97
	ICT	Tadesse et al., 2016 [33]	61 / 322	0.189	0.150	0.235	12.03
	ICT	Musa et al., 2016 [34]	86 / 324	0.265	0.220	0.316	12.11
	ICT	Mayaud et al., 2016 [37]	39 / 660	0.059	0.043	0.080	11.91
Fixed	ICT			0.173	0.159	0.188	
Random	ICT			0.128	0.076	0.206	
	PCR	Yirenya et al., 2014 [18]	12 / 191	0.063	0.036	0.108	6.25
	PCR	Obasi et al.,2001[19]	112 / 4686	0.024	0.020	0.029	6.97
	PCR	Wariso et al., 2012 [20]	44 / 400	0.110	0.083	0.145	6.81
	PCR	Buve et al., 2001 [22] B	13 / 962	0.013	0.007	0.022	6.31
	PCR	Buve et al., 2001 [22] C	96 / 1016	0.094	0.078	0.114	6.94
	PCR	Buve et al., 2001 [22] K	37 / 821	0.045	0.033	0.062	6.78
	PCR	Buve et al., 2001 [22] Z	26 / 890	0.029	0.020	0.042	6.67
	PCR	Vandepitte et al.,2007 [25]	42 / 502	0.084	0.063	0.112	6.80
	PCR	Francis et al., 2014[27]	116 / 966	0.120	0.101	0.142	6.96
	PCR	Apea-Kubi,2014 [28]	14 / 465	0.030	0.018	0.050	6.37
	PCR	Gomes et al., 2001[29]	8 / 200	0.040	0.020	0.078	5.93
	PCR	Luján et al., 2008 [30]	46 / 1119	0.041	0.031	0.054	6.83
	PCR	Maina et al., 2016 [35]	34 / 261	0.130	0.094	0.177	6.73
	PCR	Peters et al., 2014 [36]	96 / 603	0.160	0.133	0.191	6.93
	PCR	Blankhart et al., 1999 [38]	30 / 481	0.062	0.044	0.087	6.71
Fixed	PCR			0.068	0.063	0.073	
Random	PCR			0.058	0.038	0.086	
Fixed	Overall			0.096	0.091	0.101	
Random	Overall			0.078	0.056	0.106	

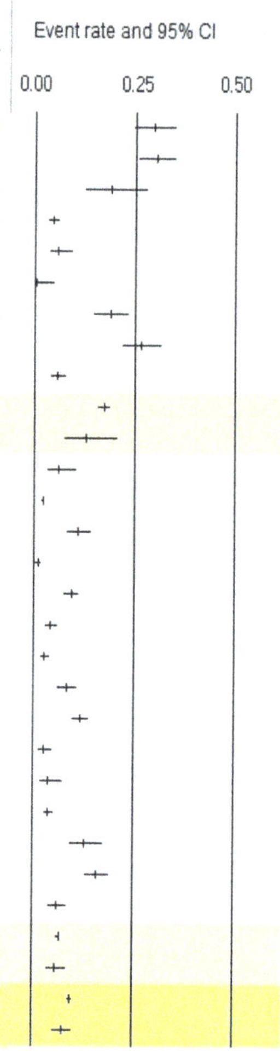

Fig. 2 The meta-analysis and forest plot presentation of *C.trachomatis* prevalence from 1997 to 2016 (Citations of studies used in the analysis from top to bottom [18–37, 50]

Table 2 Subgroup meta-analysis of C. trachomatis prevalence estimation in Sub Saharan Africa from 1997 to 2016

	Study parameters	Subgroup	Studies included	Prevalence %(95% CI)	I^2%	*P*-v
C. trachomatis	study population	Community based	9	7.0(3.2–14.7)	98.678	< 0.0001
		CFSWs	4	9.7(5.8–16.0)	93.168	< 0.0001
		Health facility based	11	7.6(4.7–12.3)	95.763	< 0.0001
	Study year	1997–2001	7	3.8(12.1–6.7)	95.289	< 0.0001
		200–2006	1	8.4(1.8–31.1)	0.000	1.000
		2007–2011	3	8.8(3.7–19.5)	98.852	< 0.0001
		2012–2016	13	11.0(7.3–16.4)	94.753	< 0.0001
	Geographical zone	Eastern	8	8.9(4.5–16.6)	98.240	< 0.0001
		Middle	2	7.2(1.8–24.6)	42.502	0.187
		Southern	3	5.9(1.9–16.8)	98.008	< 0.0001
		Western	11	7.4(4.1–13.1)	97.181	< 0.0001
	Diagnostic method	ICT	9	12.8(7.6–20.6)	97.083	< 0.0001
		PCR	15	5.8(3.8–8.6)	96.230	< 0.0001

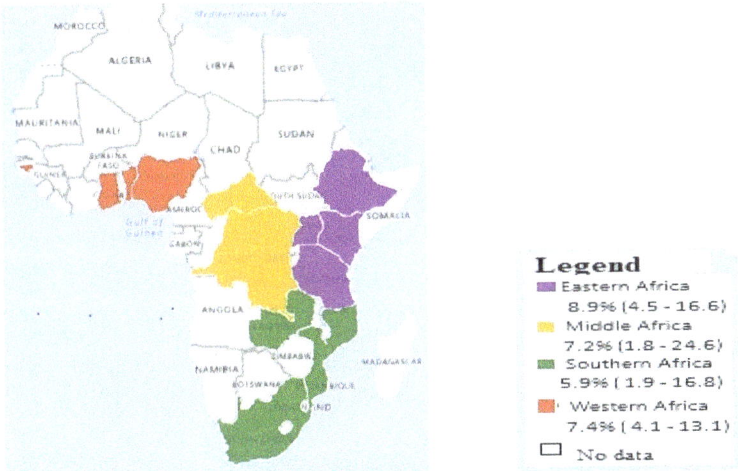

Fig. 3 Prevalence of *Chlamydia trachomatis* in different regions of Sub-Saharan Africa among reproductive age group women, 1997–2016

strategy and diagnostic method quite different from Sub-Saharan Africa.

This finding is slightly higher than over all prevalence of a systematic reviewed in Australia is 4.6%, but with similar prevalence of 5.6% among adolescent and young adults [43] and in Europe, the prevalence ranged from1.7 to 17% depending on the setting, context and country [44] and this finding also slightly higher than over all prevalence in USA is 5% [45].

Over all prevalence in Australia is slightly lower than this study might be Australia women are more educated and treated at asymptomatic stage, because in Australia there is annual chlamydial infection screening for sexual active women age < 25 years.

This finding is slightly lower than with a systematic review in prison is 12.31% (95% CI:10.61, 14.01) for chlamydial infection in women, and a systematic review and meta-analysis in Iran, the pooled prevalence of the bacterium in the female population was 12.3% (95% CI: 10.6–14.2%) [46, 47]. The difference might be sociocultural, socioeconomically, screening strategy and types of laboratory diagnostic methods.

Pooled prevalence of *Chlamydia trachomatis infection* among commercial sex workers sub group was 9.7% (95% CI: 5.8–16.0). This study is unlikely with the population based meta-analysis study conducted in Australia, for women age < 25 years reported 5.0% (95% CI: 3.1, 6.9), among women aged < 25 years attending sexual health, family planning or youth clinics, estimated prevalence was 6.2% (95% CI:5.1, 7.4; 10), and other key finding include pooled prevalence estimates of 22.1% (95% CI: 19.0, 25.3) for indigenous women < 25 years [48].

Potential limitations of this study, due to the nature of infection, most women are asymptomatic, or treated at private or traditional, self-treated and unreported or under reported, whereas *Chlamydia trachomatis is* under estimated. Another important limitation is that different diagnostic methods were used in the studies included in meta-analysis. The current estimates are limited to urogenital infections. But, chlamydial infection can be rectal and oropharyngeal infection. An important limitation is the use of reproductive age women as search term. Other limitations, among further others are the heterogeneity of data and lack of reproductive tract impact data.

Implication of this study; this review generate information on prevalence *of Chlamydia trachomatis* infection among reproductive age women in Sub-Saharan Africa. Therefore, Sub-Saharan Africa countries and their stakeholders use this information for evidence-based intervention, to establish rapid diagnostic test and to improve their national surveillance system of *Chlamydia trachomatis* infection. This systematic and meta-analysis is an input for developing countries, stakeholders and policy makers to develop diagnostic and treatment programs for *Chlamydia trachomatis* infections. *Chlamydia trachomatis* is a serious public health problem in developing countries, especially Sub Saharan Africa. STI including *Chlamydia trachomatis* over shadowed by HIV/AIDS and given less attention [20].

Conclusion

This study revealed that *chlamydia trachomatis* infection in Sub-Saharan Africa among reproductive age group women is high. This evidence suggests that the government and non-government organization shall give attention for primary prevention of this infection. Likewise, in resource limited countries policy makers, stakeholders and health care providers' due attention on *Chlamydia trachomatis* specific and rapid diagnostic test, treatment in any medical out and in patient clinics for reproductive age women.

Abbreviations

ANC: Antenatal care clinic; C.T: *Chlamydia trachomatis*; FCSWs: Female commercial sex workers; FP: Family planning; ICT: Immunochromatographic test; OB: Obstetrics; PCR: Polymerase chain reaction; PID: Pelvic inflammatory disease; STI: Sexual transmitted infection; WHO: World health organization

Acknowledgements

We don't have any person or organization to acknowledge.

Funding

There was no any funding or sponsoring organization for this paper.

Authors' contributions

SH was the principal investigator who contributed to origin, the idea and design of the study, collected, entered, analyzed, interpreted the data, prepared the manuscript and acted as corresponding author. DM, ZY and ET contributed to data analysis, interpretation and drafted the manuscript. All authors read and approved the final manuscript.

Consent for publication

Not applicable.

Competing interests

The authors declare that they have no competing interests.

Author details

[1]Department of Medical Laboratory Science, College of Medicine and Health Sciences, Hawassa University, Hawassa, Ethiopia. [2]Department of Public Health, Hawassa College of Health Sciences, South Nations and Nationalities Peoples' Region, Hawassa, Ethiopia. [3]Department of Midwifery, College of Medicine and Health Sciences, Hawassa University, Hawassa, Ethiopia.

References

1. Adachi K, Nielsen-Saines K, Klausner JD. Chlamydia trachomatis infection in pregnancy: the global challenge of preventing adverse pregnancy and infant outcomes in sub-Saharan Africa and Asia. 2016:1–21. https://doi.org/10.1155/2016/9315757.
2. World Health Organization. Prevalence and incidence of selected sexually transmitted infections, Chlamydia trachomatis, Neisseria gonorrhoeae, Syphilis and trichomonas vaginalis: methods and results used by WHO to generate 2005 estimates. Geneva; 2011.
3. Enwuru CP, Umeh SI. Asymptomatic Carriage of Chlamydia trachomatis Among Young Adults in Owerri, South East Nigeria. 2014:3:49–53.
4. Finan R, Tamim H, Almawi W. Identification of chlamydia trachomatis DNA in human papillomavirus (HPV) positive women with normal and abnormal cytology. Arch Gynecol Obstet. 2002;266(3):168–71.
5. Okoror L, Agbonlahor D, Esumeh F, Umolu P. Prevalence of chlamydia in patients attending gynecological clinics in south eastern Nigeria. Afr Health Sci. 2007;7(1):18–24.
6. Newman L, Rowley J, Vander Hoorn S, Wijesooriya NS, Unemo M, Low N, et al. Global estimates of the prevalence and incidence of four curable sexually transmitted infections in 2012 based on systematic review and global reporting. PLoS One. 2015;10(12):e0143304.
7. Land J, Van Bergen J, Morre S, Postma M. Epidemiology of chlamydia trachomatis infection in women and the cost-effectiveness of screening. Hum Reprod Update. 2009;16(2):189–204.
8. World Health Organization. Global incidence and prevalence of selected curable. Sex Transm Infect. 2008:19–20.
9. Haggerty CL, Gottlieb SL, Taylor BD, Low N, Xu F, Ness RB. Risk of sequelae after chlamydia trachomatis genital infection in women. J Infect Dis. 2010; 201(Suppl 2):S134–55.
10. World Health Organization. Global strategy for the prevention and control of sexually transmitted infections: 2006–2015: breaking the chain of transmission. Geneva; 2007.
11. World Health Organization. Sexually transmitted infections (STIs): the importance of a renewed commitment to STI prevention and control in achieving global sexual and. Reprod Health. 2013:1–2.
12. World Health Organization.Laboratory diagnosis of sexually transmitted infections, including human immunodeficiency virus. Geneva; 2013.
13. Peters RP, Nijsten N, Mutsaers J, Jansen CL, Morré SA, van Leeuwen AP. Screening of oropharynx and anorectum increases prevalence of chlamydia trachomatis and Neisseria gonorrhoeae infection in female STD clinic visitors. Sex Transm Dis. 2011;38(9):783–7.
14. Downs SH, Black N. The feasibility of creating a checklist for the assessment of the methodological quality both of randomised and non-randomised studies of health care interventions. J Epidemiol Community Health. 1998; 52(6):377–84.
15. DerSimonian R, Laird N. Meta-analysis in clinical trials. Control Clin Trials. 1986;7(3):177–88.
16. Rücker G, Schwarzer G, Carpenter JR, Schumacher M. Undue reliance on I 2 in assessing heterogeneity may mislead. BMC Med Res Methodol. 2008;8(1): 79.
17. Ioannidis JP. Interpretation of tests of heterogeneity and bias in meta-analysis. J Eval Clin Pract. 2008;14(5):951–7.
18. Yirenya-Tawiah D, Annang TN, Apea-Kubi KA, Lomo G, Mensah D, Akyeh L, et al. Chlamydia trachomatis and Neisseria gonorrhoeae prevalence among women of reproductive age living in urogenital schistosomiasis endemic area in Ghana. BMC Res Notes. 2014;7(1):349.
19. Obasi AI, Balira R, Todd J, Ross DA, Changalucha J, Mosha F, et al. Prevalence of HIV and chlamydia trachomatis infection in 15–19-year olds in rural Tanzania. Tropical Med Int Health. 2001;6(7):517–25.
20. Wariso K, Odigie J, Eyaru S. Prevalence of chlamydia trachomatis infection among female undergraduates of the University of Port Harcourt Using Strand Displacement and Amplification [SDA] technique. Nigerian Health J. 2012;12(2):35–8.
21. Ikeme A, Ezegwui H, Ikeako L, Agbata I, Agbata E. Seroprevalence of chlamydia trachomatis in Enugu, Nigeria. Niger J Clin Pract. 2011;14(2):176–80.
22. Buve A, Weiss HA, Laga M, Van Dyck E, Musonda R, Zekeng L, et al. The epidemiology of gonorrhoea, chlamydial infection and syphilis in four African cities. AIDS. 2001;15:S79–88.
23. Arinze AUH, Onyebuchi NV, Isreal J. Genital chlamydia trachomatis infection among female undergraduate students of University of Port Harcourt, Nigeria. Niger Med J. 2014;55(1):9.
24. Abubakari A, Osei-Djarbeng SN, Larbi JA, Frimpong EH. Presence of chlamydia infection among asymptomatic female commercial sex-workers (CSWs) in the Kumasi Metropolis, Ghana. Int J Curr Microbiol App Sci. 2016; 5(1):342–9.
25. Vandepitte JM, Malele F, Kivuvu D-M, Edidi S, Muwonga J, Lepira F, et al. HIV and other sexually transmitted infections among female sex workers in Kinshasa, Democratic Republic of Congo, in 2002. Sex Transm Dis. 2007; 34(4):203–8.
26. Opoku B, Sarkodie Y. Prevalence of genital chlamydia and gonococcal infections in at risk women in the Kumasi metropolis, Ghana. Ghana Med J. 2010;44(1):21–4.
27. Francis SC, Ao TT, Vanobberghen FM, Chilongani J, Hashim R, Andreasen A, et al. Epidemiology of curable sexually transmitted infections among women at increased risk for HIV in northwestern Tanzania: inadequacy of syndromic management. PLoS One. 2014;9(7):e101221.
28. Adesiji Y, Iyere S, Ogah I. Low prevalence of chlamydia trachomatis infection in women from southern Nigeria. Nitte Univ J Health Sci. 2015;5(1):4.
29. Apea-Kubi KA, Yamaguchi S, Sakyi B, Kishimoto T, Ofori-Adjei D, Hagiwara T. Neisseria gonorrhoea, chlamydia trachomatis, and Treponema pallidum infection in antenatal and gynecological patients at Korle-Bu teaching hospital, Ghana. Jpn J Infect Dis. 2014;57(6):253–6.
30. Gomes J, Tavira L, Exposto F, Prieto E, Catry M. Neisseria gonorrhoeae and chlamydia trachomatis infections in patients attending STD and family planning clinics in Bissau, Guinea-Bissau. Acta Trop. 2001;80(3):261–4.
31. Luján J, Oñate WA, Delva W, Sambola F, Claeys P, Temmerman M, et al. Prevalence of sexually transmitted infections in women attending

antenatal care in Tete province, Mozambique. SAMJ. 2008;98(1):49–51.

32. Kohli R, Konya WP, Obura T, Stones W, Revathi G. Prevalence of genital chlamydia infection in urban women of reproductive age, Nairobi, Kenya. BMC Res Notes. 2013;6(1):44.
33. Tadesse E, Teshome M, Amsalu A, Shimelis T. Genital chlamydia trachomatis infection among women of reproductive age attending the gynecology Clinic of Hawassa University Referral Hospital, southern Ethiopia. PLoS One. 2016;11(12):e0168580.
34. Musa M, Joel B, Lenard A, Joseph N, Ronald M, Julius M, et al. Prevalence and factors associated with genital chlamydial infections among women attending the Gynaecology clinic at Mbarara regional referral hospital. Prevalence. 2016;26:26–7.
35. Maina AN, Kimani J, Anzala O. Prevalence and risk factors of three curable sexually transmitted infections among women in Nairobi, Kenya. BMC Res Notes. 2016;9(1):193.
36. Peters RP, Dubbink JH, van der Eem L, Verweij SP, Bos ML, Ouburg S, et al. Cross-sectional study of genital, rectal, and pharyngeal chlamydia and gonorrhea in women in rural South Africa. Sex Transm Dis. 2014; 41(9):564–9.
37. Mayaud P, Uledi E, Cornelissen J, Todd J, Rwakatare M, West B, et al. Risk scores to detect cervical infections in urban antenatal clinic attenders in Mwanza, Tanzania. Sex Transm Infect. 2016;74:S139–46.
38. Blankhart D, Muller O, Gresenguet G, Weis P. Sexually transmitted infections in young pregnant women in Bangui, Central African Republic. Int J STD AIDS. 1999;10(9):609–14.
39. Dubbink JH, De Waaij DJ, Bos M, Van der Eem L, Bébéar C, Mbambazela N, et al. Microbiological characteristics of chlamydia trachomatis and neisseria gonorrhoeae infections in South African women. J Clin Microbiol. 2016; 54(1):200–3.
40. Low N, Cassell JA, Spencer B, Bender N, Martin Hilber A, van Bergen J, et al. Chlamydia control activities in Europe: cross-sectional survey. Eur J Public Health. 2011;22(4):556–61.
41. Chico RM, Mayaud P, Ariti C, Mabey D, Ronsmans C, Chandramohan D. Prevalence of malaria and sexually transmitted and reproductive tract infections in pregnancy in sub-Saharan Africa: a systematic review. JAMA. 2012;307(19):2079–86.
42. Dielissen PW, Teunissen DA, Lagro-Janssen AL. Chlamydia prevalence in the general population: is there a sex difference? a systematic review. BMC Infect Dis. 2013;13(1):534.
43. Vajdic CM, Middleton M, Bowden FJ, Fairley CK, Kaldor JM. The prevalence of genital chlamydia trachomatis in Australia 1997–2004: a systematic review. Sex Health. 2005;2(3):169–83.
44. Wilson J, Honey E, Templeton A, Paavonen J, Mårdh P-A, Stary A, et al. A systematic review of the prevalence of chlamydia trachomatis among European women. Hum Reprod Update. 2002;8(4):385–94.
45. Scholes D, Satterwhite CL, Yu O, Fine D, Weinstock H, Berman S. Long-term trends in chlamydia trachomatis infections and related outcomes in a US managed care population. Sex Transm Dis. 2012;39(2):81–8.
46. Kouyoumdjian F, Leto D, John S, Henein H, Bondy S. A systematic review and meta-analysis of the prevalence of chlamydia, gonorrhoea and syphilis in incarcerated persons. Int J STD AIDS. 2012;23(4):248–54.
47. Ahmadi MH, Mirsalehian A, Bahador A. Prevalence of genital chlamydia trachomatis in Iran: a systematic review and meta-analysis. Pathog Glob Health. 2015;109(6):290–9.
48. Lewis D, Newton DC, Guy RJ, Ali H, Chen MY, Fairley CK, et al. The prevalence of chlamydia trachomatis infection in Australia: a systematic review and meta-analysis. BMC Infect Dis. 2012;12:113.
49. Control CfD, Prevention. Sexually Transmitted Infections in Developing Countries. Current Concepts and Strategies on Improving STI Prevention, Treatment, and Control. 2008. http://documents.worldbank.org/curated/en/867421468313772326/Sexually.
50. Mayaud P, Uledi E, Cornelissen J, Todd J, Rwakatare M, West B, et al. Risk scores to detect cervical infections in urban antenatal clinic attenders in Mwanza, Tanzania. Sex Transm Infect. 1998;74:S139–46.

Prevalence of *Chlamydia trachomatis* and *Neisseria gonorrhoeae* infections among pregnant women and eye colonization of their neonates at birth time, Shiraz, Southern Iran

Bahman Pourabbas[1], Zahra Rezaei[1], Jalal Mardaneh[2], Mozhgan Shahian[1] and Abdolvahab Alborzi[1*]

Abstract

Background: *Chlamydia trachomatis* and *Neisseria gonorrhoeae* are the two common transmissible pathogens from pregnant women to their neonates. Given the lack of routine screening and treatment of pregnant women in some areas, the possibility of transmission rises. This study seeks to determine the prevalence of *C. trachomatis* and *N. gonorrhoeae* in the pregnant women with no clinical symptoms and the vertical transmission rate to their neonates.

Methods: The study was conducted on endocervical and eye swab samples of 239 pregnant women and their neonates. Identification was based on PCR method.

Results: The prevalence rates of *C.trachomatis* in women and neonates were 37/239 (15.5%) and 28/239 (11.7%), and for *N. gonorrhoeae* 3/239 (1.3%), 1/239 (0.4%), respectively. The vertical transmission rates to the neonates were 28/37(75.6%) for *C. trachomatis* and 1/3 for *N. gonorrhoeae*.

Conclusions: In the areas with a high prevalence of chlamydial or gonococcal infections, and in the absence of screening and treatment of the pregnant women, ocular prophylaxis with antibiotics is suggested as a part of routine neonatal care program for the prevention of chlamydial and gonococcal ophthalmia.

Keywords: *C. Trachomatis, N. Gonorrhoeae*, Pregnant women, Vertical transmission, Eye colonization

Background

C. trachomatis and *N. gonorrhoeae* are the common prevalent sexually transmitted bacteria capable of infecting men, women and neonates worldwide, especially in developing nations [1, 2]. The estimated global prevalence in 2012 was 131 million cases of *C. trachomatis* and 78 million cases of *N. gonorrhoeae* in adults between the age of 15 and 49 years [2]. The annual estimation indicates different rates of infection in various parts of the world, ranging between 1.9–30.6% in pregnant women [2] and 1.6–18% in the neonates [3, 4] for *C. trachomatis* and for *N. gonorrhoeae* 0.08–7% [2] and 0.06–0.4% [3, 5], respectively. In Iran, the results of a meta-analysis showed that the pooled prevalence rates of *C. trachomatis* in males and females were 10.9% (95% CI, range: 7.6–15.4%) and 12.3% (95% CI, range: 10.6–14.2%), respectively [6]. Also, studies reported that prevalence of *C. trachomatis* in pregnant women was 2.2% to 14.79% [7–9]. As for *N. gonorrhoeae,* studies in Iran showed that its prevalence is 0 to 2.4% in people at low risk without symptoms [10]. One study on pregnant women revealed that 1.18% samples were positive for *N. gonorrhoeae* by PCR [11]. Infection with these organisms can cause a range of serious problems in mothers and newborns and can be asymptomatic in a significant proportion of the affected individuals [12, 13]. *C. trachomatis* is the most frequent infectious agent accounting for 18% to 50% of all neonatal conjunctivitis and 3% to 20% of infantile

* Correspondence: Alborziiraj2004@yahoo.com
[1]Professor Alborzi Clinical Microbiology Research Center, Shiraz University of Medical Sciences, Shiraz, Iran
Full list of author information is available at the end of the article

pneumonia [14, 15]. About half of the neonates born from infected mothers with *N. gonorrhoeae* will develop neonatal conjunctivitis [16]. Untreated gonococcal conjunctivitis may lead to corneal scarring and blindness, whereas the risk of severe ocular damage is low with chlamydial infection which can cause purulent mucous, edema on the eyelids, papillary conjunctivitis, and the formation of pseudomembranes [16]. The transmission of these two organisms is usually through direct contact of the neonates with infected vagina at the time of delivery during vaginal birth but rarely occurs during Caesarean section [17].

Prenatal screening and treatment of pregnant women are highly recommended, but in Iran, the routine prenatal and prophylactic care to prevent these diseases in newborns is lacking, unlike some other countries in the developing world. The aim of this study is to determine the prevalence of *C. trachomatis* and *N. gonorrhoeae* in pregnant women admitted to the hospitals before delivery and respective vertical transmission rates to the neonates, using PCR method.

Methods

A total of 239 pregnant women referred to Hafez and Zeinabiye hospitals for delivery were enrolled in the study during 3 months. Over 50% of all the deliveries in Shiraz are performed in these two hospitals, with more than 60% vaginal delivery. Pregnant women from different regions and of various socioeconomic statuses are admitted. This study includes the women with vaginal delivery with no history of antibiotics prepartum and their neonates had not received prophylactic ophthalmic antibiotics, either. Endocervical and eye swab samples were obtained from the mothers and their neonates, respectively. The former were taken by a sterile cotton swab from endocervix before delivery and the latter by the scraping of upper lid conjunctiva, using a sterile cotton swab immediately after delivery. Both swabs were placed in separate tubes containing 500 µl of sucrose phosphate transport medium (8 mM KH_2PO_4, 12 mM K_2HPO_4 and 0.2 mM sucrose) supplemented with antibiotics (amphotricin B 2.5 µg/ml, streptomycin 50 µg/ml and vancomycin 100 µg/ml) and transported to Professor Alborzi Clinical Microbiology Research Center, the same day for DNA extraction. The sample tubes were vortexed, swabs removed, and then, 250 µl of the sample transferred to a 1.5 ml tube containing 250 µl 10 mM Tris-HCl, pH 8.0 and 1 mM EDTA (TE). Each sample supplemented with 4 µl proteinase K (10 µg/ml) and 250 µl TNNT buffer (0.5% Tween 20, 0.5% Nonidet P-40, 10 mM NaOH, 10 mM Tris,pH 7.2), was incubated at 56 °C overnight and then, DNA extraction was performed using phenol chloroform method and finally, DNA resolved in 50 µl TE buffer and stored at -20 °C. Detection of *N. gonorrhoeae* and *C. trachomatis* was through two single-plex conventional PCR kits (Sacace Biothecnologies co. Italy) with specific primers for cryptic plasmid and amino acyltransferase gene. Five µl of DNA was amplified in a epgradiant thermocycler (eppendorf, Germany) using the following protocol: an initial denaturation (94 °C, 5 min), followed by 42 cycles of denaturation (94 °C, 1 min), annealing (54 °C, 1 min) and extension (72 °C, 1 min), and a single final extension of 1 min at 72 °C for both *C. trachomatis* and *N. gonorrhoeae*, according to the manufacturer's instructions. These kits allow detecting DNA in 100% of the tests with a sensitivity of not less than 1000 copies/ml and a specificity of 100%.

The collected data were entered into SPSS, version 18. The statistical relationship between the demographic data and infection was assessed using the chi-square and t-test.

Results

Subjects

Of the 239 studied women with vaginal delivery (mean age 27.7; range: 18–45 years), 31.7% were illiterate or had primary education, 65% with secondary education, and 3.3% with university degrees. In total, 98% of them were housewives. The median gestational age was 39 weeks with a range of 32 to 44 weeks. Of the 239 studied neonates, 55% were male and 45% were female.

Diagnosis of *C. trachomatis* and *N. gonorrhoeae* infection in pregnant women

From 239 endocervical swabs, DNAs of *C. trachomatis* and *N. gonorrhoeae* were detected in 37 (15.4%) and 3 (1.3%), respectively. No case of co-infection with *N. gonorrhoeae* and *C. trachomatis* was observed.

No significant association was found between *C.trachomatis*, *N. gonorrhoeae* prevalence and age and educational status in the pregnant women in this study (P-value > 0.05).

Diagnosis of *C. trachomatis* and *N. gonorrhoeae* infection in neonates

Of the 239 samples from neonatal eyes, DNAs of *C. trachomatis* and *N. gonorrhoeae* were detected in 28 (11.7%) and 1 (0.4%), respectively. Transmission rates of infection in the neonates for *N. gonorrhoeae* and *C. trachomatis*, born to the infected mothers, were 28/37 (75.6%) and 1/3, respectively. No case of co-infection with *N. gonorrhoeae* and *C. trachomatis* was detected in the neonates, as was the case with mothers.

Discussion

C. trachomatis and *N. gonorrhoeae* are the most common causes of sexually transmitted infections leading to serious conditions in pregnant women and their neonates. Prior to this study, limited data existed on *C. trachomatis* and *N. gonorrhoeae* prevalence among the Iranian pregnant women with no clinical symptoms and their neonates. Therefore, the present study provides documented data for the first time in Iran on the vertical transmission rates of these two organisms in the neonates. A PCR assay which is more sensitive and specific, compared to other methods such as culture as gold standard, was used [18, 19].

The results revealed that 37 (15.5%) pregnant women were infected with *C. trachomatis.* Previous studies showed that the frequency of *C. trachomatis* among women varies in different countries, and even within the same country.

Previous studies have reported that the frequency of *C. trachomatis* infection among pregnant women is 2.5 to 4.74% in the United States [20, 21], 1.9 to 14.9% in Asia [2], 1.6 to 16.4% in Europe [2, 22], 5.2 to 18.6% in Africa [2], and 10.9 to 30.6% in Oceania [2]. Differences in frequency could be explained by sociodemographic factors; different sensitivities of the diagnostic methods used and specimen types collected. Unlike in some previous studies, no association was found between *C.trachomatis* prevalence and age and educational status in the pregnant women in the present study [23, 24].

The prevalence of eye colonization with *C. trachomatis* in the neonates was found to be 11.7% in this study, which varies in different studies, ranging between 1.6 to 18% [3, 4]. This difference is probably due to the different sensitivity of the methods used in such studies and varying prevalence of infections among mothers throughout the world.

The vertical transmission rate of *C. trachomatis* was 75.6% which is in agreement with reported rates in other studies [3, 4] but in contrast to a study by Jilian et al., which reported a lower rate of vertical transmission [25]. The discrepancy in these two findings may be due to different target populations [25].

Consistent with other studies, *N. gonorrhoeae* had a low prevalence of 1.3% in the pregnant women [26, 27]. Similar to *C. trachomatis*, there was no significant relationship between the prevalence of *N. gonorrhoeae* and the mothers' educational status and age. The prevalence of eye infection and rate of vertical transmission with *N. gonorrhoeae* in the neonates were 0.4% and 1/3 respectively, consistent with some other studies [3, 28]. No concomitant *C. trachomatis* and *N. gonorrhoeae* infection was detected in mothers or neonates while all positive neonates were born to the infected mothers.

Studies show that ocular prophylaxis in neonates was effective against gonoccocal eye infection, whereas it may not be the case for chlamydial conjunctivitis [29, 30]. Neither can it prohibit colonization or infection at other sites like nasopharynx, rectum, and vagina; conversely, it may increase antimicrobial resistance and cause some level of toxicity [31, 32]. Overall, ocular prophylaxis may help to prevent chlamydial neonatal conjunctivitis, but not that much to help to prevent gonococcal neonatal conjunctivitis [29].

In Iran, prenatal screening and treatment is not a part of the routine program for mothers care and consequently there is a chance of transmitted *C. trachomatis* and *N. gonorrhoeae* as a common cause of neonatal conjunctivitis.

Conclusion

Prenatal screening and treatment of pregnant women have been demonstrated to be very effective for the prevention of neonatal chlamydial and gonococcal infections. Given the above mentioned findings, we can conclude that in the absence of a program for screening and treatment of pregnant women and in areas with a considerable prevalence of such organisms, it is suggested that at least ocular prophylaxis with antibiotics be incorporated in the routine neonatal care program for the prevention of chlamydial and gonococcal ophthalmia.

Abbreviations

C. trachomatis: *Chlamydia trachomatis*; *N. gonorrhoeae*: *Neisseria gonorrhoeae*

Acknowledgements

We express our deep thanks to H. Khajehei, PhD for linguistic editing of the manuscript.

Funding

The study was financially supported by Professor Alborzi Clinical Microbiology Research Center of Shiraz University of Medical Sciences. The funders had no role in study design, data collection and the decision to submit the work for publication.

Author's contributions

BP, co-ordination and supervision of LAB work and critical reading of the manuscript. MS, study conception and design. ZR and JM, data analysis and interpretation, LAB work and manuscript preparation. AA, co-ordination and design of the study and critical reading of the manuscript. All authors read and approved the final manuscript.

Consent for publication

Not applicable.

Competing interests

The authors declare that they have no competing interests.

Author details
[1]Professor Alborzi Clinical Microbiology Research Center, Shiraz University of Medical Sciences, Shiraz, Iran. [2]Departments of Microbiology, School of Medicine, Gonabad University of Medical Sciences, Gonabad, Iran.

References

1. Darville T. *Chlamydia trachomatis* infections in neonates and young children. Semin Pediatr Infect Dis. 2005;16(4):235–44.
2. Newman L, Rowley J, Vander Hoorn S, et al. Global estimates of the prevalence and incidence of four curable sexually transmitted infections in 2012 based on systematic review and global reporting. PLoS One. 2015; 10(12):e0143304.
3. Justel M, Alexandre I, Martínez P, et al. Vertical transmission of bacterial eye infections, Angola, 2011–2012. Emerg Infect Dis. 2015;21(3):471–3.
4. Schachter J, Grossman M, Sweet RL, et al. Prospective study of perinatal transmission of chlamydia trachomatis. JAMA. 1986;255:3374–7.
5. Hammerschlag MR. Chlamydial and gonococcal infections in infants and children. Clin Infect Dis. 2011;53(Suppl 3):S99–102.
6. Ahmadi MH, Mirsalehian A, Bahador A. Prevalence of genital chlamydia trachomatis in Iran: a systematic review and meta-analysis. Pathog Glob Health. 2015;109(6):290–9.
7. Haghighi Hasanabad M, Mohammadzadeh M, Bahador A, Fazel N, Rakhshani H, Majnooni A. Prevalence of Chlamydia trachomatis and Mycoplasma genitalium in. pregnant women of Sabzevar-Iran. Iran J Microbiol. 2011;3(3):123–8.
8. Rashidi B, Chamani L, Haghollahi F, et al. Prevalence of *Chlamydia trachomatis* infection in fertile and infertile women; a molecular and serological study. J Reprod Infertil. 2009;10:32–41.
9. Jahromi AS, Farjam MR, Mogharrab F, Amiryan M, Makiani MJ, Madani A, et al. *Chlamydia trachomatis* in women with full-term deliveries and women with abortion. Am J Infect Dis. 2010;3:66–9.
10. Janghorban R, Azarkish F. An overview on sexually transmitted infections in Iran. Int J Reprod Contracept Obstet Gynecol. 2016;5(3):585–95.
11. Hassanzadeh P, Mardaneh J, Motamedifar M. Conventional agar-based culture method, and nucleic acid amplification test (NAAT) of the cppB gene for detection of Neisseria gonorrhea in pregnant women Endocervical swab specimens. Iran Red Crescent Med J. 2013;15(3):207–11.
12. Wager GP, Martin DH, Koutsky L, et al. Puerperal infectious morbidity: relationship to route of delivery and to antepartum chlamydia trachomatis infection. Am J Obstet Gynecol. 1980;138:1028–33.
13. Gencay M, Koskiniemi M, Ammäläa P, et al. Chlamydia trachomatis seropositivity is associated both with stillbirth and preterm delivery. APMIS. 2000;108:584–8.
14. Hammerschlag MR, Chandler JW, Alexander ER, et al. Longitudinal studies of chlamydial infection in the first year of life. Pediatr Infect Dis. 1982;1:395–401.
15. American Academy of Pediatrics. Chlamydial infections. In: Pickering LK, Baker CJ, Long SS, eds. Red Book: 2006 Report of the Committee on Infectious Diseases. 27th ed. Elk Grove Village, Ill: Am Acad Pediatr. 2006; 249–257.
16. Zuppa AA, D'Andrea V, Catenazzi P, et al. Ophthalmia neonatorum: what kind of prophylaxis? J Matern Fetal Neonatal Med. 2011;24(6):769–73.
17. Bell TA, Stamm WE, Kuo CC, et al. Risk of perinatal transmission of chlamydia trachomatis by mode of delivery. J Inf Secur. 1994;29(2):165–9.
18. Watson EJ, Templeton A, Russell I, et al. The accuracy and efficacy of screening tests for chlamydia trachomatis: a systematic review. J Med Microbiol. 2002;51(12):1021–31.
19. Centers for Disease Control and Prevention. Recommendations for the laboratory-based detection of Chlamydia trachomatis and Neisseria gonorrhoeae--2014. MMWR Recomm Rep. 2014;63(RR-02):1-19.
20. Datta SD, Sternberg M, Johnson RE, et al. Gonorrhea and chlamydia in the United States among persons 14 to 39 years of age, 1999 to 2002. Ann Intern Med. 2007;147(2):89–96.
21. Miller WC, Ford CA, Morris M, Handcock MS, et al. Prevalence of chlamydial and gonococcal infections among young adults in the United States. JAMA. 2004;291(18):2229–36.
22. Goulet V, de Barbeyrac B, Raherison S, et al. Prevalence of chlamydia trachomatis: results from the first national population-based survey in France. Sex Transm Infect. 2010;86(4):263–70.
23. Romoren M, Sundby J, Velauthapillai M, et al. Chlamydia and gonorrhoea in pregnant Batswana women: time to discard the syndromic approach? BMC Infect Dis. 2007;7:27.
24. Harrison HR, Alexander ER, Weinstein L, et al. Cervical chlamydia trachomatis and mycoplasmal infections in pregnancy. Epidemiology and outcomes. JAMA. 1983;250(13):1721–7.
25. Yu J, Wu H, Li F, et al. Vertical transmission of chlamydia trachomatis in Chongqingn China. Curr Microbiol. 2009;58:315–20.
26. Borges-Costa J, Matos C, Pereira F. Sexually transmitted infections in pregnant adolescents: prevalence and association with maternal and foetal morbidity. J Eur Acad Dermatol Venereol. 2012;26(8):972–5.
27. Panaretto KS, Lee HM, Mitchell MR, et al. Prevalence of sexually transmitted infections in pregnant urban aboriginal and Torres Strait islander women in northern Australia. Aust N Z J Obstet Gynaecol. 2006;46(3):217–24.
28. Laga M, Plummer FA, Nzanze H, et al. Epidemiology of ophthalmia neonatorum in Kenya. Lancet. 1986;2(8516):1145–9.
29. Darling EK, McDonald H. A meta-analysis of the efficacy of ocular prophylactic agents used for the prevention of gonococcal and chlamydial ophthalmia neonatorum. J Midwifery Womens Health. 2010;55(4):319–27.
30. Ramirez-Ortiz MA, Rodriguez-Almaraz M, Ochoa-Diazlopez H, et al. Randomised equivalency trial comparing 2.5% povidone-iodine drops and ophthalmic chloramphenicol for preventing neonatal conjunctivitis in a trachoma endemic area in southern Mexico. Br J Ophthalmol. 2007;91(11): 1430–4.
31. Hammerschlag MR, Chandler JW, Alexander ER, et al. Erythromycin ointment for ocular prophylaxis of neonatal chlamydial infection. JAMA. 1980;244(20):2291–3.
32. Public Health Agency of Canada, National Microbiology Laboratory. National surveillance of antimicrobial susceptibilities of Neisseria gonorrhoeae. Annual Summary 2012: http://publications. gc.ca/collections/collection_ 2014/aspc-phac/HP57-3-2012-eng.pdf.

22

Differences in *Chlamydia trachomatis* seroprevalence between ethnic groups cannot be fully explained by socioeconomic status, sexual healthcare seeking behavior or sexual risk behavior: a cross-sectional analysis in the HEalthy LIfe in an Urban Setting (HELIUS) study

Sebastiaan H. Hulstein[1,2*], Amy Matser[1], Catharina J. Alberts[1], Marieke B. Snijder[3,4], Martina Willhauck-Fleckenstein[5], Katrin Hufnagel[5], Maria Prins[1,2], Henry J. C. de Vries[1,6], Maarten F. Schim van der Loeff[1,2] and Tim Waterboer[5]

Abstract

Background: In the Netherlands, there are strong disparities in *Chlamydia trachomatis* (CT) prevalence between ethnic groups. The current study aims to identify whether socioeconomic status, sexual risk behavior and sexual healthcare seeking behavior may explain differences in CT seroprevalence between ethnic groups.

Methods: We used 2011–2014 baseline data of the HELIUS (HEalthy LIfe in an Urban Setting) study, a multi-ethnic population-based cohort study in Amsterdam, the Netherlands, including participants from Dutch, African Surinamese, South-Asian Surinamese, Ghanaian, Moroccan and Turkish origin. For this analysis, we selected sexually active, heterosexual participants aged 18–34 years old. CT seroprevalence was determined using a multiplex serology assay. The CT seroprevalence ratios between different ethnicities are calculated and adjusted for potential indicators of socioeconomic status, sexual risk behavior and sexual healthcare seeking behavior.

Results: The study population consisted of 2001 individuals (52.8% female) with a median age of 28 years (IQR 24–31). CT seropositivity differed by ethnicities and ranged from 71.6% (African Surinamese), and 67.9% (Ghanaian) to 31.1% (Turkish). The CT seroprevalence ratio of African Surinamese was 1.72 (95% CI 1.43–2.06) and 1.52 (95% CI 1.16–1.99) of Ghanaian as compared to the Dutch reference group, after adjustment for socioeconomic status, sexual risk behavior and sexual healthcare seeking behavior.

(Continued on next page)

* Correspondence: bhulstein@ggd.amsterdam.nl; s.h.hulstein@amc.nl
[1]Department of Infectious Diseases, Public Health Service of Amsterdam (GGD Amsterdam), Nieuwe Achtergracht 100, 1018, WT, Amsterdam, The Netherlands
[2]Department of Internal Medicine, Amsterdam Institute for Infection and Immunity (AI&II), Academic Medical Center, Meibergdreef 9, 1105, AZ, Amsterdam, The Netherlands
Full list of author information is available at the end of the article

(Continued from previous page)
Conclusions: Indicators of socioeconomic status, sexual risk behavior, and sexual health seeking behavior could not explain the higher CT seroprevalence among African Surinamese and Ghanaian residents of Amsterdam.

Keywords: Ethnicity, *Chlamydia trachomatis*, Sexual healthcare seeking behavior, Socioeconomic status, Sexual risk behavior

Short summary

A multi-ethnic cohort in Amsterdam, the Netherlands, showed that the disparate *Chlamydia trachomatis* seroprevalence between ethnic groups was not explained by socioeconomic status, sexual healthcare seeking behavior and sexual behavior.

Background

Chlamydia trachomatis (CT) infections are a major public health concern. In many high income countries, including the Netherlands, CT prevalence, incidence and test positivity differs substantially across ethnic groups [1–5]. Urogenital CT infection is associated with sexual risk behavior (SRB) such as condomless sexual contact and higher number of sex partners [6, 7]. Some studies reported differences in these risk behaviors between ethnic groups [2, 8]. However, differences in individual risk behaviors fail to explain the differences in CT prevalence across ethnic groups [9–11]. Evidence from several population-based and STI clinic studies in the Netherlands suggested that sexual healthcare seeking behavior (sHSB) may play an important role in explaining the ethnic differences in CT infection rates [4]. Diagnosis and treatment of, especially asymptomatic, CT infections may be delayed by reduced sHSB, prolonging the time during which CT transmission is possible. This might lead to a higher CT prevalence in (sub)populations where members are characterized by low sHSB, high risk of CT infection, and have sex predominantly with members of the same group. Lower socioeconomic status (SES) is associated with lower sHSB [12]. In one study, CT infection was found to be associated with non-Dutch ethnicity and low SES [13]. In another study the uptake of CT screening tests was different between individuals with different ethnic backgrounds [4].

To better understand the contribution and interplay of SES, SRB and sHSB in their associations with CT and whether differences in these factors may explain differences in CT prevalence between ethnic groups, we performed a retrospective analysis of baseline data of a large multi-ethnic study: the HELIUS study. We examined whether SES, SRB and sHSB could explain the difference in heterosexual CT seroprevalence between ethnic groups in Amsterdam, the Netherlands.

Material and methods

Study population

The current study is based on baseline data from the HELIUS (HEalthy LIfe in an Urban Setting) study. The goals and design of the HELIUS study have been described before [14, 15]. In brief, HELIUS is a population-based study that includes individuals aged 18–70 years from the major ethnic groups living in Amsterdam (Surinamese, Turkish, Moroccan, Ghanaian and Dutch). Individuals were randomly selected, stratified by ethnicity, from the municipal registry of the city of Amsterdam and invited to participate in the study. The aim was to include similarly sized samples for each ethnic group, oversampling smaller groups to ensure this goal. Among each ethnic group, women were more likely to participate than men, and those who participated were slightly older than those who did not. Non--response analyses also indicated that, for each ethnic group, respondents and non-respondents did not differ regarding several SES indicators, suggesting representative samples for each ethnic group [15]. Baseline data collection took place from 2011 to 2015. Data were obtained by questionnaire and a physical examination, including collection of biological samples. Written informed consent was obtained from all participants. All HELIUS study protocols have been approved by the Ethics Review Board of the Academic Medical Center and are in accordance with the revised Declaration of Helsinki of 2000.

For the current study, a subset of the HELIUS baseline data and samples that were collected until June 2014 was used, on which CT serologic tests were performed. The selection procedure of the subsample has been described previously [16]. In short, among participants aged 18 to 44 years who gave informed consent for additional blood analyses and of whom an adequate volume of blood was available, a random sample per life year from each gender and ethnic group (Dutch, South-Asian Surinamese, African Surinamese, Ghanaian, Moroccan and Turkish ethnicity) was taken, resulting in a dataset of 4682 participants (Fig. 1) [16]. From this dataset we excluded men who have sex with men (MSM) and women who have sex with women (WSW) (based on self-reported behavior) and participants who had not yet had their sexual debut, because their Chlamydia infection risk differs from the general heterosexual population. All participants over 35 years old were excluded, as

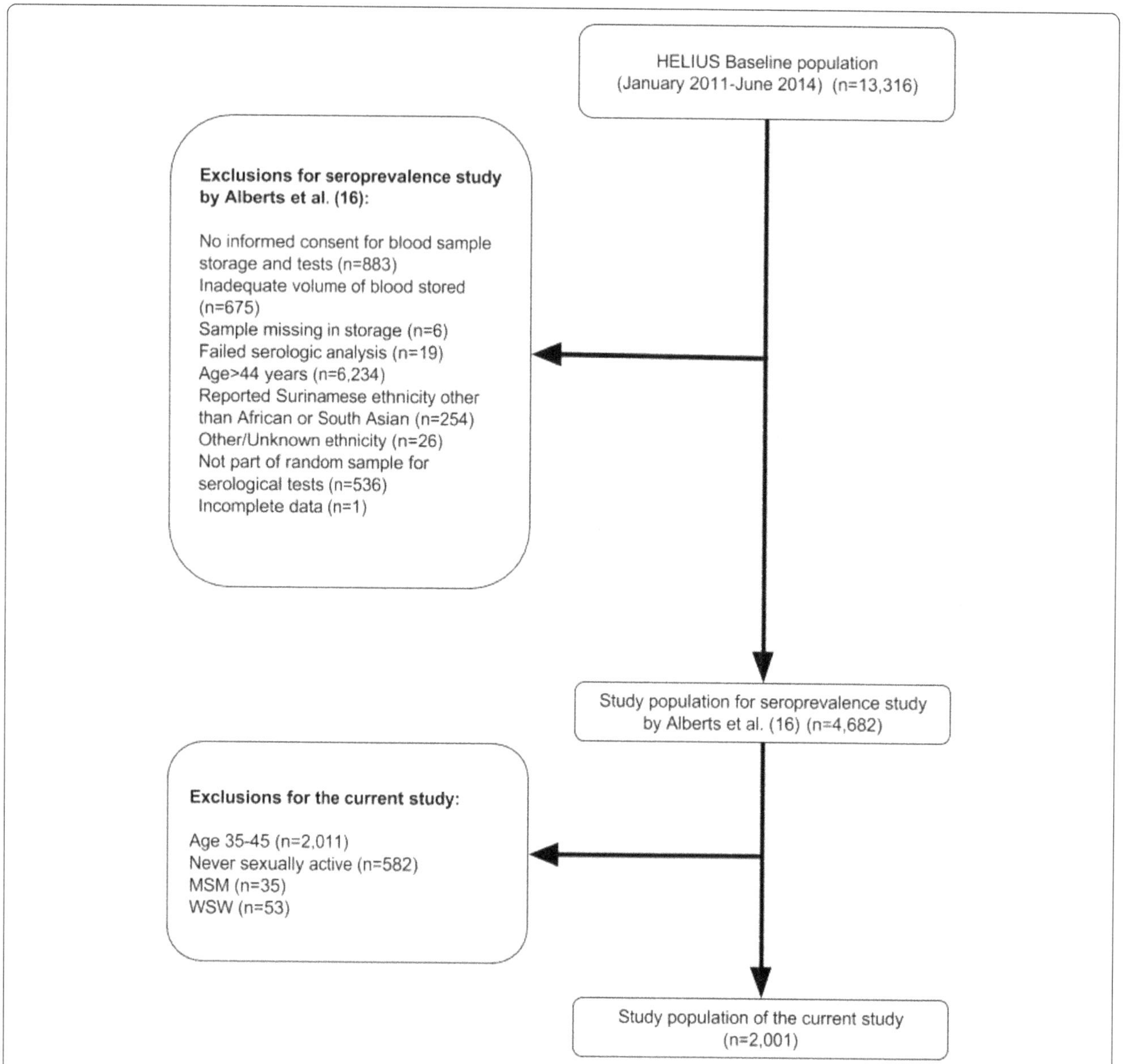

Fig. 1 Flowchart of the selection process of participants for the current study

completion of questions on SRB was optional in this group and hence data were incomplete (Fig. 1).

Ethnicity and migration status

Ethnicity was defined according to the country of birth of the participant as well as that of his/her parents [17]. Specifically, the HELIUS study invited participants of non-Dutch ethnic origin if the following criteria were met: 1) the participant and at least one parent were born abroad (first generation), or 2) the participant was born in the Netherlands, but both parents were born abroad (second generation). For participants of Surinamese origin, ethnicity was further classified according to self-reported ethnic origin (e.g. South-Asian, African, Javanese, or other). For the Dutch sample, people were invited who were born in the Netherlands and whose parents were born in the Netherlands.

Chlamydia serological assay

To be able to take past CT infections into account, CT seroprevalence was determined as a proxy for lifetime CT exposure. Serum samples of fasting blood samples were tested for the presence of CT antibodies using a multiplex serology assay, developed at the German Cancer Research Center (DKFZ) in Heidelberg, Germany. This assay detects antibodies that bind to 7 CT antigens: the Major Outer Membrane Protein (MOMP) of serovars A, D, and L2, Translocated actin-recruiting phosphoprotein (Tarp, split into its N- and C-terminal fractions based on its size), and Porin B and Heat shock Protein-60 (Hsp60). The assay was validated against serum samples with known CT DNA status and a commercial ELISA (CT-ELISA, Medac, Wedel, Germany). The maximum of the 3 MOMP responses (MOMPmax) was used as a combined variable, and CT seropositivity was classified as an antibody response to 2 or more of the following antigens: Tarp-N, Tarp-C, PorB, and MOMPmax, or a median fluorescence intensity (MFI) > 1000 to MOMPmax alone, resulting in a sensitivity of 83% and a specificity of 87% for classification as CT seropositive (indicating CT exposure). Antibody cross-reactivity of *Chlamydia trachomatis* and *Chlamydophila pneumonia* was only minor, as indicated by correlation analyses ($R^2 < 0.05$, data not shown) (Additional file 1: Appendix 1).

SES, SRB, sHSB and other measurements

Information on demographics, SES, SRB, and sHSB were obtained by questionnaire. SES was determined by occupational level and educational level. Occupational level was classified according to the Standard Classification of Occupations of 2010 by Statistics Netherlands (CBS) [18]. This document provides an extensive systematic list of all professions in the Dutch system. Based on this document, occupational level was classified into (1) elementary, or lower, (2) intermediate and (3) higher or (4) academic, based on job title and job description, including a question on fulfilling an executive function (directing personnel). Educational level was based on the highest qualification attained, either in the Netherlands or in the country of origin, and it was categorized into three groups, namely (1) no or elementary schooling, or lower vocational or lower secondary schooling, (2) intermediate vocational, or intermediate or higher secondary schooling and (3) higher vocational schooling or university.

sHSB was based on self-reports of having been tested for HIV or other STIs in the preceding 6 months. SRB characteristics were the lifetime number of sex partners, age of sexual debut and self-reported condom use in the preceding 6 months with casual and steady sex partners, categorized as (1) no sexual contact in the past 6 months, (2) sex exclusively with a steady partner in the past 6 months (regardless of condom use), (3) consistent condom use with casual sex partners (regardless of sex with a steady partner), and (4) inconsistent or no condom use with casual sex partners (regardless of sex with a steady partner). Self-reported consistent condom use is defined as having always used a condom with a sexual partner. All degrees of self-reported inconsistency with condom use were defined as inconsistent condom use.

Statistical analyses

The characteristics of the study population were described and differences between ethnic groups evaluated with χ^2 tests for categorical variables or Kruskal-Wallis tests for continuous variables. The seroprevalence ratio (PR) of CT between the different ethnicities, and adjustments for potential explanatory indicators of SES, SRB, sHSB was calculated by Poisson regression analyses with robust variance [19].

For Poisson regression analyses, age was categorized into three strata: 18–24 years, 25–29 years and 30–34 years. The distribution of the number of lifetime sex partners was positively skewed and therefore transformed to its natural logarithm.

In univariable Poisson regression analyses with robust variance, we assessed the association of CT seropositivity with the variables selected in our theoretical model. These variables were age, sex and the indicators of SRB, SES and sHSB. Analyses were done overall, and stratified by ethnicity.

We assessed the CT seroprevalence ratios of the different ethnicities compared to the Dutch reference group, adjusting for potential explanatory indicators of SES, SRB, sHSB and the confounders age and gender in five steps. The first model included age and gender, the second age, gender and indicators of SRB, the third age, gender and indicators of SES, the fourth age, gender, and indicators of sHSB and the final model included age, gender and indicators of SRB, SES, and sHSB. In case of a PR > 1, a decrease of the CT seroprevalence ratio after adjustment with an indicator suggests an explanatory effect of that specific indicator for differences in CT seroprevalence between the compared groups. In case of a PR < 1, the same goes for an increase of CT seroprevalence ratio.

To assess the effect of migration generation on CT seroprevalence after adjustments for all indicators of SRB, SES and sHSB, we have performed a multivariable analysis stratified by ethnicity and migration generation.

Data were missing for some variables; as this was occurring in less than 5% of records per variable, we performed complete case analyses.

A statistical significance level of $P < 0.05$ was used. Statistical analyses were performed in STATA Intercooled 13.1 (College Station, Texas, USA).

Results

Study population selection and baseline characteristics including SES

Serological data were available for 4682 HELIUS participants. For the current analysis, 2011 participants aged 35 years or above, 582 participants who never had sexual intercourse, 35 MSM and 53 WSW were excluded. The resulting 2001 participants were included in the current study (Fig. 1).

In our study sample, the median age (28 years) of participants was similar across all ethnicities, and participants were mostly female (Table 1). Most participants of non-Dutch origin in the subsample were second generation migrants, except for Ghanaian participants who were mostly first generation migrants (78.2%). Overall, Dutch participants were higher educated and had higher occupational levels (Table 1).

Sexual risk behavior (SRB) and sexual healthcare seeking behavior (sHSB) between the different ethnicities

Several differences in SRB between the ethnic groups were observed. The median age at sexual debut was lowest among African Surinamese participants (16 years, IQR 15–18) and highest among Turkish and Moroccan participants (both 18 years, IQR 16–22).The median lifetime number of sex partners was highest among Dutch participants (7 sex partners, IQR 3–13), and lowest among Turkish participants (1 sex partner, IQR 1–7). Most individuals reported exclusive sexual contact with a steady partner (regardless of condom use). Compared to other participants, inconsistent condom use with casual sex partners was most frequent among Dutch and African Surinamese participants (Table 1).

sHSB was also dissimilar across the different ethnic groups. 13.2% of the study population reported having been tested for HIV and 17.1% for STI both in the preceding 6 months. The proportions that had been tested in the preceding 6 months for HIV (26.4%) and STI (33.1%) were highest among African Surinamese participants, and lowest among those of Turkish origin (Table 1).

Chlamydia seroprevalence

In the overall population, CT seroprevalence was 44.6%. CT seroprevalence was highest among African Surinamese (71.6%), followed by Ghanaian participants (67.9%). Overall CT seropositivity among male participants (42.0%) was slightly lower than among female participants (47.0%; $P = 0.03$).

CT seroprevalence ratios without adjustments

In the total study population the risk of CT seropositivity was increased by being female, a higher lifetime number of sex partners, a lower age at sexual debut, and in the preceding 6 months: inconsistent condom use with casual sex partners, STI testing and HIV testing. Second generation migrants were less likely to having been exposed to CT than first generation migrants. A high level of education and a high level of occupation were significantly associated with not having been exposed to CT (Table 2).

Adjusted seroprevalence ratios of CT

The CT seroprevalence ratios (reference group: Dutch participants) were highest among African Surinamese (PR: 1.99; 95% CI 1.65–2.21) and Ghanaian participants (PR: 1.81; 95% CI 1.54–2.13) (Table 3). African Surinamese (adjusted PR (aPR): 1.72; 95% CI 1.43–2.06) and Ghanaians (aPR: 1.52; 95% CI 1.16–1.99) remained significantly more likely to be CT seropositive when adjusted for (1) age and gender, (2) age, gender and indicators of SRB, (3) age, gender and indicators of SES, (4) age, gender, and indicators of sHSB and (5) age, gender and indicators of SRB, SES, and sHSB .

Being of Turkish and Moroccan origin did not significantly increase the risk of CT seropositivity in univariable analysis, and the additional, stepwise, adjustments had little effect on the risk. In univariable analysis, South Asian Surinamese were as likely to be CT seropositive as the Dutch. When adjusted for age, gender, SRB, SES and sHSB (Step 5), the CT seroprevalence was significantly higher than in the Dutch (Table 3).

The multivariable analysis stratified by migration generation showed that among South Asian Surinamese second generation migration status, among Ghanaians first, among African Surinamese first and second was statistically associated with CT seropositivity, as compared to the Dutch. Of note, among South Surinamese first generation migration status and among Ghanaian second was not significantly associated with CT seropositivity compared to the Dutch (Table 4).

Discussion

In this study we assessed the disparate CT seroprevalence and aimed to explain the observed differences among various ethnic groups in the Netherlands. The current study showed a higher seroprevalence of CT among participants of African Surinamese and Ghanaian ethnic origin compared to the Dutch population. The seroprevalence of CT among three ethnicities (South-Asian Surinamese, Turkish and Moroccan participants) did not differ from that in the Dutch. Our study showed that SRB, SES and sHSB could not explain the disparate CT seroprevalence between the African Surinamese and Ghanaian groups and the Dutch. Being first or second generation migrant may play a role in explaining the ethnic differences in CT seroprevalence, especially among Ghanaians.

This is the first study to investigate the role of sHSB on disparate CT seroprevalence between ethnic groups. Other studies observed similar differences in CT between ethnic groups [3, 4, 9, 13], but were not based on diagnosis of CT by serology. Like in other studies [9–11] SRB failed to explain the discrepancies, but unlike a study performed by Matser et al. [9], SES was not explanatory for differences in CT between ethnicities.

The strength of this study, based on data from the large scale, population-based HELIUS study, lies in the sample sizes of the major ethnic groups of interest and data availability on demographics, SES, sHSB and SRB. These factors enabled us to assess whether these

Table 1 Characteristics of the study population ($n = 2001$)[a], stratified by ethnicity

	Dutch ($n = 392$)		South Asian Surinamese ($n = 373$)		African Surinamese ($n = 317$)		Ghanaian ($n = 193$)		Turkish ($n = 389$)		Moroccan ($n = 337$)		Total ($n = 2001$)	
Demographics														
Sex [n,%] ($n = 2001$)														
Female	214	54.6%	185	49.6%	193	60.9%	121	62.7%	167	43.4%	174	51.6%	1056	52.8%
Migration generation [n,%] ($n = 1609$)														
First generation	N/A	N/A	82	22.0%	136	42.9%	151	78.2%	137	35.2%	117	34.7%	623	38.7%
Age in years [median, IQR] ($n = 2001$)	28	25–31	28	23–31	27	23–31	27	23–32	29	25–32	29	25–32	28	24–31
Socioeconomic status														
Educational level [n,%] ($n = 1995$)														
Low	21	5.4%	79	21.2%	51	16.1%	68	35.4%	143	36.9%	88	26.3%	450	22.6%
Intermediate	94	24.0%	163	43.5%	178	56.3%	89	46.4%	166	42.8%	157	46.8%	847	42.5%
High	277	70.7%	130	35.0%	87	27.5%	35	18.2%	79	20.4%	90	26.8%	698	35.0%
Occupational level [n,%] ($n = 1717$)														
Low	53	15.2%	125	38.1%	112	44.1%	94	64.0%	172	49.3%	112	38.6%	668	38.9%
Intermediate	64	18.3%	104	31.7%	90	35.4%	37	25.2%	110	31.5%	114	39.3%	519	30.2%
High	232	66.5%	99	30.2%	52	20.5%	16	10.9%	67	19.2%	64	22.1%	530	30.9%
Sexual risk behavior														
Lifetime number of sex partners [median, IQR] ($n = 1901$)	7	3–13	3	1–6	5	3–10	4	2–6	1	1–7	2	1–7	4	1–10
Age in years at sexual debut [median, IQR] ($n = 1844$)	17	16–19	17	16–19	16	15–18	17	16–19	18	16–22	18	16–22	17	16–19
Sexual contacts and condom use (preceding 6 months) [n,%] ($n = 1836$)														
No sexual contact	48	12.5%	67	18.8%	40	13.2%	43	26.5%	63	18.5%	61	19.7%	322	17.3%
Steady partner only[b]	239	62.1%	236	66.3%	185	61.1%	93	57.4%	215	63.1%	200	64.5%	1168	62.9%
Consistent condom use with casual partners[c]	30	7.8%	31	8.7%	37	12.2%	11	6.8%	32	9.4%	29	9.4%	170	9.2%
Inconsistent condom use with casual partners[c]	68	17.7%	22	6.2%	41	13.5%	15	9.3%	31	9.1%	20	6.5%	197	10.6%
Sexual health seeking behavior														
HIV testing (preceding 6 months) [n,%] ($n = 1952$)														
Yes	44	11.3%	37	10.0%	83	26.4%	41	21.8%	26	6.9%	29	8.7%	260	13.2%
STI testing (preceding 6 months) [n,%] ($n = 1951$)														
Yes	70	17.9%	49	13.2%	104	33.1%	40	21.2%	29	7.7%	45	13.5%	337	17.1%
Primary outcome														
C. trachomatis seropositivity [n,%] ($n = 2001$)														
Overall	147	37.5%	150	40.2%	227	71.6%	131	67.9%	121	31.1%	117	34.7%	893	44.6%
Female	79	36.9%	77	41.6%	147	76.2%	81	66.9%	46	27.2%	66	37.9%	496	47.0%
Male	68	38.2%	73	38.8%	80	64.5%	50	69.4%	75	34.1%	51	31.3%	397	42.0%

IQR Interquartile range, *N/A* Not available, *HIV* Human immunodeficiency virus, *STI* Sexually transmitted infection
Data are presented as n (%) or median (IQR)
[a]Numbers may not add up due to missing values
[b]Sex exclusively with one partner, regardless of condom use
[c]Has had a casual sex partner, irrespective of having had a steady partner

variables may explain in part the association between ethnicity and CT infection.

Another strength of this study is that similar ethnic group sizes were ensured during inclusion of HELIUS and only very small differences exist between participants and non-participants. Thus, the study sample is well suited for comparison of seroprevalence between the different ethnic groups. As no attempt is made to

Table 2 (Sero) prevalence ratios of CT for potential determinants, by ethnic group. Results of stratified unadjusted Poisson regression with robust variance

	Dutch ($n = 392$)	South Asian Surinamese ($n = 373$)	African Surinamese ($n = 317$)	Ghanaian ($n = 193$)	Turkish ($n = 389$)	Moroccan ($n = 337$)	Total ($n = 2001$)
	PR (95% CI)	PR (95% CI)	PR (95% CI)	PR (95% CI)	PR (95% CI)	PR (95% CI)	PR (95% CI)
Demographics							
Gender							
Male	1	1	1*	1	1	1	1*
Female	0.97 (0.75–1.25)	1.08 (0.84–1.37)	1.18 (1.01–1.38)	0.96 (0.79–1.18)	0.80 (0.59–1.09)	1.21 (0.90–1.63)	1.12 (1.01–1.23)
Migration generation							
First	N/A	1	1	1*	1	1	1***
Second	N/A	1.00 (0.74–1.35)	0.97 (0.85–1.12)	0.73 (0.53–0.99)	1.06 (0.77–1.45)	0.95 (0.70–1.29)	0.82 (0.74–0.91)
Age							
18–24 years	1	1	1	1	1	1	1
25–29 years	0.98 (0.70–1.36)	1.31 (0.93–1.83)	1.03 (0.87–1.22)	0.96 (0.73–1.27)	1.11 (0.73–1.68)	0.88 (0.58–1.32)	0.98 (0.86–1.11)
30–34 years	0.99 (0.70–1.38)	1.45 (1.05–2.00)*	1.03 (0.87–1.23)	1.17 (0.93–1.47)	1.08 (0.72–1.63)	0.96 (0.65–1.41)	1.01 (0.89–1.14)
Socioeconomic status							
Educational level							
Low	1	1	1	1	1	1	1
Intermediate	1.24 (0.65–2.39)	1.05 (0.76–1.44)	0.97 (0.81–1.17)	0.76 (0.62–0.94)*	0.83 (0.60–1.14)	1.01 (0.71–1.44)	0.99 (0.87–1.11)
High	1.09 (0.59–2.04)	0.93 (0.66–1.32)	0.91 (0.73–1.13)	0.79 (0.60–1.05)	0.66 (0.42–1.04)	0.95 (0.63–1.42)	0.84 (0.74–0.96)*
Occupational level							
Low	1	1	1	1	1	1	1
Intermediate	0.69 (0.43–1.10)	1.13 (0.83–1.53)	1.09 (0.92–1.28)	0.74 (0.53–1.02)	0.86 (0.61–1.21)	0.99 (0.68–1.36)	0.91 (0.80–1.03)
High	0.82 (0.58–1.15)	1.11 (0.81–1.52)	0.90 (0.71–1.14)	0.77 (0.49–1.20)	0.62 (0.38–1.01)	0.81 (0.52–1.27)	0.80 (0.70–0.91)**
Sexual risk behavior							
Number of lifetime sex partners[a]	1.32 (1.17–1.50)***	1.19 (1.06–1.33)**	1.05 (0.97–1.13)	1.02 (0.90–1.17)	1.12 (1.00–1.25)	1.12 (1.00–1.25)	1.16 (1.11–1.21)***
Age at sexual debut[b]	0.90 (0.84–0.98)*	0.97 (0.93–1.01)	0.99 (0.96–1.02)	0.96 (0.93–1.00)*	0.96 (0.92–1.00)*	0.96 (0.93–1.00)*	0.95 (0.93–0.96)***
Sexual partners and condom use (preceding 6 months)							
No sexual contact	1	1	1	1	1	1	1
Steady partner[c]	0.97 (0.64–1.48)	1.02 (0.72–1.43)	1.16 (0.89–1.52)	1.11 (0.86–1.43)	1.16 (0.75–1.79)	1.53 (0.95–2.45)	1.11 (0.96–1.29)
Consistent condom use[d]	1.32 (0.77–2.26)	1.16 (0.71–1.90)	1.40 (1.04–1.87)*	0.42 (0.16–1.13)	0.88 (0.43–1.79)	0.56 (0.20–1.54)	1.10 (0.88–1.36)
Inconsistent condom use [d]	1.37 (0.87–2.16)	1.41 (0.86–2.29)	1.34 (1.00–1.80)	0.92 (0.58–1.47)	1.35 (0.75–2.45)	2.44 (1.38–4.30)**	1.42 (1.18–1.70)***
Sexual health seeking behavior							
HIV testing (preceding 6 months)							
No	1	1	1*	1	1*	1*	1***

Table 2 (Sero) prevalence ratios of CT for potential determinants, by ethnic group. Results of stratified unadjusted Poisson regression with robust variance *(Continued)*

	Dutch ($n = 392$)	South Asian Surinamese ($n = 373$)	African Surinamese ($n = 317$)	Ghanaian ($n = 193$)	Turkish ($n = 389$)	Moroccan ($n = 337$)	Total ($n = 2001$)
	PR (95% CI)	PR (95% CI)	PR (95% CI)	PR (95% CI)	PR (95% CI)	PR (95% CI)	PR (95% CI)
Yes	1.24 (0.87–1.77)	1.38 (1.00–1.92)	1.16 (1.00–1.33)	1.12 (0.90–1.40)	1.68 (1.10–2.54)	1.56 (1.06–2.30)	1.51 (1.35–1.68)
STI testing (preceding 6 months)							
No	1*	1***	1	1	1	1	1***
Yes	1.38 (1.04–1.83)	1.64 (1.26–2.13)	1.07 (0.93–1.24)	1.15 (0.93–1.43)	1.48 (0.96–2.29)	1.18 (0.80–1.75)	1.45 (1.31–1.61)

OR Odds ratio, *CI* Confidence intervals, *N/A* not applicable, *HIV* Human immunodeficiency virus, *STI* Sexually transmitted infection, *CT Chlamydia trachomatis*

[a]Per increase of 1 natural log

[b]Per 1 year increase

[c]Sex with exclusive sex partner, regardless of condom use

[d]Has had a casual partner, irrespective of having had a steady partner

*overall $p < 0.05$

**overall $p < 0.01$

***overall $p < 0.001$

Table 3 Adjusted (sero)prevalence ratios (PR) of CT by ethnicity, as compared to the Dutch reference group

Adjustments	South Asian Surinamese PR (95% CI)	African Surinamese PR (95% CI)	Ghanaian PR (95% CI)	Turkish PR (95% CI)	Moroccan PR (95% CI)
Unadjusted*	1.07 (0.90–1.28)	1.99 (1.65–2.21)	1.81 (1.54–2.13)	0.83 (0.68–1.01)	0.93 (0.76–1.12)
Model 1: Adjusted for age and gender	1.09 (0.91–1.30)	1.90 (1.64–2.20)	1.81 (1.54–2.13)	0.82 (0.67–1.00)	0.93 (0.76–1.13)
Model 2: Adjusted for age, gender and sexual risk behavior (SRB)[a]	1.29 (1.07–1.56)	1.87 (1.61–2.17)	1.83 (1.51–2.21)	1.01 (0.81–1.26)	1.13 (0.91–1.40)
Model 3: Adjusted for age, gender, and socioeconomic status (SES)[b]	1.11 (0.90–1.36)	1.76 (1.47–2.12)	1.58 (1.24–2.01)	0.75 (0.59–0.97)	0.89 (0.70–1.13)
Model 4: Adjusted for age, gender and sexual healthcare seeking behavior (sHSB)[c]	1.11 (0.93–1.33)	1.85 (1.59–2.14)	1.78 (1.51–2.10)	0.86 (0.70–1.05)	0.94 (0.77–1.14)
Model 5: Adjusted for age, gender, SRB, SES and sHSB[a, b, c]	1.27 (1.02–1.58)	1.72 (1.43–2.06)	1.52 (1.16–1.99)	0.87 (0.66–1.13)	1.09 (0.84–1.40)

PR (Sero)prevalence ratio, *CI* Confidence intervals
*Results from unadjusted Poisson regression with robust variance
[a]Sexual risk behavior includes sexual contacts and condom use in the preceding 6 months, the natural log of lifetime sex partners and age at sexual debut
[b]Socioeconomic status includes educational level and occupational level
[c]Sexual healthcare seeking behavior includes HIV testing and STI testing in the preceding 6 months

estimate the overall CT seroprevalence of Amsterdam oversampling of groups is of no concern [15].

A major limitation is the use of CT serology as a surrogate of a recent CT infection. Firstly, the specificity to detect acute infection is not optimal (87%), as it detects exposure to a (past) CT infection, rather than a recent infection. Moreover, CT seropositivity can also be induced by other CT infections like trachoma, which is a relatively common eye disease in West Africa [20] and in rare cases by pneumonia and inclusion conjunctivitis [21]. It may be that first generation migrants of Western African origin (i.e. Ghanaian participants) have been exposed to eye infections caused by CT, inflating the CT seroprevalence of the Ghanaian study group. Cross reactivity with *C. pneumoniae*, a well known issue with ELISA based CT tests, was only minor (details in Additional file 1: Appendix 1).

Table 4 Adjusted CT seropositivity ratios of different ethnic groups (stratified by migration generation), as compared to Dutch. The analyses were adjusted for SRB, SES and sHSB

Ethnicity	PR + 95% CI
South Asian Surinamese- first generation	1.26 (0.89–1.79)
South Asian Surinamese- second generation	1.27 (1.02–1.59)*
African Surinamese- first generation	1.80 (1.47–2.20)*
African Surinamese- second generation	1.66 (1.36–2.02)*
Ghanaian- first generation	1.73 (1.31–2.29)*
Ghanaian- second generation	1.04 (0.67–1.63)
Turkish- first generation	0.91 (0.64–1.31)
Turkish- second generation	0.85 (0.64–1.13)
Moroccan- first generation	1.22 (0.86–1.71)
Moroccan- second generation	1.04 (0.79–1.38)

* Indicates a statistically significant result (p <0.05)

A specificity of less than 100% means that some participants are wrongly regarded as CT-exposed. There is no reason to believe that this misclassification differs by ethnicity or sHSB. Such random misclassification of CT status dilutes the strength of the effect of a risk factor with the outcome, but does not lead to the false identification of risk factors [22]. The use of Pgp3 based CT serological assays may improve the inherent properties of a serological CT test, as it has a higher specificity for CT [23, 24]. Lastly, the sensitivity of the CT serology may be affected by waning antibodies to CT overtime. For the current serological test the degree of waning is unknown. However, very recently Horner et al. [23] have shown that the waning of CT Pgp3 antibodies is less than 5% over 12 years, which suggests only a very modest effect of waning of CT antibodies. Use of NAAT based diagnosis of CT, might have alleviated some of these limitations caused by the suboptimal sensitivity and specificity of serological tests, but such results were not available [25].

Another limitation of the study is that no assessment could be performed on other areas of health care seeking behavior than sHSB. This might introduce a selection bias as low sHSB can either be appropriate or inappropriate depending on CT risk, but the difference between the two types of low sHSB cannot be discerned independently without an indication of healthcare seeking behavior in general. Likewise, if information on healthcare seeking behavior in general was available, but on sHSB was lacking, a similar selection would occur. In the multivariable models, adjustment for SRB was performed which minimizes the risk of selection bias due to this mechanism in the current study.

The cross-sectional design of the current study limits the possibilities to establish the causal role of SES, SRB, and sHSB in the association between ethnicity and CT.

Follow-up data of CT infections and risk could establish temporal, etiologic causations of ethnicity with CT.

Another potential limitation concerns the representativeness of the HELIUS cohort with regards to health seeking behavior. It might be that HELIUS study participants differ from the general population in terms of health awareness and consequently health seeking behavior. Unfortunately, no information on these variables was available from the HELIUS (non)-response analysis, so no reasonable conclusion can be made [15].

Studies performed in the United States suggest that differences in sexual mixing patterns (e.g. assortative and disassortative mixing) between African-American and the Caucasian population as well as sexual concurrency play major roles in establishing and maintaining STI rate disparities [26, 27]. It may be that factors associated with the sexual network structure, such as assortative mixing patterns and concurrency, contribute to the increased CT risk among individuals of African Surinamese and Ghanaian ethnic origin in the Netherlands [8, 9, 26–29]. HELIUS does not collect sexual network data, so we were unable to evaluate the role of (dis)assortative mixing or concurrency, which limits the study in its potential to examine possible explanations of disparities in CT prevalence between different ethnicities in the Netherlands.

A last potential limitation is the lack of data on vaginal microbiota composition in the current study. The composition of vaginal microbiota differs between ethnicities [30–32], and might explain differences in CT prevalence as vaginal dysbiosis increases susceptibility to STIs [33–35]. Dysbiosis may partially or completely be responsible for the differences between ethnicities.

Conclusions

In conclusion, the current study shows that CT seroprevalence differs between ethnic groups in Amsterdam, the Netherlands. CT seropositivity is most common among people of African Surinamese and Ghanaian origin. The differences in CT seroprevalence could not be explained by differences in SRB, SES or sHSB between ethnic groups. To gain a better understanding of the factors that drive CT (sero)disparities in Amsterdam, additional research should be performed, directed at establishing accurate estimates of CT incidence and its explanatory factors, including sexual mixing networks and concurrency and possible biologic mechanisms.

Abbreviations

(a)PR: (adjusted) Seroprevalence ratio; CBS: Statistics Netherlands; CI: Confidence interval; CT: *Chlamydia trachomatis*; DKFZ: German Cancer Research Center; HELIUS: HEalthy Life In an Urban Setting; Hsp60: Heat shock protein 60; MOMP: Major outer membrane protein; MSM: Men who have sex with men; SES: Socioeconomic status; sHSB: Sexual health seeking behavior; SRB: Sexual risk behavior; Tarp: Translocated actin-recruiting phosphoprotein; WSW: Women who have sex with women

Acknowledgements

The HELIUS study is conducted by the Academic Medical Center Amsterdam and the Public Health Service of Amsterdam. Both organisations provided core support for HELIUS. The HELIUS study is also funded by the Dutch Heart Foundation, the Netherlands Organization for Health Research and Development (ZonMw), and the European Union (FP-7). We gratefully acknowledge the AMC Biobank for their support in biobank management and high-quality storage of collected samples. We are most grateful to the participants of the HELIUS study and the management team, research nurses, interviewers, research assistants and other staff who have taken part in gathering the data of this study. The study reported here was additionally supported by an additional grant from the Public Health Service of Amsterdam.

Funding

The Academic Medical Center (AMC) of Amsterdam and the Public Health Service of Amsterdam (GGD Amsterdam) provided core financial support for HELIUS. The HELIUS study is also funded by research grants of the Dutch Heart Foundation (Hartstichting; grant no. 2010T084), the Netherlands Organization for Health Research and Development (ZonMw; grant no. 200500003), the European Integration Fund (EIF; grant no. 2013EIF013) and the European Union (Seventh Framework Programme, FP-7; grant no. 278901).

Availability of data and materials

The HELIUS data are owned by the Academic Medical Center (AMC) in Amsterdam, The Netherlands. The HELIUS study has an open policy with regard to collaboration with other research groups and welcomes collaborations from a wide variety of disciplines. Information on procedures to acquire the available data and/or samples is described in the HELIUS Collaboration Policy, which can be found at www.heliusstudy.nl/nl/researchers/collaboration. In brief, to make use of the available data for research, we request a publication proposal describing background, aim, research questions, methods (analysis plan), and time table. All proposals should be submitted to HELIUS via m.b.snijder@amc.nl, or via info@heliusstudy.nl. The proposals are discussed in the HELIUS Executive Board regarding the study aims (compatibility with the general objectives of the HELIUS study/informed consent), the quality of the research proposal, and potential overlap with on going studies. After approval, the requested data will be provided after a Data Transfer Agreement has been signed. For more information, please visit the HELIUS website or contact the Scientific Coordinator of the HELIUS study.

Authors' contributions

SHH drafted the manuscript and performed the statistical analyses. AAM, CJA, MBS, HJCdV, MP and MFSvdL kindly contributed to the manuscript and statistical analyses. MWF, KH and TW developed the multiplex serological CT assay and are the authors of Additional file 1: Appendix 1. All authors read and approved the final manuscript.

Consent for publication

Not applicable.

Competing interests

The authors declare that they have no competing interests.

Author details

[1]Department of Infectious Diseases, Public Health Service of Amsterdam (GGD Amsterdam), Nieuwe Achtergracht 100, 1018, WT, Amsterdam, The Netherlands. [2]Department of Internal Medicine, Amsterdam Institute for Infection and Immunity (AI&II), Academic Medical Center, Meibergdreef 9, 1105, AZ, Amsterdam, The Netherlands. [3]Department of Public Health, Amsterdam Public Health Research Institute, Academic Medical Center,

Meibergdreef 9, 1105, AZ, Amsterdam, The Netherlands. [4]Department of Clinical Epidemiology, Biostatistics and Bioinformatics, Amsterdam Public Health Research Institute, Academic Medical Center, Meibergdreef 9, 1105, AZ, Amsterdam, The Netherlands. [5]Molecular Diagnostics of Oncogenic Infections Division, German Cancer Research Center (Deutsches Krebsforschungszentrum DKFZ), Im Neuenheimer Feld 280, 69120 Heidelberg, Germany. [6]Department of Dermatology, Academic Medical Center, Meibergdreef 9, 1105, AZ, Amsterdam, The Netherlands.

References

1. Low N, Sterne JA, Barlow D. Inequalities in rates of gonorrhoea and chlamydia between black ethnic groups in south East London: cross sectional study. Sex Transm Infect. 2001;77(1):15–20.
2. Fenton KA, Mercer CH, McManus S, Erens B, Wellings K, Macdowall W, Byron CL, Copas AJ, Nanchahal K, Field J, et al. Ethnic variations in sexual behaviour in Great Britain and risk of sexually transmitted infections: a probability survey. Lancet. 2005;365(9466):1246–55.
3. Gotz HM, van Bergen JE, Veldhuijzen IK, Broer J, Hoebe CJ, Steyerberg EW, Coenen AJ, de Groot F, Verhooren MJ, van Schaik DT, et al. A prediction rule for selective screening of chlamydia trachomatis infection. Sex Transm Infect. 2005;81(1):24–30.
4. Op de Coul EL, Gotz HM, van Bergen JE, Fennema JS, Hoebe CJ, Koekenbier RH, Pars LL, van Ravesteijn SM, van der Sande MA, van den Broek IV. Who participates in the Dutch chlamydia screening? A study on demographic and behavioral correlates of participation and positivity. Sex Transm Dis. 2012;39(2):97–103.
5. Van den Broek IVF, Van Aar F, Van Oeffelen A. Sexually transmitted infections in the Netherlands 2015. Bilthoven: National Institute of Health and the Enviroment (RIVM); 2016.
6. Navarro C, Jolly A, Nair R, Chen Y. Risk factors for genital chlamydial infection. Can J Infect Dis. 2002;13(3):195–207.
7. Bebear C, de Barbeyrac B. Genital chlamydia trachomatis infections. Clin Microbiol Infect. 2009;15(1):4–10.
8. Gras MJ, Weide JF, Langendam MW, Coutinho RA, van den Hoek A. HIV prevalence, sexual risk behaviour and sexual mixing patterns among migrants in Amsterdam, The Netherlands. AIDS. 1999;13(14):1953–62.
9. Matser A, Luu N, Geskus R, Heijman T, Heiligenberg M, van Veen M, Schim van der Loeff M. Higher chlamydia trachomatis prevalence in ethnic minorities does not always reflect higher sexual risk behaviour. PLoS One. 2013;8(6):e67287.
10. Hallfors DD, Iritani BJ, Miller WC, Bauer DJ. Sexual and drug behavior patterns and HIV and STD racial disparities: the need for new directions. Am J Public Health. 2007;97(1):125–32.
11. Ellen JM, Aral SO, Madger LS. Do differences in sexual behaviors account for the racial/ethnic differences in adolescents' self-reported history of a sexually transmitted disease? Sex Transm Dis. 1998;25(3):125–9.
12. Ward H, Mertens TE, Thomas C. Health seeking behaviour and the control of sexually transmitted disease. Health Policy Plan. 1997;12(1):19–28.
13. van den Broek IV, van Bergen JE, Brouwers EE, Fennema JS, Gotz HM, Hoebe CJ, Koekenbier RH, Kretzschmar M, Over EA, Schmid BV, et al. Effectiveness of yearly, register based screening for chlamydia in the Netherlands: controlled trial with randomised stepped wedge implementation. BMJ. 2012;345:e4316.
14. Stronks K, Snijder MB, Peters RJ, Prins M, Schene AH, Zwinderman AH. Unravelling the impact of ethnicity on health in Europe: the HELIUS study. BMC Public Health. 2013;13:402.
15. Snijder MB, Galenkamp H, Prins M, Derks EM, Peters RJ, Zwinderman AH, Stronks K. Cohort profile: the Healthy Life in an Urban Setting (HELIUS) study. BMJ Open. 2017.
16. Alberts CJ, Michel A, Bruisten S, Snijder MB, Prins M, Waterboer T, Schim van der Loeff MF. High-risk human papillomavirus seroprevalence in men and women of six different ethnicities in Amsterdam, the Netherlands: the HELIUS study. Papillomavirus Res. 2017;3:57–65.
17. Stronks K, Kulu-Glasgow I, Agyemang C. The utility of 'country of birth' for the classification of ethnic groups in health research: the Dutch experience. Ethn Health. 2009;14(3):255–69.
18. (CBS) SN: Standard Classification of Occupations. https://www.cbs.nl/nl-nl/onze-diensten/methoden/classificaties/onderwijs-en-beroepen/beroepenclassificatie%2D%2Disco-en-sbc--. Accessed 10 Sept 2017.
19. Barros AJ, Hirakata VN. Alternatives for logistic regression in cross-sectional studies: an empirical comparison of models that directly estimate the prevalence ratio. BMC Med Res Methodol. 2003;3:21.
20. West SK, Munoz B, Weaver J, Mrango Z, Dize L, Gaydos C, Quinn TC, Martin DL. Can we use antibodies to chlamydia trachomatis as a surveillance tool for National Trachoma Control Programs? Results from a District Survey. PLoS Negl Trop Dis. 2016;10(1):e0004352.
21. Schachter J, Grossman M, Azimi PH. Serology of chlamydia trachomatis in infants. J Infect Dis. 1982;146(4):530–5.
22. Gordis L. Epidemiology. 5th ed. Philadelphia, PA: Elsevier; 2014. p. 265.
23. Horner PJ, Wills GS, Righarts A, Vieira S, Kounali D, Samuel D, Winston A, Muir D, Dickson NP, McClure MO. Chlamydia trachomatis Pgp3 antibody persists and correlates with self-reported infection and Behavioural risks in a blinded cohort study. PLoS One. 2016;11(3):e0151497.
24. Woodhall SC, Wills GS, Horner PJ, Craig R, Mindell JS, Murphy G, McClure MO, Soldan K, Nardone A, Johnson AM. Chlamydia trachomatis Pgp3 antibody population Seroprevalence before and during an era of widespread opportunistic chlamydia screening in England (1994-2012). PLoS One. 2017;12(1):e0152810.
25. Geisler WM. Diagnosis and Management of Uncomplicated Chlamydia trachomatis infections in adolescents and adults: summary of evidence reviewed for the 2015 Centers for Disease Control and Prevention sexually transmitted diseases treatment guidelines. Clin Infect Dis. 2015;61(Suppl 8): S774–84.
26. Morris M, Kurth AE, Hamilton DT, Moody J, Wakefield S. Concurrent partnerships and HIV prevalence disparities by race: linking science and public health practice. Am J Public Health. 2009;99(6):1023–31.
27. Laumann EO, Youm Y. Racial/ethnic group differences in the prevalence of sexually transmitted diseases in the United States: a network explanation. Sex Transm Dis. 1999;26(5):250–61.
28. Aral SO, Adimora AA, Fenton KA. Understanding and responding to disparities in HIV and other sexually transmitted infections in African Americans. Lancet. 2008;372(9635):337–40.
29. van Veen MG, Kramer MA, Op de Coul EL, van Leeuwen AP, de Zwart O, van de Laar MJ, Coutinho RA, Prins M. Disassortative sexual mixing among migrant populations in the Netherlands: a potential for HIV/STI transmission? AIDS Care. 2009;21(6):683–91.
30. Ravel J, Gajer P, Abdo Z, Schneider GM, Koenig SS, McCulle SL, Karlebach S, Gorle R, Russell J, Tacket CO, et al. Vaginal microbiome of reproductive-age women. Proc Natl Acad Sci U S A. 2011;108(Suppl 1):4680–7.
31. van Houdt R, Ma B, Bruisten SM, Speksnijder A, Ravel J, de Vries HJC. Lactobacillus iners-dominated vaginal microbiota is associated with increased susceptibility to chlamydia trachomatis infection in Dutch women: a case-control study. Sex Transm Infect. 2018;94(2):117–23.
32. Borgdorff H, van der Veer C, van Houdt R, Alberts CJ, de Vries HJ, Bruisten SM, Snijder MB, Prins M, Geerlings SE, Schim van der Loeff MF, et al. The association between ethnicity and vaginal microbiota composition in Amsterdam, the Netherlands. PLoS One. 2017;12(7):e0181135.
33. Brotman RM. Vaginal microbiome and sexually transmitted infections: an epidemiologic perspective. J Clin Invest. 2011;121(12):4610–7.
34. Schwebke JR. Abnormal vaginal flora as a biological risk factor for acquisition of HIV infection and sexually transmitted diseases. J Infect Dis. 2005;192(8):1315–7.
35. van de Wijgert JH, Borgdorff H, Verhelst R, Crucitti T, Francis S, Verstraelen H, Jespers V. The vaginal microbiota: what have we learned after a decade of molecular characterization? PLoS One. 2014;9(8):e105998.

Gonorrhea and chlamydia prevalence in different anatomical sites among men who have sex with men

Li-Gang Yang[1,2*], Xiao-Hui Zhang[1,2], Pei-Zhen Zhao[1,2], Zheng-Yu Chen[1,2], Wu-Jian Ke[1,2], Xu-Qi Ren[1,2], Liu-Yuan Wang[1,2], Wei-Ying Chen[1,2] and Joseph D. Tucker[1,2,3,4]

Abstract

Background: A high rectal and oropharyngeal sexually transmitted infection (STI) burden has been reported among men who have sex with men (MSM) in many regions, but little data exists on rectal and oropharyngeal STIs among MSM in China. The purpose of this study was to determine the prevalence of gonorrhea and chlamydia at different anatomic sites among MSM in Guangzhou, China.

Methods: We recruited a cross-sectional sample of MSM in one Chinese city and collected detailed information about socio-demographic characteristics and sexual behaviors. Men had urine, rectal, and pharyngeal swab samples tested for gonorrhea and chlamydia using nucleic acid amplification tests (NAAT). Univariate and multivariate logistic regressions were used to evaluate factors associated with gonorrhea and chlamydia. Among men without any STI symptoms, we also examined the prevalence of gonorrhea and chlamydia by anatomical site.

Results: We enrolled 463 men between January 2015 and March 2017. A total of 58/463 (12.5%) of men had gonorrhea and 84/463 (18.1%) had chlamydia. MSM with gonorrhea were more likely to have been recruited from the STI clinic (OR 3.41, 95% CI 1.94–5.99), living with HIV (OR 2.41, 95% CI 1.18–4.92), diagnosed had STI co-infection (OR 2.55, 95% CI 1.39–4.69). MSM with chlamydia were more likely to be students (OR 1.8, 95% CI 0.99–3.39). Most gonorrhea (34/58, 59%) and chlamydia (64/84, 76%) infections were not associated with STI symptoms.

Conclusion: Asymptomatic gonorrhea and chlamydia infection were common in this sample of Chinese MSM. Further research is necessary to determine optimal STI screening programs.

Keywords: MSM, Chlamydia, Gonorrhea, Rectal, Pharyngeal

Background

Gonorrhea and chlamydia infections are the most common curable sexually transmitted infections (STIs). In 2012 there were an estimated 78 million (53–110 million) new gonorrhea infections and 131 million (100–166 million) chlamydia infections respectively, in 2012 [1]. Men who have sex with men (MSM) have particularly high rates of gonorrhea and chlamydia [2–7].

* Correspondence: yanglg3@hotmail.com
[1]Department of Sexually Transmitted Diseases, Dermatology Hospital, Southern Medical University, Guangzhou 510091, China
[2]Guangdong Provincial Dermatology Hospital, Guangzhou 510091, China
Full list of author information is available at the end of the article

Extragenital gonorrhea and chlamydia are major public health problems among MSM. Compared with genital infections, rectal and pharyngeal gonorrhea and chlamydia infections are more likely to be asymptomatic [5] and can easily be missed without screening. Several high-income countries recommend regular screening of extragenital sites (rectum and pharynx) among sexually active MSM [8–10]. World Health Organization MSM preventive guidelines also support gonorrhea and chlamydia screening among MSM with a higher burden of asymptomatic disease [11]. This suggests the need for research to understand the burden of extragenital gonorrhea and chlamydia among MSM in different settings.

Despite high HIV prevalence and frequent condomless sex among MSM in China, [12–18] there are limited data on MSM extragenital gonorrhea and chlamydia. [19, 20] Better understanding the burden of rectal and pharyngeal gonorrhea and chlamydia can provide useful information for research and screening pilots. We undertook this study in Guangzhou, China. Guangzhou is a provincial capital city in south China with a concentrated HIV infection in MSM [21] and a strong STI network. The purpose of this study was to determine the prevalence of gonorrhea and chlamydia at different anatomic sites among MSM in Guangzhou, China.

Methods

Study population and procedure

We recruited a cross-sectional convenience sample of MSM between January 2015 and March 2017. Enrollment criteria included being male, currently living in Guangzhou, being at least 18 years of age, self-identifying as gay or bisexual, and receiving no antibiotics in the past month.

We recruited patients from two clinics at the Dermatology Hospital of Southern Medical University, a tertiary care center with experience serving MSM. The first was an STI clinic run by the hospital, through which any patient who had STI complaints or concerns could request to see a doctor. Patients meeting enrollment criteria who agreed to participate were asked to join the research study. The second was a weekend community clinic sponsored by the Zhitong Guangzhou LGBT (lesbian, gay, bisexual, and transgender) Center, an MSM community organization. This community clinic provides free HIV and syphilis testing services for MSM. During this study, Zhitong also advertised our project on their website and social media account.

Data collection

At enrollment, we collected baseline socio-demographic information, sexual behavior, and STI history. Information about symptoms was collected as a single item. If men had symptoms consistent with an STI, this was noted. There was no effort to attribute symptoms to a particular pathogen in cases of co-infection. All participants underwent physical examination, and any abnormal findings (i.e. warts) were recorded. Urine, rectal and pharyngeal swab samples were collected for gonorrhea and chlamydia testing. Venous blood samples were collected for HIV and syphilis testing. Men with positive tests were treated according to Chinese STI clinical management guidelines.

Laboratory methods

Oropharyngeal, rectal, and urine specimens were tested for gonorrhea and chlamydia using the Cobas 4800 system (Roche Moleculer Systems, Inc. New Jersey, USA). Blood samples were tested for syphilis using a toluidine red unheated serum test (TRUST, Rongsheng Bio-technology Limited Corporation, Shanghai, China) and *Treponema pallidum* particle agglutination test (TPPA, Fujirebio Inc., Japan). Blood samples were tested for HIV using two antibody tests - a rapid HIV antibody test (Wantai, Beijing, China) and a second antibody test (Abon Biopharm, Hangzhou, China). If both were positive, another blood sample was collected for Western blot confirmation (MP Biomedical, Singapore).

Men were considered infected with gonorrhea and chlamydia if respective tests were positive. Men with positive TRUST and TPPA tests were considered to have syphilis infection, unless a documented history of previously treated syphilis was available. Men with positive HIV screening and confirmatory tests were considered to have HIV infection. Anogenital warts and anogenital herpes were diagnosed according to the diagnostic criteria for China's notifiable diseases reporting system (Version 2008). These diagnoses are mainly based on exposure history and consistent clinical findings.

Data analysis

We described socio-demographic characteristics, sexual risk behaviors, and STI (by anatomic site) among men. We compared men presenting to the STI clinic and men presenting to the MSM community clinic. Chi-square tests were used to compare gonorrhea/chlamydia prevalence between the STI clinic and MSM community groups. Univariate and multivariate logistic regressions were used to evaluate factors associated gonorrhea and chlamydia, respectively. We also calculated the frequency of men with gonorrhea and chlamydia who were asymptomatic. All data were analyzed using SAS 9.2 (SAS, Cary, USA).

Ethics, consent and permissions

Ethical approval for this study was obtained from the Science Research Ethical Committee of the Dermatology Hospital of Southern Medical University (GDDHLS-201502). Written informed consent was waived because the risk associated with participating in this study was deemed minimal and involved no procedures requiring consent outside of the context of participating in the study. This was approved by the Chinese IRB. It is also in accordance with DHHS (45 CFR 46.117). Verbal consent was obtained before participants were enrolled.

Results

We recruited 463 MSM to join the study. One-hundred and fifty-three men were from the STI clinic and 310 men were from the MSM community clinic. Most men were young, Han ethnicity, unmarried, non-students, and had a higher education level. Socio-demographic characteristics are shown in Table 1.

Among 463 men, a total of 58 (12.5%) men had gonorrhea infection. The gonorrhea prevalence at urethral, rectal, and pharyngeal sites was 5.2% (24/463), 6.1% (28/463), and 3.9% (18/463), respectively (Table 2). Among all men with gonorrhea, most men (34/58, 59%) did not have STI symptoms. MSM with asymptomatic extragenital gonorrhea were common (Fig. 1). MSM with gonorrhea were more likely to have been recruited from the STI clinic (OR 3.41, 95% CI 1.94–5.99), living with HIV (OR 2.41, 95% CI 1.18–4.92), and diagnosed with STI co-infection (OR 2.55, 95% CI 1.39–4.69) (Table 3).

A total of 84 men (18.1%) had chlamydia infection at any site. The chlamydia prevalence at the urethral, rectal and oropharyngeal sites was 6.7% (31/463), 11.2% (52/463), and 1.3% (6/463), respectively. Among all men with chlamydia, most men (64/84, 76%) did not have STI symptoms. 61.3% of urethral infections, 83.3% of rectal infections and 83.3% of pharyngeal infections were asymptomatic (Fig. 1). There was a trend towards MSM with chlamydia being more likely to be students (OR 1.8, 95% CI 0.99–3.39).

The chlamydia and gonorrhea coinfection rate was 5.6% ($n = 26$). Sixty men (13.0%) were living with HIV infection. Eighty-four men (18.1%) had other STIs, including syphilis, anogenital wards, or herpes.

Discussion

Our study evaluated the prevalence of urethral, anal, and pharyngeal gonorrhea and chlamydia among MSM in Guangzhou, China. This study expands the limited literature on MSM extragenital gonorrhea and chlamydia

Table 1 Demographic and behavioral characteristics of participants from the hospital STI clinic and the community-based MSM clinic ($n = 463$), 2015–2017

	STI Clinic n (frequency)	Community clinic n (frequency)	*P-value*
Age(years)			0.159
< 25	50/153 (32.7%)	128/310 (41.3%)	
25~35	68/153 (44.4%)	113/310 (36.4%)	
> 35	35/153 (22.9%)	69/310 (22.3%)	
Ethnicity			0.088
Han	146/153 (95.4%)	282/310 (91.0%)	
Others	7/153 (4.6%)	28/310 (9.0%)	
Marital status			< 0.0001
Unmarried	101/153 (66.0%)	265/310 (86.6%)	
Married	50/153 (32.7%)	35/310 (11.4%)	
Other	2/153 (1.3%)	6/310 (2.0%)	
Student			0.049
Yes	14/153 (9.2%)	49/310 (15.8%)	
No	139/153 (90.8%)	261/310 (84.2%)	
Local residence time			0.854
0–6 months	22/153 (14.4%)	44/310 (14.5%)	
6–12 months	9/153 (5.9%)	22/310 (7.3%)	
Over 1 year	122/153 (79.7%)	237/310 (78.2%)	
Education level			0.065
Junior middle school and below	22/153 (14.4%)	24/310 (7.8%)	
Senior middle school	22/153 (14.4%)	41/310 (13.2%)	
Senior middle school above	109/153 (71.2%)	245 (79.0%)	
Any STI related symptoms			< 0.001
Yes	49/153 (32.0%)	31/310 (10.0%)	
No	104/153 (68.0%)	279/310 (90.0%)	
Condom use in the last 6 months			< 0.001
Any condom less sex	141/153 (92.8)	305/310 (99.3%)	
Consistent condom use	11/153 (7.2%)	2/310 (0.7%)	

Table 2 Gonorrhea and chlamydia infection by anatomic sites among 463 MSM in an STI clinic and a community-based clinic in Guangzhou China, 2015–2017

Variables	STI clinic n (frequency)	Community clinic n (frequency)	Total n (frequency)	*p**
Gonorrhea	34/153(22.2%)	24/310 (7.7%)	58/463 (12.5%)	< 0.001
Urethral	22/153 (14.4%)	2/310 (0.7%)	24/463 (5.2%)	< 0.001
Rectal	11/153 (7.2%)	17/310 (5.5%)	28/463 (6.1%)	0.469
Pharyngeal	6/153 (3.9%)	12/310 (3.9%)	18/463 (3.9%)	0.979
Chlamydia	29/153 (19.0%)	55/310(17.7%)	84/463 (18.1%)	0.750
Urethral	18/153 (11.8%)	13/310 (4.2%)	31/463 (6.7%)	0.002
Rectal	10/153 (6.5%)	42/310 (13.6%)	52/463 (11.2%)	0.025
Pharyngeal	1/153 (0.7%)	5/310 (1.6%)	6/463 (1.3%)	0.391
HIV	20/153 (13.1%)	40/310 (12.9%)	60/463 (13.0%)	0.959
[a]Other STIs	49/153 (32.0%)	35/310 (11.3%)	84/463 (18.1%)	< 0.001

*Chi-squared test
[a]Other STIs refers to syphilis, ano-genital warts and herpes
26 participants were co-infected with gonorrhea and chlamydia

prevalence in an low and middle income country context. This study also compares two different populations of MSM within the same city, providing insight about risk in these groups.

The overall chlamydia prevalence was 18.1%, and the gonorrhea prevalence was 12.5%. The burden of chlamydia and gonorrhea are similar to findings from other Chinese studies in Shenzhen [19] and Kunming [20]. Over half of all STIs were asymptomatic, consistent with other studies. Given that World Health Organization Guidelines recommend MSM screening for asymptomatic urethral and rectal gonorrhea/chlamydia if prevalence is greater than 1–2% [11], our data suggest that screening would be indicated in this population.

We found that the majority of MSM STI infections were asymptomatic. This is consistent with a previous study from the United States [5]. This trend is more pronounced for rectal and pharyngeal infections [22]. The high burden of extra-genital STIs among MSM may help researchers and policy makers making decisions about routine screening guidelines.

Our data suggest that more MSM with symptoms seek care at the STI clinic compared to the MSM community clinic. This is consistent with the STI literature on MSM seeking care at STI clinics compared to community clinics [5]. Asymptomatic infections were especially common in the MSM community clinic. This suggests that asymptomatic screening programs may be more appropriate for MSM community clinics and related settings.

Our study has implications for STI research priorities among MSM. Better understanding the burden of asymptomatic extragenital STIs may be helpful in designing prospective screening studies or modelling research. Despite the fact that many guidelines recommend periodic STI screening among MSM, there are also barriers to screening (cost. Feasibility, logistics). The US Preventive Service Task Force found insufficient evidence to recommend gonorrhea and chlamydia testing among men when it last reviewed

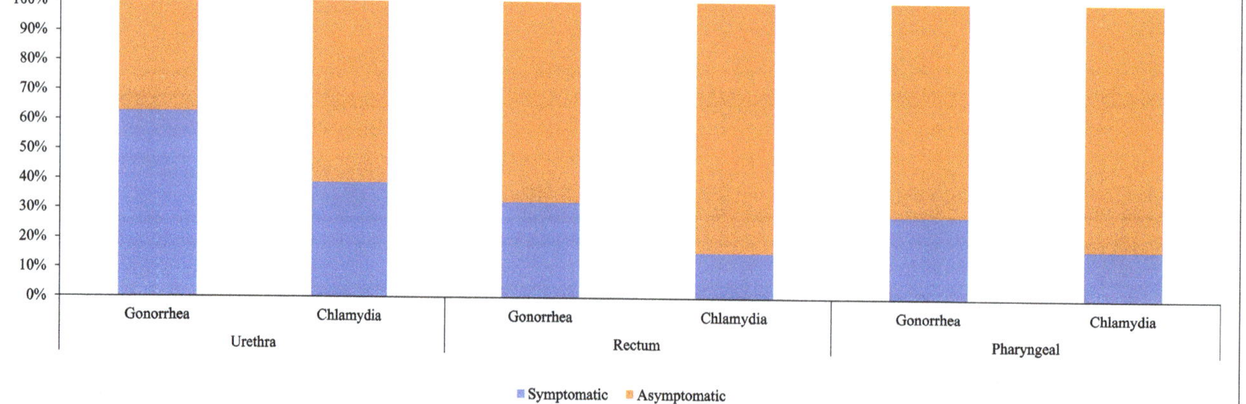

Fig. 1 Proportion of symptomatic and asymptomatic urethral, rectal and pharyngeal chlamydia and gonococcal infections

Table 3 Factors associated with gonorrhea and chlamydia infections among 463 MSM in Guangzhou China, 2015–2017

	gonorrhea(%)	*OR (95%CI)*	*P*	AOR	chlamydia(%)	*OR(95%CI)*	*P*	AOR
Age(years)								
< 25	26/178 (14.6%)	1.81 (0.81,4.02)	0.148	–	37/178 (20.8%)	1.34 (0.71,2.53)	0.362	
25~35	23/181 (12.7%)	1.54 (0.68,3.46)	0.299	–	30/181 (16.6%)	1.02 (0.53,1.95)	0.960	
> 35	9/104 (8.7%)	1.00		–	17/104 (16.4%)	1.00		
Ethnicity								
Han	52/428 (12.2%)	0.67(0.27,1.69)	0.394	–	76/428 (17.8%)	0.73(0.32,1.67)	0.453	
Others	6/35 (17.1%)	1.00		–	8/35 (22.9%)	1.00		
Marital status								
Unmarried	45/366 (12.3%)	0.98(0.12,8.16)	0.986	–	63/366 (17.2%)	0.62(0.12,3.16)	0.568	
Married	12/85 (14.1%)	1.15(0.13,10.20)	0.899	–	17/85 (20.0%)	0.75(0.14,4.05)	0.737	
Other	1/8 (12.5%)	1.00		–	2/8 (25.0%)	1.00		
Student								
Yes	11/63 (17.5%)	1.59(0.78,3.26)	0.206	–	17/63 (27.0%)	1.84(0.99,3.39)	0.053	
No	47/400 (11.8%)	1.00		–	67/400 (16.8%)	1.00		
Local residence time								
0–6 months	12/66 (18.2%)	1.59(0.79,3.21)	0.194	–	12/66 (18.2%)	0.99(0.50,1.95)	0.969	
6–12 months	2/31(6.5%%)	0.49(0.11,2.14)	0.346	–	4/31 (12.9%)	0.66(0.22,1.94)	0.449	
Over 1 year	44/359 (12.3%)	1.00		–	66/359 (18.4%)	1.00		
Education level								
Junior middle school and below	6/46 (13.0%)	1.03(0.41,2.57)	0.949	–	7/46 (15.2%)	0.74(0.32,1.73)	0.488	
Senior middle school	7/63 (11.1%)	0.86(0.39,2.00)	0.723		8/63 (12.7%)	0.60(0.27,1.32)	0.204	
Senior middle school above	45/354 (12.7%)	1.00			69/354 (19.5%)	1.00		
Recruited from								
STI clinic	34/153 (22.2%)	3.41(1.94,5.99)	< 0.01	2.71(1.49,4.96)	29/153 (19.0%)	1.08(0.66,1.79)	0.750	–
Community clinic	24/310 (7.7%)	1.00		1.00	55/310 (17.7%)	1.00		–
Any STI related symptoms								
Yes	24/80 (30.0%)	4.40(2.43,7.97)	< 0.01	2.89(1.53,5.47)	20/80 (25.0%)	1.66(0.94,2.95)	0.082	–
No	34/383 (8.9%)	1.00		1.00	64/383 (16.7%)	1.00		–
Condom use in the last 6 months								
Any condom less sex	56/446 (12.6%)	0.79(0.17,3.66)	0.763	–	82/446 (18.4%)	1.23(0.27,5.70)		–
Consistent condom use	2/13 (15.4%)	1.00		–	2/13 (15.4%)	1.00		–
No. of sex partners in last 6 months	–	1.04(0.94,1.15)	0.424	–	–	1.09(1.01,1,18)	0.0495	1.09(1.01,1,18)
HIV positive								
Yes	15/60 (25.0%)	2.79(1.44,5.42)	0.0025	2.41(1.18,4.92)	15/60 (25.0%)	1.61(0.85,3.06)	0.1424	–
No	43/403 (10.7%)	1.00		1.00	69/403 (17.1%)	1.00		–
Other STIs#								
Yes	19/84 (22.6%)	2.55(1.39,4.69)	0.0026	–	18/84 (21.4%)	1.29(0.72,2.32)	0.3885	–
No	39/379 (10.3%)	1.00		–	66/379 (17.4%)	1.00		–

#: other STIs refers to syphilis, ano-genital warts and ano-genital herpes

the evidence [23]. Accurate assessment of asymptomatic extragenital MSM STIs will also be helpful for the development of local policies and practice guidelines.

Our study has several limitations. First, our study was limited to two clinics taking place in the same hospital in Guangzhou. This study is not representative of MSM in China and caution should be used in making generalizations to other settings. Second, the study was cross-sectional in nature, so we cannot draw conclusions regarding causality. Third, although we asked patients about their symptoms, the main purpose of the survey instrument was not to better understand co-existing symptoms. In addition, symptoms may not have been related to an STI. Pharyngeal symptoms have a wide differential diagnosis, so our estimate of asymptomatic cases of pharyngeal chlamydia and gonorrhea are likely underestimates.

Conclusions

Our findings show that chlamydia and gonorrhea prevalence are high among Chinese MSM. Enhanced screening and treatment of rectal chlamydia and gonorrhea among MSM is necessary to improve sexual health.

Abbreviations

DHHS: Department of Health and Human Services; LGBT: Lesbian, gay, bisexual, and transgender; MSM: Men who have sex with men; NAAT: Nucleic acid amplification tests; STI: Sexually transmitted infection; STIs: Sexually transmitted infections; TPPA: Treponema pallidum particle agglutination test; TRUST: Toluidine red unheated serum test

Acknowledgements

The authors gratefully acknowledge the support of the Guangzhou LGBT Center and thank the many study participants who made this work possible.

Funding

This work was supported by Medical Science and Technology Foundation of Guangdong Province (C2013010) and Research Fund of the Bureau of Science and Information Technology of Guangzhou Municipality (201704020219). This funding resources had no role in the design of the study and collection, analysis, interpretation of data, and in writing the manuscript.

Authors' contributions

YLG, ZXH, ZPZ and JDT designed the study and wrote the initial manuscript. YLG, ZXH, ZPZ, CZY, KWJ, RXQ,WLY and CWY did the data collection and analysis. YLG, ZXH, ZPZ, CZY, KWJ, RXQ, WLY, CWY and JDT edited the manuscript and completed the final revisions. All authors read and approved the final manuscript.

Consent for publication

Not Applicable.

Competing interests

The authors declare that they have no competing interests.

Author details

[1]Department of Sexually Transmitted Diseases, Dermatology Hospital, Southern Medical University, Guangzhou 510091, China. [2]Guangdong Provincial Dermatology Hospital, Guangzhou 510091, China. [3]Institute for Global Health and Infectious Diseases, University of North Carolina at Chapel Hill, Raleigh, USA. [4]Faculty of Infectious and Tropical Diseases, London School of Hygiene and Tropical Medicine, London, UK.

References

1. Newman L, Rowley J, Vander Hoorn S, Wijesooriya NS, Unemo M, Low N, Stevens G, Gottlieb S, Kiarie J, Temmerman M. Global estimates of the prevalence and incidence of four curable sexually transmitted infections in 2012 based on systematic review and global reporting. PLoS One. 2015; 10(12):e0143304.
2. Leon SR, Segura ER, Konda KA, Flores JA, Silva-Santisteban A, Galea JT, Coates TJ, Klausner JD, Caceres CF. High prevalence of chlamydia trachomatis and Neisseria gonorrhoeae infections in anal and pharyngeal sites among a community-based sample of men who have sex with men and transgender women in Lima, Peru. BMJ Open. 2016;6(1):e008245.
3. Tongtoyai J, Todd CS, Chonwattana W, Pattanasin S, Chaikummao S, Varangrat A, Lokpichart S, Holtz TH, van Griensven F, Curlin ME. Prevalence and correlates of chlamydia trachomatis and Neisseria gonorrhoeae by anatomic site among urban Thai men who have sex with men. Sex Transm Dis. 2015;42(8):440–9.
4. Vodstrcil LA, Fairley CK, Fehler G, Leslie D, Walker J, Bradshaw CS, Hocking JS. Trends in chlamydia and gonorrhea positivity among heterosexual men and men who have sex with men attending a large urban sexual health service in Australia, 2002-2009. BMC Infect Dis. 2011;11:158.
5. Kent CK, Chaw JK, Wong W, Liska S, Gibson S, Hubbard G, Klausner JD. Prevalence of rectal, urethral, and pharyngeal chlamydia and gonorrhea detected in 2 clinical settings among men who have sex with men: San Francisco, California, 2003. Clin Infect Dis. 2005;41(1):67–74.
6. Rebe K, Lewis D, Myer L, de Swardt G, Struthers H, Kamkuemah M, McIntyre J. A Cross Sectional Analysis of gonococcal and chlamydial infections among men-who-have-sex-with-men in Cape Town, South Africa. PLoS One. 2015;10(9):e0138315.
7. Dudareva-Vizule S, Haar K, Sailer A, Wisplinghoff H, Wisplinghoff F, Marcus U. Group Ps: prevalence of pharyngeal and rectal chlamydia trachomatis and Neisseria gonorrhoeae infections among men who have sex with men in Germany. Sex Transm Infect. 2014;90(1):46–51.
8. Workowski KA. Bolan GA, centers for disease C, prevention: sexually transmitted diseases treatment guidelines, 2015. MMWR Recomm Rep. 2015; 64(RR-03):1–137.
9. Bourne C, Edwards B, Shaw M, Gowers A, Rodgers C, Ferson M. Sexually transmissible infection testing guidelines for men who have sex with men. Sex Health. 2008;5(2):189–91.
10. Patel RR, Patel S, Clarke E, Khan AW, Doshi B, Radcliffe KW. European collaborative clinical G: guidance and practice on frequency of HIV and sexually transmitted infection testing in men who have sex with men - what is the European situation? Int J STD AIDS. 2014;25(3):213–8.
11. Gerbase A. Prevention and treatment of HIV and other sexually transmitted infections among men who have sex with men and transgender People: Recommendations for a public health approach. Geneva: WHO, Programme HIV/AIDS; 2011. Report No.: ISBN 978 92 4 150175 0.
12. Dai W, Luo Z, Xu R, Zhao G, Tu D, Yang L, Wang F, Cai Y, Lan L, Hong F, et al. Prevalence of HIV and syphilis co-infection and associated factors among non-commercial men who have sex with men attending a sexually transmitted disease clinic in Shenzhen, China. BMC Infect Dis. 2017;17(1):86.
13. Zhao J, Chen L, Chaillon A, Zheng C, Cai W, Yang Z, Li G, Gan Y, Wang X, Hu Y, et al. The dynamics of the HIV epidemic among men who have sex with men (MSM) from 2005 to 2012 in Shenzhen, China. Sci Rep. 2016;6: 28703.
14. Zeng X, Zhong X, Peng B, Zhang Y, Kong C, Liu X, Huang A. Prevalence and associated risk characteristics of HIV infection based on anal sexual role among men who have sex with men: a multi-city cross-sectional study in Western China. Int J Infect Dis. 2016;49:111–8.
15. Yang Z, Huang Z, Dong Z, Li J, Zhang S, Wu N, Jin M. Risk factors for HIV diagnosis among men who have sex with men: results of a case-control study in one sample of eastern China. AIDS Res Hum Retrovir. 2016;32(12): 1163–8.
16. Li R, Wang H, Pan X, Ma Q, Chen L, Zhou X, Jiang T, He L, Chen J, Zhang X, et al. Prevalence of condomless anal intercourse and recent HIV testing and their associated factors among men who have sex with men in Hangzhou, China: a respondent-driven sampling survey. PLoS One. 2017;12(3):e0167730.
17. Qin Q, Tang W, Ge L, Li D, Mahapatra T, Wang L, Guo W, Cui Y, Sun J. Changing trend of HIV, syphilis and hepatitis C among men who have sex with men in China. Sci Rep. 2016;6:31081.

18. Qin Q, Guo W, Tang W, Mahapatra T, Wang L, Zhang N, Ding Z, Cai C, Cui Y, Sun J. Spatial analysis of the human immunodeficiency virus epidemic among men who have sex with men in China, 2006-2015. Clin Infect Dis. 2017;64(7):956–63.
19. Li JH, Cai YM, Yin YP, Hong FC, Shi MQ, Feng TJ, Peng RR, Wang BX, Chen XS. Prevalence of anorectal chlamydia trachomatis infection and its genotype distribution among men who have sex with men in Shenzhen, China. Jpn J Infect Dis. 2011;64(2):143–6.
20. Zhang X, Jia M, Chen M, Luo H, Chen H, Luo W, Zhang W, Ma Y, Yang C, Yang Y, et al. Prevalence and the associated risk factors of HIV, STIs and HBV among men who have sex with men in Kunming, China. Int J STD AIDS. 2017;28(11):1115–23.
21. Zhong F, Liang B, Xu H, Cheng W, Fan L, Han Z, Liang C, Gao K, Mai H, Qin F, et al. Increasing HIV and decreasing syphilis prevalence in a context of persistently high unprotected anal intercourse, six consecutive annual surveys among men who have sex with men in Guangzhou, China, 2008 to 2013. PLoS One. 2014;9(7):e103136.
22. Chan PA, Robinette A, Montgomery M, Almonte A, Cu-Uvin S, Lonks JR, Chapin KC, Kojic EM, Hardy EJ. Extragenital infections caused by chlamydia trachomatis and Neisseria gonorrhoeae: a review of the literature. Infect Dis Obstet Gynecol. 2016;2016:5758387.
23. LeFevre ML, Force USPST. Screening for chlamydia and gonorrhea: U.S. preventive services task Force recommendation statement. Ann Intern Med. 2014;161(12):902–10.

24

Prevalence, risk factors, and medical costs of *Chlamydia trachomatis* infections in Shandong Province, China

Pengcheng Huai[1,2,3], Furong Li[2], Zhen Li[2], Lele Sun[2,4], Xi'an Fu[2,4], Qing Pan[2,4], Gongqi Yu[2,4], Zemin Chai[2,4], Tongsheng Chu[2], Zihao Mi[2,4], Fangfang Bao[2,4], Honglei Wang[2,4], Bingni Zhou[2,4], Chuan Wang[2,4], Yonghu Sun[2,4], Guiye Niu[2,4], Yuan Zhang[2,4], Fanghui Fu[2,4], Xiaoqiao Lang[2,4], Xiaoling Wang[2,4], Hui Zhao[2,4], Daina Liu[2,4], Hong Liu[2,4], Dianchang Liu[2], Jian Liu[2], Aiqiang Xu[3,5] and Furen Zhang[2,4*]

Abstract

Background: A population-based study of *Chlamydia trachomatis* (CT) infections is essential in designing a specific control program; however, no large investigation of CT infections among the general population in mainland China has been conducted since 2000. We aimed to determine the prevalence, risk factors, and associated medical costs of CT among residents, 18–49 years of age, in Shandong, China.

Methods: From May to August 2016, a multistage probability sampling survey involving 8074 individuals was distributed. Data were collected via face-to-face interviews, followed by self-administered questionnaire surveys. First-void urines were collected and tested for CT and *Neisseria gonorrhoeae* (NG) using nucleic acid amplification.

Results: The weighted prevalence of CT infection was 2.3% (95% confidence interval [CI], 1.5–3.2) in females and 2.7% (1.6–3.8) in males. Women, 30–34 years of age, had the highest prevalence of CT infections (3.5%, 2.6–4.4), while the highest prevalence of CT infections in males was in those 18–24 years of age (4.3%, 0.0–8.8). *Neisseria gonorrhoeae* infection had a prevalence of 0.1% (0.0–0.3) in women and 0.03% (0.0–0.1) in men. Risk factors for CT infections among females included being unmarried, divorced, or widowed (odds ratio [OR], 95% CI 3.57, 1.54–8.24) and having two or more lifetime sex partners (3.72, 1.14–12.16). Among males, first intercourse before 20 years of age (1.83, 1.10–3.02) and having two or more lifetime sex partners (1.85, 1.14–3.02) were associated with CT infections. The estimated lifetime cost of CT infections in patients 18–49 years of age in Shandong was 273 million (range, 172–374 million) China Renminbi in 2016.

Conclusions: This study demonstrated a high burden of CT infections among females < 35 years of age and males < 25 years of age in Shandong. Thus, a CT infection control program should focus on this population, as well as others with identified risk factors.

Keywords: *Chlamydia trachomatis*, *Neisseria gonorrhea*, Prevalence, Risk factor, Medical cost, General population, China

* Correspondence: zhangfuren@hotmail.com
[2]Shandong Provincial Institute of Dermatology and Venereology, Shandong Academy of Medical Sciences, 27397 Jingshi Road, Jinan 250022, China
[4]Shandong Provincial Key Laboratory for Dermatovenereology, Jinan, China
Full list of author information is available at the end of the article

Background

Chlamydia trachomatis (CT) is the most commonly diagnosed bacterial sexually transmitted infection (STI) worldwide [1]. According to the 2015 global STI surveillance report from the World Health Organization (WHO), global estimates of new CT infections in 2012 were approximately 131 million [2]. Legally notifiable STIs, such as syphilis and HIV, have increased significantly in China from 2004 to 2013, with annual percentage changes of 16.3% for both STIs [3]; however, little information is available regarding the incidence or prevalence of CT infections among the general population in mainland China over the past decade. The current estimated burden of CT infections in China is based primarily on national or regional STIs surveillance sites; however, surveillance data does not measure the true burden of CT infections among the general population because infections are often asymptomatic and undiagnosed. Furthermore, the reported data are frequently misclassified or duplicated [4, 5]. A population-based survey of STIs provided an estimate of the prevalence, determinants, and economic burden of CT infections, which facilitate the design and delivery of a CT infection control program [4]. Because the first national population-based CT infection investigation conducted in China was in 1999–2000, more than 18 years ago, the information for CT infection control and prevention strategies is outdated [6]. Another population-based CT infection survey was conducted in Shanxi Province of China in 2004, but the sample size was small ($n = 399$) [7]. Therefore, a population-based CT infection study with a large sample size is needed in China.

The Chinese government replaced the one-child policy with a universal two-child policy in October 2015, implying that more couples have opportunity to have their second child [8]. Thus, more CT infections involving couples may suffer from infertility and adverse pregnancy outcomes, such as ectopic pregnancy, without early screening [9]. The complication burden due to CT infection may be higher after the introduction of the universal two-child policy. Furthermore, CT infections and other STIs could facilitate transmission of HIV [10]. Fortunately, most of the bacterial STIs, including CT infections are treatable, so screening among high-risk populations enables early identification and treatment, which reduce the disease burden and adverse outcomes [11].

A number of population-based studies of CT infections have been conducted, including the United States and European and Oceania countries [4, 5, 12, 13]. Several strategies to improve sexual health have been implemented in a number of developed countries or regions based on findings from these population-based studies [14, 15]. Thus, it is essential to conduct a population-based CT infection investigation and provide official recommendations for CT infection-specific control interventions in China.

Shandong Province is a coastal province located in eastern China, with a population of 98.5 million in 2015, accounting for 7% of the total population in China. This study was a population-based, cross-sectional study conducted from 9 May to 25 August 2016 in Shandong Province. We undertook this study to determine the prevalence, risk factors, and associated medical costs of CT infections among the general population 18–49 years of age in China.

Methods

Study design and participants

The population was sampled to represent the general population of Shandong Province, China (18–49 years of age). General population refers to males and females who had lived in their current residence for at least the past 6 months. The estimated sample size was 8074 individuals based on the national survey conducted in 1999–2000 [6]. (Additional file 1) The multi-stage sampling process included four steps, as follows: Shandong Province was divided into four strata based on geographic region (east, northwest, south, and middle); 2–4 urban districts or counties were randomly extracted from each stratum, producing 12 primary sampling units (PSUs; Fig. 1); 4–7 subunits (rural townships and urban street districts) were selected from each PSU using the probability proportionate to size sampling (PPS) method; a total of 59 subunits were selected; 3–12 rural villages or urban communities were selected from each subunit using the aforementioned sampling method, with more populated subunits having a higher probability of selection; villages and communities were selected with a proportion of 1:1; a total of 184 rural villages and 183 urban communities were included; residents, 18–49 years of age, who had lived in their current residence for at least the past 6 months were selected and arrayed in order by age and gender; systematic sampling was performed based on the gender and age distribution of the Shandong Province population to produce the sample; Thus, 22 persons were drawn from each village or community according to sample size and number of selected villages or communities.

The inclusion criteria were as follows: participants born between 1 January 1966 and 31 September 1997; continuous residence at the study site for at least the past 6 months; consent to provide urine specimens for testing; and willing to participate in the study and complete the questionnaires. The exclusion criteria were as follows: individuals denying sexual debut (including oral sex); and inability to provide correct information, such as individuals with a mental illness or alcohol abusers.

This study was approved by the Ethics Committee of Shandong Provincial Institute of Dermatology and Venereology (approval number: 2016–04). Oral informed consent was obtained from each participant by interviewers before interview.

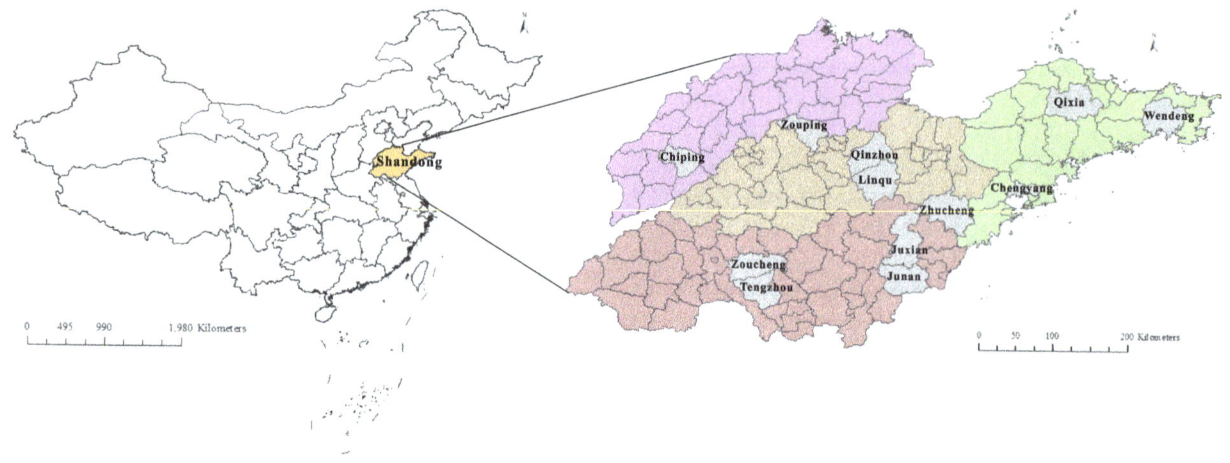

Fig. 1 Geographic locations of Shandong Province and 12 primary sampling units

Procedures

Before implementation of this survey, 3 days of training on fieldwork staff was provided by epidemiology and clinical laboratory professionals in each of the PSUs. One laboratory technician for urine collection and coding, one male and one female questionnaire interviewers, and one financial staff for providing rewards to participants were selected on the basis of course performance for each field team. A trained supervisor from the study group was also assigned to each field team for ethics and quality control of the interview.

Before sampling, individuals who continuously lived in their current residences for at least the past 6 months were identified by village/community committee staff or physicians by 3 steps. First, they referred to the official registers of household or health record of local residents for eligible individuals. Second, they inquired and recorded unregistered migrants who had lived in the local village/community for 6 months or more. Third, these two groups of people were combined in a roster for sampling. The sampled participants were informed to be interviewed in the village/community clinic or meeting room in private. For individuals who could not be reached via telephone, staff or physicians would visit them in their home. Individuals who could not be reached after repeated visits were excluded from the study. To retain privacy, questionnaire interviews were performed in a private room, and interviewers were the same gender as the respondent. Most of the selected respondents worked during the daytime, so the interviews were usually performed early in the morning or in the evening. Computer-based interviews were not performed because the pilot investigation showed that many participants could not use the computer to navigate the questionnaire, especially in villages. We adopted questionnaire-based interviews to collect information. Face-to-face interviews addressed demographic information, including gender, age, marital status (unmarried, married, divorced, or widowed), educational level (elementary school or below, middle school, senior high school or technical school, and university or above), and location of residence (rural or urban). Other information on the questionnaires was completed by the respondents themselves. The structured questionnaires included information regarding occupation, income, living status (living with family, living with roommates, or living alone), living with a spouse (yes or no), smoking (a smoker was defined as someone who had smoked > 100 cigarettes during their lifetime), number of episodes of intoxication in the past year (0, 1–3, 4–6, and > 6), STIs (including syphilis, gonorrhea, CT infection, condyloma acuminatum, genital herpes, and HIV infection) in the past 5 years (yes or no), quality of sex life (satisfied or not satisfied), sexual behaviors, such as age at first intercourse (≤ 20 years and > 20 years), number of sex partners (1 and ≥ 2), and number of new sex partners in the past year ($\leq$ 1 and ≥ 2). After the interview, the supervisor checked the questionnaires for missing values and logical errors and wrote a unique alphanumeric code on the questionnaires instead of the individual's name.

Every respondent was instructed not to urinate for at least 1 h before they participated in the interview. Approximately 30–50 ml of first-void urine was collected into a urine cup. Laboratory technicians promptly transferred the urine into Cobas PCR Media tubes (Roche Molecular Systems, Inc., Branchburg, New Jersey, USA) using a disposable pipette and the tube was inverted 5 times to mix. Each specimen was labeled with a unique alphanumeric code, which was the same as on the questionnaire. Urine was transported inside a Styrofoam cooler to the local laboratory within 3 h of collection and was stored 4 °C as soon as the staff received the specimen. Urine was transported inside the cooler to the laboratory of Shandong Provincial Institute of Dermatology and Venereology in Jinan within 2 weeks.

Chlamydia trachomatis and *Neisseria gonorrhoeae* (NG) DNA in urine specimens were detected with a Roche Cobas 4800 CT/NG Assay (Roche Molecular Systems, Inc.), which had a sensitivity of 96.6% and a specificity of 100% [16]. Only participants with positive results were notified, then referred to a local STI clinic or general hospital for treatment.

Statistical analysis

Questionnaire information, as well as testing results, was double-entered into Epidata 3.1 (EpiData association, Odense, Denmark); discrepancies were checked against raw data. We applied selection probability weights which were inversely proportional to the selection probabilities for the number of units at each sampling step to balance differences in the probabilities of selection. Non-response weighting was made by adjustment among those who participated in this survey with those who did not. Post-stratification weighting was made by adjusting data according to age and gender distribution of the Shandong census data. We analyzed data with *surveyfreq* and *surveylogistic* methods using SAS 9.3 (SAS Institute, Inc., Cary, NC, USA). The prevalence with 95% confidence interval (CI) of CT and NG was calculated based on total population weights and Taylor series linearization. We determined the association between CT infection and demographic and behavioral variables with logistic regression and reported crude odds ratio (ORs) in univariate analysis. Risk factors with a p value < 0.20 in univariate analysis were applied into the multivariate logistic model. Adjusted ORs and 95% CIs are presented. The variance inflation factor (VIF), condition index, and variance proportions were calculated to examine multicollinearity among risk factors. Maximal variance inflation factor values ≥ 10 or maximal condition index values ≥ 10 and a corresponding variance proportion value > 0.5 indicated multicollinearity among variables. All tests were two-sided, and a p value < 0.05 was considered statistically significant.

Proportion of symptomatic and treatment, incidences of various complications after CT infection were on the basis of our primary data as well as previous published studies [17, 18] (Figs. 2 and 3, Additional file 2). Medical costs for CT infections were based on diagnosis and treatment of the infection and complications; costs related to transportation, lodging, and time missed from work were not included into analysis. According to guidelines for STI treatment and control in China, we assumed that the diagnosis of CT infections was established with PCR testing and the treatment of CT infections involved a single 1 g dose of oral azithromycin [19]. Medical costs of cases with complications were estimated based on published research in Shandong Province [17]. The discounted rate of medical costs was assumed to be 3%. Sensitivity analysis was performed by adding uncertainty factors, such as the prevalence of CT infections, proportion of asymptomatic CT infections [20], and diagnostic method (antigen detection), into the computation.

Results

Of the 8074 individuals originally sampled, 184 could not be reached via telephone and were not at home on repeated visits. Among the 7890 individuals who were contacted, 231 declined to participate in this survey, 391 denied a sexual debut, and 5 had mental illnesses, leaving 7263 (90.0%) individuals who participated in the study and provided a urine sample. In addition, 60 urine samples were excluded due to mislabeling or insufficient urine, leaving 7203 (89.2%) satisfactory urine sample with test results for analysis (Fig. 4).

Prevalence of CT and NG infections

The weighted age-specific prevalence of CT and NG infections is shown in Table 1. Of the 7203 urine samples tested, 167 participants (90 females and 77 males) tested positive for CT. The estimated prevalence of CT in the

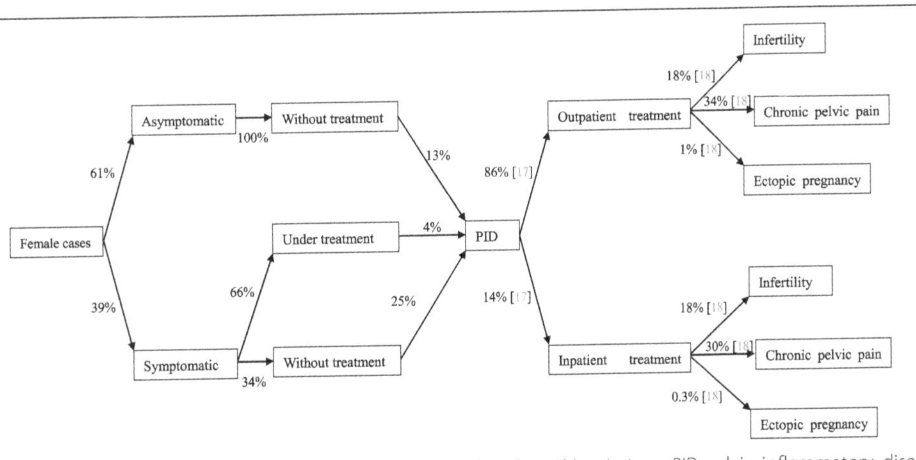

Fig. 2 The method of calculating the medical costs of CT infection for females. *Abbreviations: PID* pelvic inflammatory disease, *CT* *Chlamydia trachomatis*

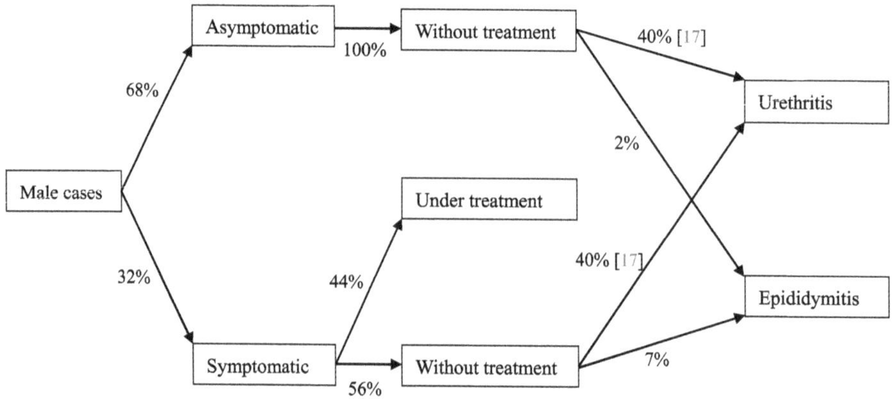

Fig. 3 The method of calculating the medical costs of CT infection for males. *Abbreviations: CT Chlamydia trachomatis*

general population, 18–49 years of age, in 2016 was 2.3% (95% CI, 1.5–3.2) for females and 2.7% (95% CI, 1.6–3.8) for males, corresponding to approximately 1,263,000 infections (95% CI, 774,000-1,753,000) in Shandong. No significant difference in the prevalence of CT infections existed between females and males ($p = 0.52$). The highest prevalence of CT infections occurred in females 30–34 years of age (3.5%; 95% CI, 2.6–4.4), followed by females 18–24 (3.2%; 95% CI, 0.4–6.1) and 25–29 years of age (2.9%; 95% CI, 1.9–3.8). The prevalence of CT infections in females 18–34 years of age (3.2%; 95% CI, 1.8–4.6) was significantly higher than females 35–49 years of age (1.5%; 95% CI, 0.8–2.2 [OR, 2.16; 95% CI, 1.14–4.08]); however, the highest prevalence of CT infections

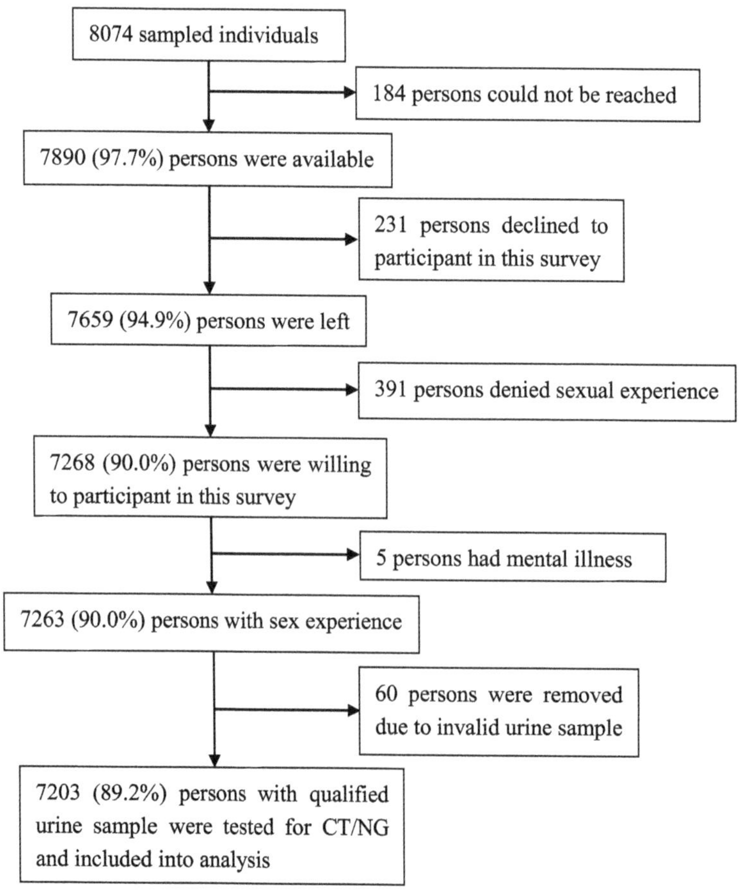

Fig. 4 Flow chart for participant selection. *Abbreviations: CT Chlamydia trachomatis, NG neisseria gonorrhoeae*

Table 1 The weighted prevalence of CT and NG in participants 18–49 years of age in Shandong, China

	Male [n, %(95%CI)]		Female [n, %(95%CI)]		Denominator[a] (unweighted, weighted[b])	
	CT	NG	CT	NG	Male	Female
Age(years)						
18–24	11, 4.3% (0.0–8.8)	0, 0.0%	7, 3.2% (0.4–6.1)	1, 0.2% (0.0–0.6)	253, 851	194, 825
25–29	18, 2.3% (0.5–4.1)	0, 0.0%	24, 2.9% (1.9–3.8)	0, 0.0%	780, 496	914, 499
30–34	13, 2.8% (1.3–4.2)	0, 0.0%	20, 3.5% (2.6–4.4)	1, 0.1% (0.0–0.2)	500, 469	555, 461
35–39	13, 2.7% (1.1–4.2)	0, 0.0%	8, 1.4% (0.4–2.4)	1, 0.1% (0.0–0.3)	557, 567	588, 559
40–44	15, 2.4% (1.3–3.5)	0, 0.0%	14, 1.5% (0.4–2.6)	1, 0.1% (0.0–0.4)	713, 667	735, 659
45–49	7, 0.8% (0.2–1.3)	1, 0.2% (0.0–0.5)	17, 1.6% (0.9–2.4)	1, 0.1% (0.0–0.3)	692, 572	722, 578
Region						
Northwest	4, 3.0% (0.0–7.7)	0, 0.0%	7, 1.6% (0.6–2.5)	0, 0.0%	338, 390	348, 356
Middle	28, 3.0% (1.1–4.9)	0, 0.0%	17, 2.0% (0.0–4.6)	0, 0.0%	895, 941	907, 851
South	29, 2.7% (1.7–3.8)	1, 0.1% (0.0–0.2)	46, 3.0% (2.2–3.9)	2, 0.1% (0.0–0.5)	1489, 1456	1567, 1479
East	16, 2.0% (1.3–2.7)	0, 0.0%	20, 1.8% (1.1–2.5)	3, 0.2% (0.0–0.5)	773, 835	886, 895
Total	77, 2.7% (1.6–3.8)	1, 0.03% (0.0–0.1)	90, 2.3% (1.5–3.2)	5, 0.1% (0.0–0.3)	3495, 3622	3708, 3581

Abbreviations: CI confidence interval, *CT* chlamydia trachomatis, *NG* neisseria gonorrhoeae
[a]Denominator was participants with sex experience and a urine test result
[b]Selection probability weighting, non-response weighting, and post-stratification weighting were applied to calculate the weighted denominator

occurred in males 18–24 years of age (4.3%; 95% CI, 0.0–8.8). For females, the highest prevalence was in those from South region (3.0%, 95%CI, 2.2–3.9) of Shandong. By contrast, for males, the highest prevalence was in those from Northwest (3.0%, 95%CI, 0.0–7.7) and Middle region (3.0%, 95%CI, 1.1–4.9) of Shandong. The prevalence of CT infections for urban and rural residents was 2.8% (95% CI, 1.5–4.0) and 2.2% (95% CI, 1.4–2.9), respectively, but the difference was not statistically significant ($p = 0.42$).

Of the 7203 urine samples tested, 6 participants (5 females and 1 male) tested positive for gonorrhoea. The estimated prevalence of gonorrhoea in the target population in 2016 was 0.1% (95% CI, 0.0–0.3) for females and 0.03% (95% CI, 0.0–0.1) for males, but the difference was not significant between female and male residents ($p = 0.25$). The estimated number of NG infections in Shandong corresponded to approximately 35,000 cases (95% CI, 0–83,000). The prevalence of NG infections among urban residents (0.10%; 95% CI, 0.0–0.2) was significantly higher than rural residents (0.03%; 95% CI, 0.0–0.1 [OR, 3.58; 95% CI, 1.08–11.83]). Because of the limited number of NG-positive cases, the following analysis focused on CT infections.

Risk factors for CT infections

Based on univariate analyses, risk variables associated with CT infections for both males and females 18–49 years of age included being unmarried/divorced/widowed, first sexual intercourse before 20 years of age, and having ≥2 sex partners. For females, an increased prevalence of CT infections was also associated with a higher level of education. For males, an increased prevalence of CT infections was associated with living alone, living separated from their spouse, and having been infected with a STI in the past 5 years, while a decreased prevalence of CT infections was associated with increasing age (Table 2).

In the multivariate logistic model, factors remaining significantly associated with CT infection for women were being unmarried/divorced/widowed (OR, 3.57; 95% CI, 1.54–8.24) and having ≥2 sex partners (OR, 3.72; 95% CI, 1.14–12.16). A higher level of education was marginally associated with CT infections in females. In males, first sexual intercourse before 20 years of age (OR, 1.83; 95% CI, 1.10–3.02) and having ≥2 sex partners (OR, 1.85; 95% CI, 1.14–3.02) remained significantly associated with CT infections (Table 2).

In the collinearity diagnosis, the maximal VIF was 1.17 and the maximal condition index was 1.55 for the female regression model, while the maximal VIF was 1.29 and the maximal condition index was 1.87 for the male regression model, which indicated no multicollinearity in the multivariate logistic analysis.

Medical costs for CT infections

Based on calculated costs for treatment of CT complications in 2016 (Additional file 2), we estimated that the lifetime total costs for CT infections for patients 18–49 years of age in Shandong Province was 273 million Renminbi (RMB), which corresponds to 348 RMB for each CT infection in females and 102 RMB for each CT infection in males.

Table 2 Risk factors for CT in urine specimens from participants 18–49 years of age in Shandong, China

	Male				Female				Denominator[c] unweighted, weighted	
	% (95% CI)	Crude OR	Adjusted OR[a]	95% CI	% (95% CI)	Crude OR	Adjusted OR[b]	95% CI	Male	Female
All ages	2.7% (1.6–3.8)				2.3% (1.5–3.2)				3495, 3622	3708, 3581
Age(years)		$P = 0.02$	$P = 0.48$			$P = 0.08$	$P = 0.57$			
18–24	4.3% (0.0–8.8)	1.00	1.00	1.00–1.00	3.2% (0.4–6.1)	1.00	1.00	1.00–1.00	253, 851	194, 825
25–29	2.3% (0.5–4.1)	0.52	0.91	0.24–3.48	2.9% (1.9–3.8)	0.88	2.23	0.72–6.86	780, 496	914, 499
30–34	2.8% (1.3–4.2)	0.63	1.40	0.37–5.35	3.5% (2.6–4.4)	1.08	3.74	1.09–12.83	500, 469	555, 461
35–39	2.7% (1.1–4.2)	0.61	1.40	0.37–5.21	1.4% (0.4–2.4)	0.42	1.54	0.58–4.06	557, 567	588, 559
40–44	2.4% (1.3–3.5)	0.54	1.32	0.54–3.24	1.5% (0.4–2.6)	0.46	1.48	0.45–4.86	713, 667	735, 659
45–49	0.8% (0.2–1.3)	0.17	0.40	0.15–1.03	1.6% (0.9–2.4)	0.50	1.81	0.60–5.45	692, 572	722, 578
Education		$P = 0.70$				$P = 0.02$	$P = 0.07$			
Elementary school, or below	3.2% (0.0–8.3)	1.00	–	–	1.6% (1.1–2.2)	1.00	1.00	1.00–1.00	367, 330	806, 697
Middle school	2.5% (1.4–3.5)	0.75	–	–	1.8% (1.2–2.3)	1.08	1.04	0.69–1.55	1906, 1830	1935, 1788
Senior high school or technical school	3.3% (1.6–5.0)	1.02	–	–	3.1% (0.8–5.3)	1.90	1.52	0.80–2.92	920, 1040	669, 752
College, university, or above	1.4% (0.0–3.1)	0.44	–	–	5.2% (0.0–10.6)	3.32	2.11	0.93–4.81	302, 422	298, 344
Marital status		$P = 0.01$	$P = 0.45$			$P < 0.01$	$P < 0.01$			
Married	2.1% (1.5–2.8)	1.00	1.00	1.00–1.00	1.8% (1.2–2.4)	1.00	1.00	1.00–1.00	3164, 3043	3528, 3253
Unmarried, divorced or widowed	5.4% (0.9–9.9)	2.61	1.45	0.55–3.84	7.8% (1.4–14.3)	4.65	3.64	1.63–8.13	331, 579	180, 328
Location of residence		$P = 0.80$				$P = 0.22$				
urban	2.8% (1.1–4.5)	1.00	–	–	2.8% (1.0–4.5)	1.00	–	–	1708, 2063	1824, 2040
rural	2.5% (1.2–3.9)	0.91	–	–	1.8% (1.3–2.2)	0.64	–	–	1787, 1559	1884, 3581
Living status		$P = 0.01$	$P = 0.17$			$P = 0.75$				
living with family	2.3% (1.5–3.1)	1.00	1.00	1.00–1.00	2.3% (1.4–3.2)	1.00	–	–	3279, 3327	3538, 3320
living with roommates	6.5% (0.0–17.8)	2.99	2.20	0.53–9.19	2.9% (0.0–9.3)	1.29	–	–	69, 99	54, 108
living alone	7.3% (0.0–16.4)	3.38	1.77	0.50–6.22	2.8% (0.0–6.0)	1.21	–	–	147, 196	116, 153
Living with spouse[d]		$P = 0.01$				$P = 0.92$				
Yes	1.9% (1.5–2.3)	1.00	–	–	1.8% (1.1–2.5)	1.00	–	–	3080, 3149	3309, 3213
No	10.4% (0.0–24.6)	5.93	–	–	1.9% (0.3–3.5)	1.06	–	–	84, 86	219, 244

Table 2 Risk factors for CT in urine specimens from participants 18–49 years of age in Shandong, China *(Continued)*

	Male				Female				Denominator[c] unweighted, weighted	
	% (95% CI)	Crude OR	Adjusted OR[a]	95% CI	% (95% CI)	Crude OR	Adjusted OR[b]	95% CI	Male	Female
Smoking		$P = 0.18$	$P = 0.42$			$P = 0.31$				
No	2.1% (0.9–3.3)	1.00	1.00	1.00–1.00	2.3% (1.5–3.1)	1.00	–	–	1747, 1785	3309, 3527
Yes	3.2% (1.5–4.9)	1.58	1.36	0.65–2.86	5.9% (0.0–16.5)	2.68	–	–	1748, 1837	70, 54
STI in the past 5 years[e]		$P = 0.01$	$P = 0.08$			$P = 0.19$	$P = 0.13$			
No	2.5% (1.4–3.6)	1.00	1.00	1.00–1.00	2.3% (1.5–3.1)	1.00	1.00	1.00–1.00	3467, 3595	3697, 3572
Yes	21.1% (0.0–54.8)	10.3	7.65	0.79–73.84	9.0% (0.0–28.4)	4.15	6.21	0.58–66.18	19, 27	11, 9
Age at first intercourse (years)		$P = 0.01$	$P = 0.03$			$P < 0.01$	$P = 0.24$			
>20	1.8% (1.4–2.3)	1.00	1.00	1.00–1.00	1.9% (1.2–2.6)	1.00	1.00	1.00–1.00	2698, 2549	3308, 3000
≤ 20	4.6% (1.0–8.2)	2.58	1.76	1.05–2.94	4.7% (2.5–7.0)	2.59	1.94	0.64–5.90	797, 1073	400, 581
Number of sex partners		$P < 0.01$	$P = 0.02$			$P < 0.01$	$P = 0.04$			
1	2.1% (1.5–2.8)	1.00	1.00	1.00–1.00	2.0% (1.2–2.7)	1.00	1.00	1.00–1.00	3086, 3107	3597, 3441
≥ 2	6.0% (1.5–10.4)	2.92	2.09	1.10–3.94	11.5% (0.0–23.3)	6.47	3.66	1.07–12.48	409, 515	111, 140
Number of new sex partners in the past year		$P = 0.14$	$P = 0.40$			$P = 0.44$				
≤ 1	2.5% (1.4–3.7)	1.00	1.00	1.00–1.00	2.3% (1.5–3.1)	1.00	–	–	3375, 3459	3678, 3549
≥ 2	5.2% (0.5–9.8)	2.08	0.56	0.15–2.16	5.0% (0.0–12.0)	2.21	–	–	120, 163	30, 32

Abbreviations: *CT* Chlamydia trachomatis, *CI* confidence interval, *OR* odds ratio, *AOR* adjusted odds ratio, *STI* sexually transmitted infection
[a]Adjusted for age, marital status, living status, smoking, STI in the past 5 years, age at first intercourse, number of sex partners, number of new sex partners in the past year and smoking
[b]Adjusted for age, education, marital status, STI in the past 5 years, age at first intercourse and number of sex partners
[c]Denominator was participants with sex experience and a urine test result
[d]This variable included those who have been married
[e]STIs included syphilis, gonorrhea, chlamydia trachomatis infection, condyloma acuminatum, genital herpes, and HIV infection

In sensitivity analysis, the estimated range for the total lifetime costs of CT infections in patients 18–49 years of age in Shandong was 172–374 million RMB in 2016. The estimated range of medical costs for each female and male patient was 339–361 RMB and 97–108 RMB, respectively. (Additional file 2).

Discussion

This is the first representative population-based cross-sectional study with a large sample size to determine the epidemiology of CT infections in mainland China since 1999–2000. In addition, the medical costs of CT infections and associated complications were estimated for the first time in China. Compared with the only national population-based STI prevalence study conducted in China (1999–2000), which reported a CT prevalence of 0.6% for females and 1.1% for males 20–24 years of age in China, the results from this study showed that the prevalence of CT infections has now increased 5-fold for females and 3-fold for males in this age group [6]. This change appears to be influenced by increased premarital and extramarital sexual activity in China, especially among youth [21]. According to a study conducted in 1999, approximately 15% of male and 9% of female university students had participated in premarital sexual activity [22]; however, another study concluded that 26% of college students had sexual intercourse in 2010 [21]. The rate of premarital sexual activity was even higher among out of school/community young adults than among those in school [23].

We compared our study with other population-based cross-sectional surveys that have used a complex sampling design and urine tests of infection. In 2014–2016, Wong

WC et al. performed a survey of 733 sexually experienced individuals in Hong Kong, China [24]. Among females 18–49 years of age, prevalence of CT infections was 2.0% (95% CI, 1.0–3.7) in Hong Kong compared with 2.3% (95% CI, 1.5–3.2) in Shandong Province. Among males 18–49 years of age, the prevalence was 1.5% (95% CI, 0.6–3.6) in Hong Kong compared with 2.7% (95% CI, 1.6–3.8) in Shandong. No significant difference of CT prevalence was found between these two studies due to overlap of 95% CI. The third cycle of the National Surveys of Sexual Attitudes and Lifestyles (Natsal-3), which was conducted in the UK in 2010–2012, indicated that the prevalence of CT infections was 1.5% (95% CI, 1.1–2.0) and 1.1% (95% CI, 0.7–1.6) for females and males 16–44 years of age, respectively [4]. In this study, prevalence of CT among males 18–44 years of age (3.0%, 95% CI, 1.8–4.3) was nearly 2 times higher than that in the UK, while difference of CT prevalence for females 18–44 years of age (2.5%, 95% CI, 1.5–3.4) was not significantly. Data from the 2011–2012 American National Health and Nutrition Examination Survey (NHANES) showed that the prevalence of CT infections among females and males 14–39 years of age was 2.0% (95% CI, 1.5–2.5) and 1.4% (95% CI, 1.1–1.8), respectively [25]. The difference of CT prevalence between males 18–39 years of age (3.2%, 95% CI, 1.8–4.6) in our study and that in the United States was marginally significant, while prevalence of CT for females 18–39 years of age (2.8%, 95% CI, 1.6–3.9) was as high as that in the US. Therefore, males in Shandong Province may suffer a higher burden of CT infection than that in the UK and US.

Our study also indicated that CT infections were more prevalent among females < 35 years of age and males < 25 years of age. Thus, these young adults need to be prioritized when implementing a CT infection control program. A previous study showed that screening for CT infections is cost-effective when the prevalence of CT infections among the female population ranged from 3.1 to 10.0% [26]. This finding indicated that the female population < 35 years of age in Shandong should be screened regularly for CT infections; however, the effectiveness of CT screening to control transmission and prevent complications of CT infection is controversial. In the UK, The National Chlamydia Screening Programme (NCSP), implemented in September 2002, offers opportunistic screening for CT infections among males and females < 25 years of age [15]; however, according to the Natsal-2 (conducted in 1999–2000) compared with Natsal-3, the prevalence of CT infections in young people 18–24 years of age was similar in females (3.1% vs. 3.2%), and males (2.9% vs. 2.6%) [4]. In 2001, the United States Preventive Services Task Force (USPSTF) recommended that clinicians routinely screen all sexually-active females ≤25 years of age, and other asymptomatic females at increased risk for CT infections [27]; however, NHANES reported a similar prevalence of CT infections in the 1999–2000 (4.1%) and 2007–2008 cycles (3.8%) among females 14–25 years of age [28]. In addition, randomized controlled trials (RCTs) also revealed contradictory evidence on the effectiveness of a CT infection screening strategy [29, 30]. The low screening efficacy on reducing the prevalence of CT infections and associated complications may be due to several factors. First, the uptake rate of CT screening is quite low in most countries that conduct screening programs. In 2017, an estimated 28% of young females and 11% of young males were tested for CT infections in England [31]. In the US, the estimated annual CT testing rate for sexually-active females 15–25 years of age was 37.9% [32]. Second, annual screening may not be frequent enough to prevent complications of CT infections. A RCT from the UK indicated that PID over 12 months was not prevented by a single CT screen and occurred in women who were negative for CT at baseline [30]. Thus, it is critical to answer questions, such as how to increase screening coverage and how often to screen through RCT or other type of studies before performing universal CT screening in Shandong, China. In our study, women 30–34 years of age had the highest prevalence of CT infections, while the highest prevalence of CT infections in males was in those 18–24 years of age. The age differentials of CT prevalence may be associated with variation of sexual desire. For males, sexual desire significantly increased after puberty and reached its peak at about 18–30 years of age [33]. For females, the sexual desire reached its peak at around 30–40 years of age [33]. Strong desire usually accompanied with frequent sexual activity, which may contribute to the high prevalence of STIs, including CT infections.

A multivariate analysis indicated that younger age at the time of first sexual intercourse is associated with a higher risk of CT infections in men. Another study showed the same conclusion among adolescents and young adults [34]. Early initiation of sexual intercourse was shown to be associated with multiple partners, more casual or commercial sex partners, and infrequent use of condoms, resulting in a higher prevalence of STIs [35]. Therefore, sex education strategies should focus on an earlier age, advice on delaying the age of first sexual intercourse, and address other issues, such as reducing the number of partners and promoting condom use [35]. The prevalence of CT infections among unmarried, divorced, or widowed females 18–49 years of age was 7.8%, which was 4 times the prevalence among married counterparts (1.8%) in this study. Data from the NHANES in 2007–2012 showed that the risk of CT infection among divorced/widowed individuals was 3 times higher than married persons [25]. Marital status is therefore a useful marker for identifying those at increased risk for a CT infection. Compared with the national CT study in 1999–2000, the difference in prevalence of CT infections among urban and rural residents is not statistically significant, which may be due to increasing proportion of migrants among the general population in China [6, 36]. The prevalence of CT was much higher for migrants than the non-migrant population [37]. Frequently, the flow of a large number of migrants may decrease the difference in STIs between urban and rural populations.

The results of this study indicate that CT infections produce a substantial economic burden in Shandong Province. The total medical costs of CT infections in Shandong Province are mainly influenced by the variation in the prevalence of CT infections rather than different methods of detection. Thus, adequate public health financial support is required to support specific CT control strategies.

Our study had several limitations. First, individuals who left their original place of residence and had lived in their current residence for ≥6 months were not completely registered by the local government and it was difficult to select all of them for sampling; however, this unregistered population could engage in more risky behaviors leading to STIs [6], thus resulting in an underestimation of the prevalence of CT and NG in our study. Second, our estimate of economic burden of CT was partially based on previous surveys. The incidence of complications after CT infection in other populations may not precisely correspond with that in Shandong Province, China. Third, the conclusions of this study might not be applicable to all provinces in China. Fourth, the statistical power of this study might be insufficient to identify potential risk factors of CT infection that were poisson distributed among general population, such as men who have sex with men (MSM) or female sex worker (FSW).

Conclusions

In conclusion, the results indicate that the prevalence of CT infections in young adults has increased rapidly since 2000. *Chlamydia trachomatis* is highly prevalent among females < 35 years of age and males < 25 years of age. Thus, CT control programs should focus on this population, as well as other people with identified risk factors, to reduce the prevalence and economic burden of CT infections. Further studies evaluating the effectiveness of CT control interventions through RCTs or other types of study design in China are recommended.

Abbreviations

CI: Confidence interval; CT: Chlamydia trachomatis; FSW: Female sex worker; MSM: Men who have sex with men; Natsal: National surveys of sexual attitudes and lifestyles; NCSP: National chlamydia screening programme; NG: Neisseria gonorrhoeae; NHANES: National health and nutrition examination survey; OR: Odds ratio; PID: Pelvic inflammatory disease; PPS: Probability proportionate to size sampling; PSU: Primary sampling unit; RCT: Randomized controlled trial; RMB: Renminbi; STI: Sexually transmitted infection; USPSTF: United States preventive services task force; VIF: Variance inflation factor; WHO: World health organization

Acknowledgments

The authors thank the 12 implementation partners in our survey: Station of Dermatology and Venereology in Ju county, Junan county, Qingzhou county-level city, Liaocheng municipality, Tengzhou county-level city, Qixia county-level city, Zhucheng county-level city and Linqu county, Center for Disease Control and Prevention in Chengyang District and Zoucheng county-level city, Wendeng District Hospital for Skin Disease, Zouping County Hospital of Traditional Chinese Medicine. We thank International Science Editing and Beng Tin Goh from the Royal London Hospital for editing this manuscript. We thank all men and women who participated in this study.

Funding

This study was supported by the National Key Research and Development Program of China (2016YFE0201500),the Innovation Project of Shandong Academy of Medical Sciences and the Syphilis and Other Sexually Transmitted Diseases Control Research in Shandong. The funders had no roles in the design of the study, or the collection, analysis and interpretation of data, or writing the manuscript.

Authors' contributions

FZ conceived the study. FZ, AX, JL, DL, HL and PH contributed to the design of the study. PH, FL, ZL, LS, XF, ZC, TC, HW, BZ, CW, YS, GN, YZ, FF, XL, XW, HZ and DL performed the fieldwork and data collection. LS, XF, QP, GY, ZM and FB undertook the laboratory analysis of the samples. PH conducted statistical data analysis. PH drafted the manuscript with intellectual contributions from all other authors. FZ, AX, JL, DL and HL critically revised the manuscript. All authors interpreted the data, reviewed and approved the final manuscript.

Consent for publication

Not applicable.

Competing interests

The authors declare that they have no competing interests.

Author details

[1]Shandong Provincial Hospital for Skin Disease, Shandong University, Jinan, China. [2]Shandong Provincial Institute of Dermatology and Venereology, Shandong Academy of Medical Sciences, 27397 Jingshi Road, Jinan 250022, China. [3]Department of Epidemiology, School of Public Health, Shandong University, Jinan, China. [4]Shandong Provincial Key Laboratory for Dermatovenereology, Jinan, China. [5]Shandong Center for Disease Control and Prevention, Jinan, China.

References

1. Unemo M, Bradshaw CS, Hocking JS, De Vries H, Francis SC, Mabey D, et al. Sexually transmitted infections: challenges ahead. Lancet Infect Dis. 2017;17: e235–79.
2. World Health Organization. Report on global sexually transmitted infection surveillance 2015. Retrieved March 10, 2016 from [http://apps.who.int/iris/bitstream/10665/249553/1/9789241565301-eng.pdf?ua=1]. Accessed 10 Mar 2016.

3. Yang S, Wu J, Ding C, Cui Y, Zhou Y, Li Y, et al. Epidemiological features of and changes in incidence of infectious diseases in China in the first decade after the SARS outbreak: an observational trend study. Lancet Infect Dis. 2017;17:716–25.
4. Sonnenberg P, Clifton S, Beddows S, Field N, Soldan K, Tanton C, et al. Prevalence, risk factors, and uptake of interventions for sexually transmitted infections in Britain: findings from the National Surveys of sexual attitudes and lifestyles (Natsal). Lancet. 2013;382:1795–806.
5. Miller WC, Ford CA, Morris M, Handcock MS, Schmitz JL, Hobbs MM, et al. Prevalence of chlamydial and gonococcal infections among young adults in the United States. JAMA. 2004;91:2229–36.
6. Parish WL, Laumann EO, Cohen MS, Pan S, Zheng H, Hoffman I, et al. Population-based study of chlamydial infection in China: a hidden epidemic. JAMA. 2003;289:1265–73.
7. Franceschi S, Smith JS, van den Brule A, Herrero R, Arslan A, Anh PT, et al. Cervical infection with chlamydia trachomatis and Neisseria gonorrhoeae in women from ten areas in four continents. A cross-sectional study. Sex Transm Dis. 2007;34:563–9.
8. Zeng Y, Hesketh T. The effects of China's universal two-child policy. Lancet. 2016;388:1930–8.
9. Haggerty CL, Gottlieb SL, Taylor BD, Low N, Xu F, Ness RB. Risk of sequelae after chlamydia trachomatis genital infection in women. J Infect Dis. 2010; 201:S134–55.
10. Peterman TA, Newman DR, Maddox L, Schmitt K, Shiver S. Risk for HIV following a diagnosis of syphilis, gonorrhoea or chlamydia: 328,456 women in Florida, 2000-2011. Int J STD AIDS. 2015;26:113–9.
11. Workowski KA, Bolan GA. Sexually transmitted diseases treatment guidelines, 2015. MMWR Recomm Rep. 2015;64:1–137.
12. Goulet V, de Barbeyrac B, Raherison S, Prudhomme M, Semaille C, Warszawski J. Prevalence of chlamydia trachomatis: results from the first national population-based survey in France. Sex Transm Infect. 2010;86: 263–70.
13. Hocking JS, Willis J, Tabrizi S, Fairley CK, Garland SM, Hellard M. A chlamydia prevalence survey of young women living in Melbourne. Victoria Sex Health. 2006;3:235–40.
14. Australian Department of Health and Ageing. Second national sexually transmissible infections strategy 2010-2013. Retrieved March 10, 2016 from [http://www.health.gov.au/internet/main/publishing.nsf/Content/ohp-national-strategies-2010-sti]. Accessed 10 Mar 2016.
15. LaMontagne DS, Fenton KA, Randall S, Anderson S, Carter P. Establishing the National Chlamydia Screening Programme in England: results from the first full year of screening. Sex Transm Infect. 2004;80:335–41.
16. Parra-Sanchez M, Palomares JC, Bernal S, Gonzalez MT, Sivianes N, Perez L, et al. Evaluation of the cobas 4800 CT/NG test for detecting chlamydia trachomatis and Neisseria gonorrhoeae DNA in urogenital swabs and urine specimens. Diagn Microbiol Infect Dis. 2012;74:338–42.
17. Chen S, Li J, van den Hoek A. Universal screening or prophylactic treatment for chlamydia trachomatis infection among women seeking induced abortions: which strategy is more cost-effective? Sex Transm Dis. 2007;34:230–6.
18. Ness RB, Soper DE, Holley RL, Peipert J, Randall H, Sweet RL, et al. Effectiveness of inpatient and outpatient treatment strategies for women with pelvic inflammatory disease: results from the pelvic inflammatory disease evaluation and clinical health (PEACH) randomized trial. Am J Obstet Gynecol. 2002;186:929–37.
19. Wang QQ, Liu QZ, Xu JH. Guideline for sexually transmitted infection treatment and control in China. Shanghai: Shanghai Science and Technology Press; 2014. p. 108–9.
20. Tuite AR, Jayaraman GC, Allen VG, Fisman DN. Estimation of the burden of disease and costs of genital chlamydia trachomatis infection in Canada. Sex Transm Dis. 2012;39:260–7.
21. Xiao Z, Mehrotra P, Zimmerman R. Sexual revolution in China: implications for Chinese women and society. AIDS Care. 2011;23:105–12.
22. Zhang L, Gao X, Dong Z, Tan Y, Wu Z. Premarital sexual activities among students in a university in Beijing. China Sex Transm Dis. 2002;29:212–5.
23. Yu XM, Guo SJ, Sun YY. Sexual behaviours and associated risks in Chinese young people: a meta-analysis. Sex Health. 2013;10:424–33.
24. Wong WC, Zhao Y, Wong NS, Parish WL, Miu HY, Yang LG, et al. Prevalence and risk factors of chlamydia infection in Hong Kong: a population-based geospatial household survey and testing. PLoS One. 2017;12:e172561.
25. Torrone E, Papp J, Weinstock H. Prevalence of chlamydia trachomatis genital infection among persons aged 14-39 years--United States, 2007-2012. MMWR Morb Mortal Wkly Rep. 2014;63:834–8.
26. Honey E, Augood C, Templeton A, Russell I, Paavonen J, Mardh PA, et al. Cost effectiveness of screening for chlamydia trachomatis: a review of published studies. Sex Transm Infect. 2002;78:406–12.
27. The US. Preventive services task force. Screening for chlamydial infection: recommendations and rationale. Am J Prev Med. 2001;20:90–4.
28. Datta SD, Torrone E, Kruszon-Moran D, Berman S, Johnson R, Satterwhite CL, et al. Chlamydia trachomatis trends in the United States among persons 14 to 39 years of age, 1999-2008. Sex Transm Dis. 2012;39:92–6.
29. Scholes D, Stergachis A, Heidrich FE, Andrilla H, Holmes KK, Stamm WE. Prevention of pelvic inflammatory disease by screening for cervical chlamydial infection. N Engl J Med. 1996;34:1362–6.
30. Oakeshott P, Kerry S, Aghaizu A, Atherton H, Hay S, Taylor-Robinson D, et al. Randomised controlled trial of screening for chlamydia trachomatis to prevent pelvic inflammatory disease: the POPI (prevention of pelvic infection) trial. BMJ. 2010;c1642:340.
31. Public Health England. Sexually transmitted infections and screening for Chlamydia in England, 2017. Retrieved June 6, 2018 from [https://assets.publishing.service.gov.uk/government/uploads/system/uploads/attachment_data/file/713962/hpr2018_AA-STIs_v5.pdf]. Accessed 6 June 2018.
32. Tao G, Hoover KW, Leichliter JS, Peterman TA, Kent CK. Self-reported chlamydia testing rates of sexually active women aged 15-25 years in the United States, 2006-2008. Sex Transm Dis. 2012;39:605–7.
33. Shui M, Hu PC. Influence factors of sex desire for women in China [article in Chinese]. Chin J Fam Plan Obstet Gyneco. 2016;2:14–6,27.
34. Kaestle CE, Halpern CT, Miller WC, Ford CA. Young age at first sexual intercourse and sexually transmitted infections in adolescents and young adults. Am J Epidemiol. 2005;161:774–80.
35. Ma Q, Ono-Kihara M, Cong L, Xu G, Pan X, Zamani S, et al. Early initiation of sexual activity: a risk factor for sexually transmitted diseases, HIV infection, and unwanted pregnancy among university students in China. BMC Public Health. 2009;9:111.
36. National Bureau of Statistics of China. China statistical yearbook. Retrieved March 10, 2016 from [http://www.stats.gov.cn/tjsj/ndsj/2016/indexeh.htm]. Accessed 10 Mar 2016.
37. Wang W, Wei C, Buchholz ME, Martin MC, Smith BD, Huang ZJ, et al. Prevalence and risks for sexually transmitted infections among a national sample of migrants versus non-migrants in China. Int J STD AIDS. 2010;21:410–5.

A high burden of asymptomatic genital tract infections undermines the syndromic management approach among adolescents and young adults in South Africa: implications for HIV prevention efforts

Angela Kaida[1*], Janan J. Dietrich[2], Fatima Laher[2], Mags Beksinska[3], Manjeetha Jaggernath[3], Megan Bardsley[4], Patricia Smith[1], Laura Cotton[1], Pooja Chitneni[5], Kalysha Closson[1], David A. Lewis[6,7], Jenni A. Smit[3], Thumbi Ndung'u[8,9,10], Mark Brockman[1] and Glenda Gray[2,11]

Abstract

Background: Youth in southern Africa, particularly adolescent girls and young women, are a key population for HIV prevention interventions. Untreated genital tract infections (GTIs) increase both HIV transmission and acquisition risks. South African GTI treatment guidelines employ syndromic management, which relies on individuals to report GTI signs and symptoms. Syndromic management may, however, underestimate cases, particularly among youth. We compared genital tract infection (GTI) prevalence by symptom-based and laboratory assessment among sexually-experienced youth in South Africa, overall and stratified by sex.

Methods: Interviewer-administered surveys assessed socio-demographics, behaviors, and GTI symptoms among 352 youth (16-24 yrs., HIV-negative or unknown HIV status at enrollment) enrolled in community-based cohorts in Durban and Soweto (2014–2016). Laboratory tests assessed HIV, *Chlamydia trachomatis* (CT), *Neisseria gonorrhoeae* (NG), *Mycoplasma genitalium* (MG), *Trichomonas vaginalis* (TV) infections and, among females, bacterial vaginosis (BV) and Candida species. Youth with genital ulcers were tested for HSV-2 and syphilis. We assessed sensitivity (and specificity) of symptom-based reporting in identifying laboratory-confirmed GTIs.

Results: At baseline, 16.2% of females (32/198) and < 1% (1/154) of males reported ≥1 GTI symptom. However, laboratory tests identified ≥1 GTI in 70.2% and 10.4%, respectively. Female CT prevalence was 18.2%, NG 7.1%, MG 9.6%, TV 8.1%, and 5.1% were newly diagnosed with HIV. BV prevalence was 53.0% and candidiasis 9.6%. One female case of herpes was identified (0 syphilis). Male CT prevalence was 7.8%, NG 1.3%, MG 3.3%, TV < 1%, and 2.0% were newly diagnosed with HIV. Overall, 77.8% of females and 100% of males with laboratory-diagnosed GTIs reported no symptoms or were asymptomatic. Sensitivity (and specificity) of symptom-based reporting was 14% (97%) among females and 0% (99%) among males.

(Continued on next page)

* Correspondence: kangela@sfu.ca
Faculty of Health Sciences, Simon Fraser University, Blusson Hall Rm 10522, 8888 University Drive, Burnaby B.C. V5A 1S6, Canada
Full list of author information is available at the end of the article

(Continued from previous page)
Conclusion: A high prevalence of asymptomatic GTIs and very poor sensitivity of symptom-based reporting undermines the applicability of syndromic GTI management, thus compromising GTI control and HIV prevention efforts among youth. Syndromic GTI management does not meet the sexual health needs of young people. Policy changes incorporating innovations in GTI diagnostic testing are needed to reduce GTIs and HIV-associated risks among youth.

Keywords: Adolescents and young adults, Youth, Women, Sexually transmitted infections, Genital tract infections, HIV prevention, Screening, Syndromic management, Performance analysis, South Africa

Background

Adolescents and young adults (aged 15–24 years) account for one-third of incident adult HIV infections in South Africa. Girls and young women are particularly at risk, with nearly 2000 young women acquiring HIV every week [1, 2]. Accordingly, reducing HIV risk among youth remains a pressing global public health priority [3].

Untreated genital tract infections (GTIs) increase risk of HIV acquisition and transmission through several organism-specific pathways [4, 5]. Untreated HIV can also increase GTI severity and duration through immune suppression pathways. For women, untreated GTIs are a significant cause of reproductive morbidity, including pelvic inflammatory disease, tubal factor infertility, adverse birth outcomes, and infertility [6].

The success of GTI control programs is predicated on timely and effective diagnosis and treatment [7]. South African GTI treatment guidelines employ syndromic management [8], consistent with WHO recommendations [9]. Syndromic management is based on the identification of syndromes (i.e., consistent groups of symptoms and clinical signs) associated with infection by a defined pathogen, followed by syndromic treatment for the most common causative GTI organisms.

While syndromic GTI management can be used to treat and manage symptomatic GTIs at the primary healthcare level without the need for laboratory facilities or diagnostic tests, such an approach can underestimate GTI cases, particularly among women for whom an estimated 50–75% of those with a GTI are asymptomatic [10, 11]. Few studies from high HIV-burden settings have examined GTI prevalence or diagnostic performance of syndromic management among adolescents and young adults [11]. This is concerning given the dual burdens and synergies between HIV and GTIs among youth and the potential for long-term sequelae. There are also concerns about the ability of syndromic treatment to differentiate between the etiologies of the disease, leading to the potential for over-prescription of antibiotics and attendant risks of antimicrobial resistance [5].

This analysis measured and compared GTI prevalence by syndromic-based and laboratory assessment among sexually-experienced South African adolescents and young adults, stratified by sex. We assessed the performance of syndromic GTI management compared with the 'gold standard' of laboratory diagnosis (including measurement of sensitivity, specificity, positive predictive value [PPV], and negative predictive value [NPV]. In pursuing these objectives, we seek to inform GTI control programs for youth in the context of emerging biomedical HIV prevention efforts.

Methods

Study design and participants

We used baseline data from adolescents and young adults (females and males) enrolled in the AYAZAZI study, a youth-centered, dual-site, community-based, prospective cohort study focused on understanding linked patterns of socio-behavioural and biomedical HIV risk among youth in South Africa [12].

AYAZAZI study inclusion criteria included being 16–24 years of age, residing in Soweto or Durban, self-reporting an HIV-negative or unknown HIV status, and being willing and able to provide voluntary written informed consent. Exclusion criteria included current participation in another clinical or observational HIV prevention study. The Soweto cohort was based at the Perinatal HIV Research Unit (PHRU) located at Chris Hani Baragwanath Hospital. The Durban cohort was based at the Commercial City research site led by MatCH Research Unit (MRU).

We used posters, pamphlets, word-of-mouth, and in-person community outreach to recruit 425 participants (253 females, 172 males) across both sites. In Soweto, participants were also recruited through the PHRU's HIV testing and counselling clinic while in Durban, participants were also recruited through a public sector reproductive health clinic at Commercial City. Enrolment occurred between November 2014 and April 2015 in Soweto and between September 2015 and April 2016 in Durban.

Study procedures

Participants completed a structured questionnaire (supported by DataFAX™ software) at enrolment, administered in-person by youth interviewers. The questionnaire assessed demographic characteristics, social determinants of health, healthcare-seeking behaviours, sexual behaviors, pregnancy history, substance use, experiences of violence, and self-perceived HIV risk. Questionnaires were conducted in English, isiZulu, or Sesotho, as per participant preference. Participants received a 150 ZAR (~$12 USD) reimbursement per visit to compensate for transportation costs and time.

Presence of GTI symptoms was assessed via a nurse-administered questionnaire. All participants underwent a nurse-led physical examination (including genital examination for presence of a genital ulcer), consistent with standard treatment guidelines [8].

Urine (males) and nurse-collected vaginal swab (females) specimens were collected and transported daily to the National Institute for Communicable Diseases in Johannesburg (for the Soweto site) and the Global Clinical and Viral Laboratory (for the Durban site) for analysis. Using multiplex nucleic acid amplification test (NAAT) methods, all participants were tested for *Chlamydia trachomatis* (CT), *Neisseria gonorrhoeae* (NG), *Mycoplasma genitalium* (MG), and *Trichomonas vaginalis* (TV). All females were tested for the presence of bacterial vaginosis (BV) and *Candida* species (CA) using Gram-stain techniques. Vaginal microbiota specimens were evaluated using Nugent criteria, which differentiate between BV (scores 7–10), intermediate microbiota (scores 4–6), and normal microbiota (scores 0–3) [13]. Participants with active genital ulcers identified during physical exams were tested for herpes simplex virus type 2 (HSV-2), *Treponema pallidum*, *Haemophilus ducreyi* and *C.trachomatis serovar L1-L3* via multiplex PCR using the Roche LightCycler. AYAZAZI clinical staff offered counselling and treatment (either onsite or via referral to a local clinic) to participants immediately following a syndromic diagnosis or after receipt of positive GTI laboratory results. Recent data demonstrating increased inflammation and thus HIV acquisition risk among women with asymptomatic BV informed study procedures to include asymptomatic BV cases as requiring treatment, after confirmation using Nugent criteria [14].

For female participants, research nurses performed rapid pregnancy testing using the QuickVue One-Step HCG urine test (Quidel Corporation, San Diego, CA, USA). Vaginal swabs were deferred for a week for menstruating women, and deferred until pregnancy resolution.

All participants were tested for HIV using the Abon™ HIV 1/2/0 Tri-Line HIV RDT test (Abon Biopharm Co. Ltd., Hangzhou, China) with confirmatory testing using the First Response™ HIV-1-2.0 Rapid Whole Blood Test kit (Premier Medical Corporation Private Ltd., Gujarat, India). Those who tested negative on the first rapid test were considered HIV-negative and offered standard HIV prevention counselling. Individuals who tested positive using both the rapid HIV tests were considered HIV-positive, counselled, and referred to a local clinic for further assessment, including CD4 testing, and counselling on initiation of antiretroviral therapy (ART). CD4 T cells were enumerated from whole blood using Tru-Count technology and analysed on a FACSCalibur flow cytometer (Becton Dickinson). If one rapid test was positive and the other negative, offsite confirmation was conducted using 3rd generation (i.e., antibody only) ELISA tests (MICROLISA HIV test, J.Mitra & Co. Ltd., New Delhi, India [Soweto]; Vironostika HIV Uni-Form II Plus O test, Biomerieux, Marcy L'Etoile, France [Durban]).

Measures

We measured the prevalence and types of nine self-reported GTI symptoms (for both female and male participants) and associated seven syndromes, stratified by sex [8, 9] (Additional file 1: Table S1).

We measured the prevalence of laboratory-confirmed GTIs, stratified by sex. Ulcerative STIs were analysed separately from non-ulcerative STIs, as only the etiological distribution of ulcerative STIs could be reported as opposed to prevalence. We measured the prevalence of (a) each GTI screened, (b) ≥1 GTI, (c) co-infection with ≥2 non-ulcerative STIs, (d) co-infection with ≥1 non-ulcerative STI and BV, and (e) newly-diagnosed HIV.

Statistical analysis

Of 425 participants enrolled in AYAZAZI, this GTI analysis was restricted to sexually-experienced (excluded $n = 64$) and non-pregnant (excluded $n = 9$) youth, yielding a final analytic sample of 352 (82.4% of the total cohort).

Descriptive statistics (median [IQR] for continuous variables and n [%] for categorical variables) were used to characterize baseline distributions of study variables, stratified by natal sex (female or male). Baseline differences between females and males were compared using Wilcoxon rank sum test for continuous variables and Pearson χ^2 or Fisher's exact test for categorical variables. Descriptive statistics were used to characterize (1) distribution of GTI symptoms and syndromes by sex and by study site; and (2) distribution of laboratory-confirmed infections by sex and study site.

For sensitivity, specificity, PPV, and NPV calculations [15], the gold-standard was a positive laboratory test result for any aetiological agent of the syndrome, defined as follows [8, 9]: Vaginal Discharge Syndrome (VDS): NG, CT, MG (cervical infections), or TV, BV, or CA (vaginal infections); Lower Abdominal Pain (LAP): NG, CT, or, MG; Male Urethritis Syndrome (MUS): NG, CT, MG, or TV; and Scrotal Swelling (SSW): NG or CT.

Sensitivity analysis of VDS was stratified by cervical, vaginal, and BV as the causative agent to compare performance statistics for each infection type and considering that the high BV prevalence could augment performance statistics relative to other VDS-associated organisms. Performance analysis of Genital Ulcer Disease (GUD) was not possible as only those with genital ulcers (n = 3) were tested for ulcerative-STIs. Data were analyzed with SAS version 9.1.

All participants aged 18–24 years provided voluntary informed consent at enrollment. For participants aged 16–17 years, parents/legal guardians provided voluntary written informed consent and the participant provided voluntary written informed assent. Ethical approval was provided by the Research Ethics Boards of Simon Fraser University (Canada), the University of the Witwatersrand (South Africa), and the University of KwaZulu-Natal (South Africa).

Results

Participant characteristics

Of 352 youth included in this analysis, 56% were female, 17.1% were less than 18 years old, 6.8% identified as LGBTQ (lesbian, gay, bisexual, transgender, and queer), 66.1% were currently in school and 25.9% reported high food insecurity. All participants identified as cis gender. Over one-quarter reported living in informal housing (27.6%) or having a personal monthly income < 400 ZAR (~$30 USD) (26.4%), with significant differences by sex ($p < 0.05$).

We also observed several differences in sexual and reproductive experiences by sex. While 55.6% of youth self-perceived as having no or low risk of HIV, 20.7% of females and 45.5% of males reported ≥2 sexual partners in the past 6 months ($p < 0.001$), and 80.6% of females and 51.3% of males reported inconsistent condom use ($p < 0.001$). A higher proportion of males than females reported ever having engaged (i.e., provided or received) in transactional sex (22.9% and 7.2%; respectively), while a higher proportion of females than males reported an age-disparate sex partner (i.e., ≥ 5 years older or younger) (34.9% and 12.4%; respectively) (Table 1).

GTI symptoms and associated syndromes

Among females, 16.2% (32/198) reported ≥1 GTI symptom. The most commonly reported symptoms were vaginal discharge (7.1%) and vaginal itching or irritation (4.5%). By syndrome, 10.6% of females reported symptoms of VDS, 6.6% of LAP, and 2.0% of GUD. Among males, 0.7% (1/154) reported symptoms compatible with MUS (urethral discharge); no other STI syndromes were described in males (Table 2).

Laboratory-confirmed prevalence of GTIs

Laboratory tests identified ≥1 GTI in 44.0% of study participants, including 70.2% of females and 10.4% of males ($p < 0.001$) (Table 3).

Among female participants, over one-third (34.8%; n = 69/198) were infected with at least one non-ulcerative STI, including 18.2% with CT, 7.1% with NG, 9.6% with MG, and 8.1% with TV. Of those infected with ≥1 one non-ulcerative STI (n = 69), one-fifth (20.3%; n = 14) were co-infected with other STI pathogens while nearly three-quarters (72.5%; n = 50) were co-infected with a GTI. By site, the prevalence of non-ulcerative STIs was higher among females in Soweto compared with Durban (44.1% and 25.0% respectively, $p = 0.008$). Of two young women with genital ulcers, one case of herpes was confirmed and there were no cases of laboratory-proven syphilis. Just over half (53.0%) of all females tested positive for BV, with a further 11 females having intermediate flora (5.6%). Prevalence of CA was 9.6%. One-quarter (25.3%) of females were co-infected with a non-ulcerative STI and BV or CA. Ten female participants (5.1%) were newly diagnosed with HIV (median CD4 = 301 cells/mm^3 [IQR: 197–392], with a significantly higher baseline HIV prevalence in Durban than Soweto (9.4% and 1.0%, respectively; $p = 0.008$). Overall, 90.0% (9/10) of HIV-positive females were co-infected with BV, while none had an STI.

Among male participants, one-tenth (10.4%; n = 16/154) were infected with at least one non-ulcerative STI, including 7.8% with CT, 1.3% with NG, 3.3% with MG, and 0.7% with TV. Of those infected with an MUS-associated STI, one-quarter (25.0%) were co-infected. No STI pathogen was detected in the single male participant with genital ulcers. Three male participants (2.0%) were newly diagnosed with HIV (median CD4 = 102 cells/mm^3 IQR: 85–119), with a non-statistically significant higher HIV prevalence in Durban compared to Soweto (2.4% and 1.4%, respectively, $p = 1.00$). No HIV-positive males were co-infected with an STI.

Sensitivity analysis

Overall, only 22.2% of females and 0% of males with a confirmed GTI reported at least one GTI symptom. In other words, 77.8% of females and 100% of males with laboratory-diagnosed GTIs reported no accompanying symptoms or were asymptomatic (Table 4).

Females

Sensitivity analyses revealed that VDS symptomology poorly indicated infection with associated pathological organisms (i.e., NG, CT, MG, TV, BV, or CA). Overall, 19/21 reporting VDS symptoms were infected with a VDS-associated GTI; however, of 139 females with laboratory-confirmed infections with a VDS-associated GTI, just 19 reported symptoms (sensitivity 13.7%, specificity 96.6%, PPV 90.5%, NPV 32.2%). When restricted to cervical STIs as the causative agents of VDS, sensitivity, specificity and PPV all decreased to 11.7%, 89.9%, and 33.3% (respectively), while NPV increased to 70.1%.

Table 1 Baseline characteristics of sexually-experienced and non-pregnant youth (aged 16–24 years) enrolled in the AYAZAZI study in South Africa, stratified by sex ($n = 352$)

Characteristics	Overall $n = 352$ n (%)	Total n	Females $n = 198$	Males $n = 154$	P-value
			n (%)		
Socio-demographics					
Study Site		352			0.314
Soweto	173 (49.2)		102 (51.5)	71 (46.1)	
Durban	179 (50.8)		96 (48.5)	83 (53.9)	
Age category, years		352			0.734
16 to 17	60 (17.1)		31 (15.7)	29 (18.8)	
18 to 20	187 (53.1)		107 (54.0)	80 (52.0)	
21 to 24	105 (29.8)		60 (30.3)	45 (29.2)	
Sexual orientation		351			0.533
Heterosexual	327 (93.2)		183 (92.4)	144 (94.1)	
LGBTQ[a]	24 (6.8)		15 (7.6)	9 (5.9)	
Currently in school		351			0.615
Yes	232 (66.1)		128 (65.0)	104 (67.5)	
No	119 (33.9)		69 (35.0)	50 (32.5)	
Food insecurity[b]		347			0.989
Low	257 (74.1)		143 (74.1)	114 (74.0)	
High	90 (25.9)		50 (25.9)	40 (26.0)	
Housing		352			0.006
Formal	255 (72.4)		132 (66.7)	123 (79.9)	
Informal[c]	97 (27.6)		66 (33.3)	31 (20.1)	
Monthly personal income[d]		352			0.008
< 400 ZAR	93 (26.4)		43 (21.7)	50 (32.5)	
401–1600 ZAR	174 (49.4)		112 (56.6)	62 (40.3)	
1601+ ZAR	85 (24.2)		43 (21.7)	42 (27.3)	
Sexual history and socio-structural variables					
Self-perceived HIV risk		347			0.940
None/low risk	193 (55.6)		107 (55.4)	86 (55.8)	
Medium/high risk	154 (44.4)		86 (44.6)	68 (44.2)	
≥2 Sexual partners in P6m[e]		352			< 0.001
Yes	111 (31.5)		41 (20.7)	70 (45.5)	
No	241 (68.5)		157 (79.3)	84 (54.5)	
Condom use in P6m		343			< 0.001
Consistent ("always")	111 (32.4)		37 (19.4)	74 (48.7)	
Inconsistent ("sometimes"/"never")	232 (67.6)		154 (80.6)	78 (51.3)	
Age-disparate sex partner in P6m[f]		340			< 0.001
Yes	85 (25.0)		68 (34.9)	18 (12.4)	
No	255 (75.0)		127 (65.1)	127 (87.6)	
Ever had transactional sex[g]		347			< 0.001
Yes	49 (14.1)		14 (7.2)	35 (22.9)	
No	298 (85.9)		180 (92.8)	118 (77.1)	

Table 1 Baseline characteristics of sexually-experienced and non-pregnant youth (aged 16–24 years) enrolled in the AYAZAZI study in South Africa, stratified by sex ($n = 352$) *(Continued)*

Characteristics	Overall $n = 352$ n (%)	Total n	Females $n = 198$	Males $n = 154$	*P*-value
			n (%)		
Ever been/made pregnant		352			< 0.001
Yes	118 (33.5)		93 (47.0)	25 (16.2)	
No	234 (66.5)		105 (53.0)	129 (83.8)	
Ever experienced physical/sexual violence		347			0.001
Yes	59 (17.0)		45 (23.3)	14 (9.1)	
No	288 (83.0)		148 (76.7)	140 (90.9)	

Notes: [a] LGBTQ refers to individuals who identify their sexual orientation as *Lesbian, Gay, Bisexual, Transgender, or Queer*; [b] Food insecurity was defined as high if the participant or a household member had ever slept hungry, had no food to eat because of lack of money, or ever went a day and night without eating; [c] Informal housing includes RDP housing (government subsidized housing), shacks, or hostels; [d] ZAR = South African Rand, with 400 ZAR = $25 USD and 1601 ZAR = $100 USD using the May 30, 2016 currency exchange rate of 1 ZAR = 0.063 USD; [e] P6m refers to the 6 months prior to interview; [f] Sexual partner is ≥5 years older or younger than participant; [g] Transactional sex was classified as ever having sex with someone in exchange for something (given or received)

When restricted to vaginal STIs as the causative agents of VDS or only BV, performance measures were also poor (for BV: sensitivity 13.3%, specificity 92.5, PPV 66.7%, NPV 48.6%).

Similarly, LAP symptomology poorly indicated infection with associated pathogens (i.e., NG, CT, MG), with both poor sensitivity and poor PPV. Overall, only 4/13 females reporting LAP symptoms were infected with a LAP-associated GTI; while of 57 females with confirmed infection with a LAP-associated GTI, just 4 reported symptoms (sensitivity 7.0%, specificity 93.4%, PPV 30.8%, NPV 70.6%).

Males

No MUS-associated pathogen (i.e., NG, CT, MG, and/or TV) was detected in the one male reporting urethral discharge. Of 16 males truly infected with a MUS-associated STI, none reported symptoms (sensitivity 0%, specificity 99.3%, PPV 0%, NPV 89.5%).

Discussion

GTIs, including asymptomatic infections, induce genital tract inflammation among young women, increasing HIV acquisition risk [14]. We found a high and frequently asymptomatic burden of GTI infection among South African youth, with significant differences by sex. While only 16% of young women and < 1% of young men reported GTI-related symptoms, laboratory tests identified at least one GTI in 70% of females and 10% of males. Syndromic GTI management revealed very poor sensitivity. The high burden of asymptomatic GTIs contributes to a silent GTI epidemic in youth, which requires additional attention, innovations, and resources to control. We strongly recommend policy changes to replace syndromic management with innovative public health approaches, inclusive of widespread diagnostic testing to reduce GTI burden and HIV-associated risks among youth.

The high GTI prevalence observed here is particularly notable, given that participants are young (16–24 years of age), primarily recruited from community settings, and were not enrolled due to high GTI risk. Nonetheless, over one-third of young women had at least one non-ulcerative STI and half had laboratory-detected BV. The prevalence of each non-ulcerative STI (CT: 18.2%; NG: 7.1%; MG: 9.6%; TV: 8.1%) was higher or similar to the prevalence observed among older women (18–40 years) presenting for STI care in Durban (CT: 18.4%; NG: 5.2%; MG: not assessed; TV: 3.0%) [16], high HIV-risk women enrolling in the CAPRISA 002 Acute HIV Infection study in Durban (overall STI prevalence = 25.3%; CT: 4.2%; NG: 5.4%; MG: 1.2%; TV: 20.3%) [17], women enrolled in three large clinical trials in Durban (STI prevalence = 13%) [18], "high HIV risk" Tanzanian women (CT: 12%; NG: 4%; MG: not assessed; TV: 19%) [19], and women attending antenatal care in Kenya (CT: 14.9%; NG: 1.0%; MG: not assessed; TV: 7.4%) [20]. The exception to this pattern was TV, which was lower in female youth in our study relative to older women in both the Tanzanian and South African studies. Such patterns are consistent with known biological reasons for increases in TV prevalence with age (i.e., protozoal accumulation over time). The high BV prevalence (53.0%) mirrors levels reported in other South African studies [4, 17, 18, 21, 22].

Fewer (10%) young men in our study had a laboratory-confirmed non-ulcerative STI compared to women. STI prevalence among men was driven largely by CT (7.8%). Our findings are consistent with the limited available data regarding STI prevalence for young and older heterosexual men in South Africa [23, 24].

We observed a 3.7% prevalence of HIV sero-positivity at baseline, despite study eligibility criteria aimed at enrolling HIV-negative participants. Moreover, low median CD4 cell counts at HIV diagnosis signal advanced HIV disease progression. HIV prevalence was higher among Durban

Table 2 Sex-stratified prevalence of genital tract infection (GTI) symptoms and associated syndromes reported by sexually experienced, non-pregnant South African youth (aged 16–24 years) enrolled in the AYAZAZI study, overall and by site ($n = 352$)

	Durban	Soweto	Whole cohort
	Females $n = 96$ Males $n = 83$	Females $n = 102$ Males $n = 71$	Females $n = 198$ Males $n = 154$
	n (%)	n (%)	n (%)
Female-specific symptoms:			
Vaginal discharge	6 (6.3)	8 (7.8)	14 (7.1)
Dysuria	0 (0)	4 (3.9)	4 (2.0)
Vaginal Itching or irritation	4 (4.2)	5 (4.9)	9 (4.5)
Vaginal redness or swelling	0 (0)	1 (1.0)	1 (0.5)
Lower abdominal or groin pain (with/without vaginal discharge)	1 (1.0)	4 (3.9)	5 (2.5)
Dyspareunia	0 (0)	2 (2.0)	2 (1.0)
Post-coital bleeding or metrorrhagia	2 (2.1)	4 (3.9)	6 (3.0)
Vaginal sores or skin changes	3 (3.1)	1 (1.0)	4 (2.0)
None of the above	82 (85.4)	82 (80.4)	164 (82.8)
≥ 1 symptom	12 (12.5)	20 (19.6)	32 (16.2)
Female-specific syndromes:			
Vaginal Discharge Syndrome (VDS)	8 (8.3)	13 (12.8)	21 (10.6)
Lower Abdominal Pain (LAP)	3 (3.1)	10 (9.8)	13 (6.6)
Genital Ulcer Disease (GUD)	3 (3.1)	1 (1.0)	4 (2.0)
Male-specific symptoms:			
Sores or skin changes around penis or scrotum	0 (0)	0 (0)	0 (0)
Urethral discharge	0 (0)	1 (1.4)	1 (0.7)
Dysuria	0 (0)	0 (0)	0 (0)
Pain, swelling or redness of scrotum	0 (0)	0 (0)	0 (0)
Pain in testes	0 (0)	0 (0)	0 (0)
Soreness or itching around foreskin (if uncircumcised)	0 (0)	0 (0)	0 (0)
Hot tender swelling with redness	0 (0)	0 (0)	0 (0)
None of the above	83 (100.0)	70 (98.6)	153 (99.4)
≥ 1 symptom	0 (0)	1 (1.4)	1 (0.7)
Male-specific syndromes:			
Genital Ulcer Disease (GUD)	0 (0)	0 (0)	0 (0)
Male Urethritis (MUS)	0 (0)	1 (1.4)	1 (0.7)
Scrotal Swelling (SSW)	0 (0)	0 (0)	0 (0)
Balanitis	0 (0)	0 (0)	0 (0)
Bubo	0 (0)	0 (0)	0 (0)

Notes: GTI symptoms and syndromes are classified based on WHO and South African STI management guidelines (WHO 2004, South African Department of Health 2015)

participants compared to Soweto, consistent with findings from surveillance data [1]. Given the known synergistic relationship between HIV and STI co-infection, the higher prevalence of non-ulcerative STIs but lower prevalence of HIV in Soweto is notable.

Consistent with previous reports, syndromic management was unable to detect the majority of GTIs due to their asymptomatic nature [17, 25]. Without laboratory testing, approximately 80% of prevalent GTIs among young women and 100% among young men in our study would have remained untreated. Poor sexual health knowledge and a lack of familiarity with GTI symptoms among youth may have exacerbated under-reporting of symptoms [26–28]. Both VDS and LAP had poor sensitivity (13.7% and 7.0% respectively). This is a well-documented limitation to the VDS algorithm, especially for cervical infection

Table 3 Sex-stratified prevalence of laboratory-confirmed genital tract infections (GTIs) among sexually experienced, non-pregnant South African youth (aged 16–24 years) enrolled in the AYAZAZI study, overall and by study site ($n = 352$)

Laboratory-confirmed infections	Durban			Soweto			Whole cohort		
	Female $n = 96$	Male $n = 83$	Total $n = 179$	Female $n = 102$	Male $n = 71$	Total $n = 173$	Female $n = 198$	Male $n = 154$	Total $n = 352$
≥ 1 GTI (excluding HIV)	66 (68.8)	10 (12.0)	76 (42.5)	73 (71.6)	6 (8.5)	79 (45.7)	139 (70.2)*	16 (10.4)*	155 (44.0)
Non-ulcerative STIs									
C. trachomatis (CT)	14 (14.6)	7 (8.4)	21 (11.7)	22 (21.6)	5 (7.0)	27 (15.6)	36 (18.2)*	12 (7.8)*	48 (13.6)
N. gonorrhoeae (NG)	5 (5.2)	2 (2.4)	7 (3.9)	9 (8.8)	0 (0)	9 (5.2)	14 (7.1)*	2 (1.3)*	16 (4.6)
M. genitalium (MG)	5 (5.2)	3 (3.6)	8 (4.5)	14 (13.7)	2 (2.8)	16 (9.3)	19 (9.6)*	5 (3.3)*	24 (6.8)
T. vaginalis (TV)	3 (3.1)	0 (0)	3 (1.7)	13 (12.8)	1 (1.4)	14 (8.1)	16 (8.1)*	1 (0.7)*	17 (4.8)
≥ 1 of CT/NG/MG	22 (22.9)	10 (12.0)	32 (17.9)	38 (37.3)	5 (7.0)	43 (24.9)	60 (30.3)*	15 (9.7)*	75 (21.3)
≥ 1 non-ulcerative STI	24 (25.0)	10 (12.0)	34 (19.0)	45 (44.1)	6 (8.5)	51 (29.5)	69 (34.8)*	16 (10.4)*	85 (24.1)
Female-only GTIs									
Bacterial Vaginosis (BV)	52 (54.2)			53 (52.0)			105 (53.0)		
C. albicans (CA)	7 (7.3)			12 (11.8)			19 (9.6)		
Co-infection									
≥ 2 non-ulcerative STIs	3 (3.1)	2 (2.4)	5 (2.8)	11 (10.8)	2 (2.8)	13 (7.5)	14 (7.0)*	4 (2.6)*	18 (5.0)
≥ 1 non-ulcerative STI & ≥1 GTI	16 (16.7)			34 (33.3)			50 (25.3)		
Among those with ≥ 1 non-ulcerative STI									
≥ 2 non-ulcerative STIs	3 (12.5)	2 (20.0)	5 (14.7)	11 (24.4)	2 (33.3)	13 (25.5)	14 (20.3)	4 (25.0)	18 (21.2)
≥ 1 non-ulcerative STI & ≥1 GTI	16 (66.7)			34 (75.6)			50 (72.5)		
Ulcerative STIs (among those with genital ulcers)[a]	$n = 1$	$n = 0$	$n = 1$	$n = 1$	$n = 1$	$n = 2$	$n = 2$	$n = 1$	$n = 3$
HSV-2	1 (100.0)	0 (0)	1 (100.0)	0 (0)	0 (0)	0 (0)	1 (50.0)	0 (0)	1 (33.3)
T. pallidum	0 (0)	0 (0)	0 (0)	0 (0)	0 (0)	0 (0)	0 (0)	0 (0)	0 (0)
H. ducreyi	0 (0)	0 (0)	0 (0)	0 (0)	0 (0)	0 (0)	0 (0)	0 (0)	0 (0)
LGV	0 (0)	0 (0)	0 (0)	0 (0)	0 (0)	0 (0)	0 (0)	0 (0)	0 (0)
HIV[b]	9 (9.4)	2 (2.4)	11 (6.2)	1 (1.0)	1 (1.4)	2 (1.2)	10 (5.1)	3 (2.0)	13 (3.7)

Notes: *Statistically significant difference ($p < 0.05$) between prevalence among females vs males; [a]Prevalence of ulcerative STIs restricted to the n = 3 participants who had a genital ulcer identified during physical exams, which was swabbed and tested using multiplex NAAT testing; [b]As per the study inclusion criteria, all participants reported being HIV-negative or unknown HIV status at enrollment

[17, 21, 29]. VDS had a high PPV (90.5%) indicating that most women who reported VDS-related symptoms did have a laboratory-confirmed GTI and would have been appropriately treated under syndromic management. That is, syndromic management performed appropriately in its role of detecting and managing symptomatic GTIs. However, the PPV for LAP was poor (30.8%) highlighting that a majority of young women who reported LAP-associated symptoms did not have a laboratory-confirmed GTI and may have been inappropriately treated under syndromic management guidelines. Insufficient symptomatic infection in young men in our study precluded robust sensitivity analyses of syndromic management; no men with an STI reported symptoms and no men who reported symptoms had an STI.

There are important advantages to syndromic management on a national scale; the primary being cost, and a second being that it requires a single visit, decreasing the likelihood of treatment loss-to-follow-up at a second visit, typically required with diagnostic testing [9]. These advantages must be considered against the performance of syndromic approaches for high-priority populations. Our findings suggest that in South Africa, both male and female youth have a high burden of undetected GTIs. Reliance on a syndromic management approach will continue to yield low detection of prevalent GTIs and thus poor GTI control.

Our findings suggest a need to evolve sexual health services to benefit youth. Although a test-and-treat approach to GTIs has historically posed financial and logistical challenges, recent innovations in affordable real-time STI testing, such as point-of-care (POC) diagnostics, warrant further investigation for wide-scale implementation

Table 4 Sex-stratified sensitivity analyses of syndromic screening for genital tract infections (GTIs) among sexually experienced, non-pregnant South African youth (aged 16–24 years) enrolled in the AYAZAZI study ($n = 352$)

Syndrome	Symptomatic	Laboratory test (gold standard)		Total	Sensitivity (%) [95% CI]	Specificity (%) [95% CI]	PPV (%) [95% CI]	NPV (%) [95% CI]
		Positive	Negative					
Females (n = 198)								
Vaginal discharge (VDS)[a]	Yes	19	2	21	13.7	96.6	90.5	32.2
	No	120	57	177	[8.4–20.5]	[88.2–99.6]	[69.6–98.8]	[25.4–39.6]
with cervical STIs as causative agents[b]	Yes	7	14	21	11.7	89.9	33.3	70.1
	No	53	124	177	[4.8–22.6]	[83.6–94.3]	[14.6–57.0]	[62.7–76.7]
with vaginal STIs as causative agents[c]	Yes	18	3	21	14.8	96.1	85.7	41.2
	No	104	73	177	[9.0–22.3]	[88.9–99.2]	[63.7–97.0]	[33.9–48.9]
with only BV as a causative agent	Yes	14	7	21	13.3	92.5	66.7	48.6
	No	91	86	177	[7.5–21.4]	[85.1–96.9]	[43.0–85.4]	[41.0–56.2]
Lower abdominal pain (LAP)[d]	Yes	4	9	13	7.0	93.4	30.8	70.6
	No	53	127	180	[1.9–17.0]	[87.8–97.0]	[9.1–61.4]	[63.3–77.1]
Males (n = 154)								
Male urethritis (MUS)[e]	Yes	0	1	1	0.0	99.3	0.0	89.5
	No	16	137	153	[0–20.6][g]	[96.0–100.0]	[0–97.5][g]	[83.6–93.9]
Scrotal Swelling (SSW)[f]	Yes	0	0	0	0.0	100.0	N/A	91.6
	No	13	141	154	[0–24.7][g]	[97.4–100.0][g]	[N/A]	[86.0–95.4]

Notes: GTIs included as the gold standard for VDS, LAP, MUS and SSW include (note: no sensitivity analysis was performed for GUD given testing via genital swabs and NAAT:
[a]Any STI/GTI with VDS as a syndrome: *N.gonorrhoeae, C.trachomatis, M.genitalium* (cervical infection), *T.vaginalis*, BV, or *C. albicans* (vaginal infection);
[b]Any cervical STI with VDS as a syndrome: *N.gonorrhoeae, C.trachomatis, M.genitalium*;
[c]Any vaginal STI with VDS as a syndrome: *T.vaginalis*, BV, *C. albicans;*
[d]Any STI/GTI with LAP as a syndrome: *N.gonorrhoeae, C.trachomatis, M.genitalium*
[e]Any STI with MUS as syndrome: *N.gonorrhoeae, C.trachomatis, M.genitalium, T.vaginalis;*
[f]Any STI with SSW as syndrome: *N.gonorrhoeae, C.trachomatis;*
[g]1-sided 97.5% CI

[16, 30]. By providing immediate testing results and facilitating treatment without delay, POC tests can help reduce secondary transmission and the consequences of infection progression [31]. POC testing also presents an opportunity to screen outside of traditional clinic settings, which young people infrequently access [32], and move testing into community-based and youth-friendly settings that offer comprehensive HIV and GTI services. POC testing quality is growing with improving technology [33], with good performance across several prevalent STIs, including CT, NG, TV, and syphilis [34, 35]. Recent work also suggests that POC testing for STIs is acceptable to providers [33] and to young women and their partners [16]. Additional studies are warranted to assess the cost-effectiveness of POC STI testing for youth in low- and middle-income countries.

GTI control will not be solved by diagnostic innovation alone. In addition to GTI burden, and consistent with previous studies [1], youth in our study report high behavioral, social, and structural vulnerability for GTI and HIV acquisition. Notably, over half of adolescent and young adults in this HIV hyper-endemic setting self-perceived themselves as being at low or no risk of HIV acquisition. These findings underscore the need for efforts to move beyond individual-level risk factors for promoting healthy sexuality for young people, and address the social and structural risk environments, such as gender and power inequity in relationships, coercive sex, economic inequity, violence, and poverty, which shape how young people navigate their sexual lives.

This study has limitations. First, HSV-2 and syphilis prevalence are likely to be under-estimated as the study protocol specified NAAT testing of genital ulcerative lesions only. Future work should incorporate serological testing to assess the true prevalence of both HSV-2 and syphilis in youth. Second, not all GTIs were tested (for example, anorectal samples were not taken), thus the reported GTI prevalence may be an underestimate. Third, participants were asked directly about GTI symptoms and their genital areas carefully examined by a study nurse with expertise in youth-focused care delivery, and may have been more willing to report symptoms or undergo genital examination. Thus, our assessment of the sensitivity and PPV of syndromic management of GTIs among youth, although very low, is likely higher than would be observed in a public care setting.

Conclusion

Maintaining the status quo of syndromic GTI management for youth is not acceptable. We observed a substantial burden of subclinical GTI infection alongside HIV risk behaviors and low risk-perception for HIV acquisition among South African youth. Sensitivity of symptom-based reporting was poor and offered no value in identifying the highly prevalent asymptomatic GTI infections. Syndromic management does not meet the needs of young people in this and similar settings and leaves them at increased risk of HIV acquisition. In the context of evolving and less costly GTI diagnostic capabilities, exploring new approaches to implementing youth-focused GTI services is warranted.

Abbreviations

ART: Antiretroviral therapy; BV: Bacterial Vaginosis; CT: *Chlamydia trachomatis*; ELISA: Enzyme-linked immunosorbent assay; GTI : Genital tract infection; GUD: Genital Ulcer Disease; HCG: Human Chorionic Gonadotropin; HIV: Human Immunodeficiency Virus; HSV-2 : Herpes simplex virus type 2; IQR: Interquartile Range; LAP: Lower Abdominal Pain; MG: *Mycoplasma genitalium*; MRU: MatCH Research Unit; MUS: Male Urethritis Syndrome; NAAT: Nucleic Acid Amplification Test; NG: *Neisseria gonorrhoeae*; NPV: Negative Predictive Value; PHRU: Perinatal HIV Research Unit; POC: Point-of-care; PPV: Positive Predictive Value; SSW: Scrotal Swelling; STI: Sexually Transmitted Infection; TV: *Trichomonas vaginalis*; VDS: Vaginal Discharge Syndrome; ZAR: South African Rand

Acknowledgements

The AYAZAZI Research Team would like to thank our youth participants for their contributions to this study. We also thank our international team of co-investigators, collaborators, and youth representatives, and acknowledge the Adolescent Community Advisory Boards and our partnering organizations for supporting the study. We are grateful to Nimesh Patel for his contributions to this analysis.

Funding

AYAZAZI is funded through the Canadian HIV Vaccine Initiative (CHVI) and the Canadian Institutes of Health Research (CIHR), with support from the South African Medical Research Council. AK and MB received salary support awards from the Canada Research Chair program. TN is supported by the South Africa Research Chairs Initiative and the Sub-Saharan African Network for TB/HIV Research Excellence (SANTHE), a DELTAS Africa Initiative [grant # DEL-15-006]. The DELTAS Africa Initiative is an independent funding scheme of the African Academy of Sciences (AAS)'s Alliance for Accelerating Excellence in Science in Africa (AESA) and supported by the New Partnership for Africa's Development Planning and Coordinating Agency (NEPAD Agency) with funding from the Wellcome Trust [grant # 107752/Z/15/Z] and the UK government. The views expressed in this publication are those of the author(s) and not necessarily those of AAS, NEPAD Agency, Wellcome Trust, or the UK government.

Authors' contributions

The multiple site community-based nature of this study required engagement of a large study team. Each of the listed co-authors contributed substantively to this manuscript, in accordance with ICMJE recommendations regarding authorship as follows: *Conceived and designed the study:* AK, JJD, MB, DAL, JS, TN, MB, GG. *Led the implementation of the AYAZAZI study:* AK (at SFU), JJD (at the PHRU in Soweto), MB (at the MRU in Durban), LC (at SFU), DAL (at the NICD in Johannesburg), JS (at the MRU in Durban), TD (at the HPP lab in Durban), MB (at SFU), GG (at the PHRU in Soweto). *Contributed substantially to data acquisition:* AK, JJD, FL, MB, MJ, PS, DAL, JS, TN, MB, GG. *Contributed substantially to data analysis:* MB, KC. *Contributed substantially to interpretation of the data:* AK, JJD, FL, MB, MJ, MB, PC, DAL, JS, TN, MB, GG. *Drafted the initial manuscript:* AK, MB. *Contributed critical revisions to the initial manuscript for important intellectual content:* AK, JJD, FL, MB, MJ, MB, PS, LC, PC, KC, DAL, JS, TN, MB, GG. All co-authors approved the final manuscript and agree to be accountable for all aspects of the work.

Consent for publication

All authors consent for publication.

Competing interests

The authors declare no conflicts of interest. This research was previously presented at: (1) the 2016 HIVR4P conference in Chicago, USA as a poster; and (2) the 2017 International Women and HIV Workshop in Boston, USA as a guided poster.

Author details

[1]Faculty of Health Sciences, Simon Fraser University, Blusson Hall Rm 10522, 8888 University Drive, Burnaby B.C. V5A 1S6, Canada. [2]Perinatal HIV Research Unit (PHRU), Faculty of Health Sciences, University of the Witwatersrand, Johannesburg, South Africa. [3]Maternal Adolescent and Child Health (MatCH) Research Unit (MRU), Faculty of Health Sciences, University of the Witwatersrand, Durban, South Africa. [4]London School of Hygiene and Tropical Medicine, London, UK. [5]Harvard combined Infectious Diseases Fellowship, Boston, MA, USA. [6]Centre for HIV and STIs, National Institute for Communicable Diseases, Johannesburg, South Africa. [7]Faculty of Medicine and Health & Marie Bashir Institute for Infectious Diseases and Biosecurity, University of Sydney, Sydney, Australia. [8]HIV Pathogenesis Programme and Africa Health Research Institute, University of KwaZulu-Natal, Durban, South Africa. [9]Ragon Institute of Massachusetts General Hospital, Massachusetts Institute of Technology and Harvard University, Cambridge, MA, USA. [10]Max Planck Institute for Infection Biology, Berlin, Germany. [11]South African Medical Research Council, Cape Town, South Africa.

References

1. Shisana O, Rehle T, Simbayi LC, Zuma K, Jooste S, Zungu N, et al. South African National HIV Prevalence, Incidence and Behaviour survey, 2012. Cape Town: HSRC Press; 2014.
2. UNAIDS. Global AIDS Update (2016). Geneva: UNAIDS; 2016.
3. Bekker LG, Johnson L, Wallace M, Hosek S. Building our youth for the future. J Int AIDS Soc. 2015;18(2 Suppl 1):20027.
4. Atashili J, Poole C, Ndumbe PM, Adimora AA, Smith JS. Bacterial vaginosis and HIV acquisition: a meta-analysis of published studies. AIDS. 2008;22(12): 1493–501.
5. Ward H, Ronn M. Contribution of sexually transmitted infections to the sexual transmission of HIV. Curr Opin HIV AIDS. 2010;5(4):305–10.
6. Moodley P, Sturm AW. Sexually transmitted infections, adverse pregnancy outcome and neonatal infection. Semin Neonatol. 2000;5(3):255–69.
7. Mayaud P, Mabey D. Approaches to the control of sexually transmitted infections in developing countries: old problems and modern challenges. Sex Transm Infect. 2004;80(3):174–82.
8. South African Department of Health. Sexually Transmitted Infections: Management Guidelines 2015. Pretoria: SA Department of Heatlh; 2015.
9. World Health Organization (WHO). Guidelines for the management of sexually transmitted infections. Geneva: WHO; 2004.
10. Wilkinson D, Abdool Karim SS, Harrison A, Lurie M, Colvin M, Connolly C, et al. Unrecognized sexually transmitted infections in rural south African women: a hidden epidemic. Bull World Health Organ. 1999;77(1):22–8.
11. Francis SC, Mthiyane TN, Baisley K, McHunu SL, Ferguson JB, Smit T, et al. Prevalence of sexually transmitted infections among young people in South

Africa: a nested survey in a health and demographic surveillance site. PLoS Med. 2018;15(2):e1002512.
12. Dietrich J, Smith P, Hornschuh S, Mathenjwa T, Greener L, Beksinska M, et al. "At AYAZAZI, they do something." Factors motivating participation in a youth-centred cohort study on HIV prevention in Soweto and Durban, South Africa. Durban: South African AIDS Conference; 2017.
13. Nugent RP, Krohn MA, Hillier SL. Reliability of diagnosing bacterial vaginosis is improved by a standardized method of gram stain interpretation. J Clin Microbiol. 1991;29(2):297–301.
14. Passmore JS, Jaspan HB. Vaginal microbes, inflammation, and HIV risk in African women. Lancet Infect Dis. 2018;18(5):483–4.
15. Rothman K, Greenland S, Lash T. Modern Epidemiology. 3rd ed. Philadelphia, USA: Lippincott Williams & Wilkins; 2008.
16. Garrett NJ, Osman F, Maharaj B, Naicker N, Gibbs A, Norman E, et al. Beyond syndromic management: opportunities for diagnosis-based treatment of sexually transmitted infections in low- and middle-income countries. PLoS One. 2018;13(4):e0196209.
17. Mlisana K, Naicker N, Werner L, Roberts L, van Loggerenberg F, Baxter C, et al. Symptomatic vaginal discharge is a poor predictor of sexually transmitted infections and genital tract inflammation in high-risk women in South Africa. J Infect Dis. 2012;206(1):6–14.
18. Naidoo S, Wand H, Abbai NS, Ramjee G. High prevalence and incidence of sexually transmitted infections among women living in Kwazulu-Natal, South Africa. AIDS Res Ther. 2014;11:31.
19. Francis SC, Ao TT, Vanobberghen FM, Chilongani J, Hashim R, Andreasen A, et al. Epidemiology of curable sexually transmitted infections among women at increased risk for HIV in northwestern Tanzania: inadequacy of syndromic management. PLoS One. 2014;9(7):e101221.
20. Masha SC, Wahome E, Vaneechoutte M, Cools P, Crucitti T, Sanders EJ. High prevalence of curable sexually transmitted infections among pregnant women in a rural county hospital in Kilifi, Kenya. PLoS One. 2017;12(3):e0175166.
21. Lewis DA, Chirwa TF, Msimang VM, Radebe FM, Kamb ML, Firnhaber CS. Urethritis/cervicitis pathogen prevalence and associated risk factors among asymptomatic HIV-infected patients in South Africa. Sex Transm Dis. 2012; 39(7):531–6.
22. Moodley D, Moodley P, Sebitloane M, Soowamber D, McNaughton-Reyes HL, Groves AK, et al. High prevalence and incidence of asymptomatic sexually transmitted infections during pregnancy and postdelivery in KwaZulu Natal, South Africa. Sex Transm Dis. 2015;42(1):43–7.
23. Sobngwi-Tambekou J, Taljaard D, Nieuwoudt M, Lissouba P, Puren A, Auvert B. Male circumcision and Neisseria gonorrhoeae, chlamydia trachomatis and trichomonas vaginalis: observations after a randomised controlled trial for HIV prevention. Sex Transm Infect. 2009;85(2):116–20.
24. Lewis DA, Pillay C, Mohlamonyane O, Vezi A, Mbabela S, Mzaidume Y, et al. The burden of asymptomatic sexually transmitted infections among men in Carletonville, South Africa: implications for syndromic management. Sex Transm Infect. 2008;84(5):371–6.
25. van der Eem L, Dubbink JH, Struthers HE, McIntyre JA, Ouburg S, Morre SA, et al. Evaluation of syndromic management guidelines for treatment of sexually transmitted infections in south African women. Tropical Med Int Health. 2016;21(9):1138–46.
26. Nawagi F, Mpimbaza A, Mukisa J, Serwadda P, Kyalema S, Kizza D. Knowledge and practices related to sexually transmitted infections among women of reproductive age living in Katanga slum, Kampala, Uganda. Afr Health Sci. 2016;16(1):116–22.
27. Leichliter JS, Paz-Bailey G, Friedman AL, Habel MA, Vezi A, Sello M, et al. Clinics aren't meant for men': sexual health care access and seeking behaviours among men in Gauteng province, South Africa. SAHARA J. 2011;8(2):82–8.
28. Jemmott JBI, Jemmott LS, O'Leary A, Ngwane Z, Lewis DA, Bellamy SL, et al. HIV/STI risk-reduction intervention efficacy with south African adolescents over 54 months. Health Psychol. 2015;34:610–21.
29. Pettifor A, Walsh J, Wilkins V, Raghunathan P. How effective is syndromic management of STDs?: a review of current studies. Sex Transm Dis. 2000; 27(7):371–85.
30. Cristillo AD, Bristow CC, Peeling R, Van Der Pol B, de Cortina SH, Dimov IK, et al. Point-of-care sexually transmitted infection diagnostics: Proceedings of the STAR Sexually Transmitted Infection-Clinical Trial Group Programmatic Meeting. Sex Transm Dis. 2017;44(4):211–8.
31. van Dommelen L, van Tiel FH, Ouburg S, Brouwers EE, Terporten PH, Savelkoul PH, et al. Alarmingly poor performance in chlamydia trachomatis point-of-care testing. Sex Transm Infect. 2010;86(5):355–9.
32. Otwombe K, Dietrich J, Laher F, Hornschuh S, Nkala B, Chimoyi L, et al. Health-seeking behaviours by gender among adolescents in Soweto, South Africa. Glob Health Action. 2015;8:25670.
33. Herbst de Cortina S, Bristow CC, Joseph Davey D, Klausner JD. A systematic review of point of care testing for chlamydia trachomatis, Neisseria gonorrhoeae, and trichomonas vaginalis. Infect Dis Obstet Gynecol. 2016;2016:4386127.
34. Gaydos CA, Van Der Pol B, Jett-Goheen M, Barnes M, Quinn N, Clark C, et al. Performance of the Cepheid CT/NG Xpert rapid PCR test for detection of chlamydia trachomatis and Neisseria gonorrhoeae. J Clin Microbiol. 2013; 51(6):1666–72.
35. Jafari Y, Peeling RW, Shivkumar S, Claessens C, Joseph L, Pai NP. Are Treponema pallidum specific rapid and point-of-care tests for syphilis accurate enough for screening in resource limited settings? Evidence from a meta-analysis. PLoS One. 2013;8(2):e54695.

Comparison of rRNA-based and DNA-based nucleic acid amplifications for detection of *Chlamydia trachomatis, Neisseria gonorrhoeae,* and *Ureaplasma urealyticum* in urogenital swabs

Yuying Liang[1†], Xin Jin[2†], Fang Yuan[2†], Zhanjia Li[2] and Shuiping Chen[1*]

Abstract

Background: Nucleic acid amplification tests (NAAT) are well-accepted in diagnosis and surveillance of sexually infectious pathogens worldwide. However, performance differences between a RNA-based NAAT and DNA-based NAAT are rarely reported. This study compares the performances of the RNA-based SAT (simultaneous amplification and testing) assay and the DNA-based quantitative real-time polymerase chain reaction (qPCR) assay.

Methods: A total of 123 urogenital swabs were collected from outpatients with suspected genital infections in our hospital. *Chlamydia trachomatis* (CT), *Neisseria gonorrhoeae* (NG), and *Ureaplasma urealyticum* (UU) in these swabs were simultaneously tested by SAT and qPCR. Any swabs were positive in the qPCR assay were further verified by following cloning and sequencing. All statistical analysis was performed using the SPSS software.

Results: When the concentrations of CT, NG, or UU were more than 1×10^3 copies/ml, 100% agreements between SAT and qPCR were observed regardless of the pathogen. No discrepancy was found. However, the sensitivity of SAT is significantly higher than qPCR in samples with concentration less than 1×10^3 copies/ml. When tested by SAT and qPCR, 57.14 and 28.57% were positive for CT, 46.15% and 0 were positive for NG, 80% and 0 were positive for UU, respectively.

Conclusions: The SAT assay has better agreements and higher sensitivities when compared with the qPCR assay, and thus could be a better choice for screening, diagnosis, and surveillance of sexually transmitted diseases, especially for CT and NG.

Keywords: *Chlamydia trachomatis*, *Neisseria gonorrhoeae*, *Ureaplasma urealyticum*, Simultaneous amplification and testing, qPCR

Background

Chlamydia trachomatis (CT) and *Neisseria gonorrhoeae* (NG) are two of the most prevalent sexually infectious pathogenic bacteria worldwide with 131 million chlamydia infections and 78 million gonorrhea infections out of 357 million new infections per year (http://www.who.int/mediacentre/factsheets/fs110/en/). Although *Ureaplasma urealyticum* (UU) is considered as a commensal bacterium in the urogenital tract, it has been reported to be associated with some sexually transmitted diseases including non-gonococcal urethritis (NGU) [1, 2] and patients with high UU loads are associated with acute NGU [2]. Although these infections are curable, screening still remains very important to prevent late complications caused by these pathogens.

* Correspondence: shpchen@hotmail.com
†Yuying Liang, Xin Jin and Fang Yuan contributed equally to this work.
1Department of Infection Control, Affiliated Hospital of Academy of Military Medical Sciences, Beijing, People's Republic of China
Full list of author information is available at the end of the article

Traditionally, selective culture methods are used to detect CT, NG, and UU in clinical samples, but their sensitivities are very low [3, 4]. Nucleic acid amplification tests (NAAT), which have a better performance with high sensitivity, specificity, and ease of sample transport, have been approved by the Food and Drug Administration (FDA) for the detection of CT and NG, and widely used in clinical facilities to detect the sexually infectious pathogens [5, 6]. Recently, a novel RNA-based NAAT (simultaneous amplification and testing, SAT), which is based on transcription mediated amplification (TMA) and designed to detect pathogenic bacteria by amplification of 16S rRNA, has been reported to detect some sexual, respiratory, and enteric pathogens, including CT, NG, UU, *Mycoplasma genitalium, Mycobacterium tuberculosis, Mycoplasma pneumon*niae, entervirus 71, and coxsackievirus A16 [7–11]. SAT provides a great advantage because rRNA is about 10,000 times of the copy number of genomic DNA and 1000 times of that of plasmid DNA [12]. It is noteworthy that probes in SAT are labeled with fluorescences [8–11], while probes in another TMA-based detection method, APTIMA, are labeled with chemiluminescences [13]. Performance comparison of the RNA-based SAT with DNA-based NAAT assay is unclear yet.

Here, we compared the performances of the RNA-based SAT assay with the DNA-based quantitative real-time polymerase chain reaction (qPCR) assay by simultaneous detection of CT, NG, and UU in urogenital swabs.

Methods

Samples

A total of 123 urogenital swabs were collected from 123 outpatients with suspected genital infections in our hospital, which consisted of 64 male and 59 female with a median age of 29 years old (range: 19–63). Swabs were placed into 2 ml of sterile normal saline and the tubes were vortexed. For each sample, the two NAATs were performed at the same time. RNase-free tubes and tips were used in the SAT assay.

This study was exempted from a requirement for a statement of ethical approval from ethical committee of the affiliated hospital of academy of military medical sciences.

DNA extraction and the qPCR assay

CT, NG, and UU qPCR kits (Liferiver Biotech) were used in the DNA-based NAAT. 1 ml of each sample was centrifuged at 13000 g for 5 min at room temperature. The supernatant was discarded and the pellet was washed twice with normal saline. After the second wash, the pellet was resuspended in 100 µl extraction buffer and heated at 100 °C for 10 min. After another centrifugation at 13000 g for 5 min, the supernatants were collected and used as DNA extracts.

The reaction mixtures were prepared as described by the manufacturer's instructions. The amplifications were performed on a Roche LightCycler® 480 system under the following conditions: 94 °C 2 min, 40 cycles of 93 °C 15 s and 60 °C 60 s. If the qPCR assay was positive, the amplified segments were subjected to cloning and sequencing to confirm whether they were true or not. Both negative and positive controls were included in each run.

The SAT assay

Briefly, 16S rRNA was isolated from samples by a capture oligomer via target capture by magnetic microparticles. The target rRNA was then reverse transcribed to generate cDNA fragments using Moloney murine leukemia virus reverse transcriptase and multiple RNA copies (100–1000) were produced from each cDNA copy by the T7 RNA polymerase. Afterwards, these RNA copies were transcribed into cDNA again and bound to fluorescence-labeled specific probes, which were labeled with 6-carboxyfluorescein (FAM) phosphoramidite at the 5′ end and with 4-[4-(dimethylamino) phenylazo] benzoic acid N-succinimidyl ester (DABCYL) at the 3′ end [10]. The SAT assay was performed according to the manufacturer's instructions (Shanghai Rendu Biotechnology Co, Ltd). 400 µl of samples and 100 µl RNA nucleic acid extraction buffer were mixed in a 1.5 ml microcentrifuge tube and heated at 60 °C for 5 min. After incubation at room temperature for 10 min, RNA extraction was performed by magnetic beads. 30 µl of RNA extracts and 40 µl of amplification detection buffer were mixed as the final reaction mixture. After incubation at 60 °C for 10 min, the reaction mixture was immediately placed at 42 °C for 5 min. 10 µl of pre-heated (42 °C) enzyme reagent was then added. The tubes were immediately placed on a Roche LightCycler® 480 system and subjected to amplification with the following conditions: 40 cycles of 42 °C for 1 min. Both negative and positive controls were included in each run.

To evaluate the reproducibility of SAT, high (original) and low (100-fold diluted) concentrations of the positive controls in the kits (CT: 10^4 and 10^2 copies/µl; NG: 10^4 and 10^2 copies/µl; UU: 2×10^5 and 2×10^3 cfu/ml) were tested, respectively. Each control sample was tested five times.

Statistical analysis

All statistical analysis was performed using the SPSS software package version 20.0. Frequencies were compared using Fisher's exact test. *p* values less than 0.05 were considered statistically significant.

Results

All swabs were firstly detected by the qPCR assay. Of the 123 urogenital swabs, 33 swabs were positive for CT, 32 swabs were positive for NG, and 29 swabs were positive for UU after confirmation by the qPCR assay and sequencing. All positive swabs had a concentration of more than 1×10^3 copies/ml. The remaining 29 swabs were negative for CT, NG, and UU.

Excellent agreements between the SAT assay and the qPCR assay

After 19 of the 33 CT-positive, 19 of the 32 NG-positive, 19 of the 29 UU-positive, and 29 pathogen-negative samples were tested by SAT, 100% agreements between the SAT assay and the qPCR assay were observed in samples with a concentration more than 1×10^3 copies/ml, as shown in Table 1. Specifically, the sensitivity and specificity were 100% (19/19) and 100% (10/10) for CT, 100% (19/19) and 100% (10/10) for NG, and 100% (19/19) and 100% (10/10) for UU, respectively. No discrepancy was found. In addition, SAT exhibited a good reproducibility. Specifically, the coefficient of variations (CV) of CT, NG, and UU were 1.91, 2.94, and 1.25% for high concentration of positive controls, and 3.14, 0.28, and 2.28% for low concentration of positive controls, respectively.

The SAT assay had higher sensitivity than the qPCR assay

Because the minimum quantification limits of CT, NG, and UU qPCR kits (Liferiver Biotech) were 1×10^3 copies/ml, samples with concentrations less than the limit could not be accurately quantified or might be detected as negative. Thus, samples with concentrations less than 1×10^3 copies/ml would be ideal to evaluate the sensitivities. However, due to less availability of this kind of samples, especially NG samples, diluted samples were used here. The remaining 14 of the 33 CT-positive, 13 of the 32 NG-positive, and 10 of the 29 UU-positive were diluted to 1×10^2 copies/ml. Then, nucleic acids (DNA and RNA) of these diluted samples were simultaneously isolated and tested using both of the SAT assay and the qPCR assay.

Among the 14 CT samples, 28.57% (4/14) was positive in the qPCR assay, while 57.14% (8/14) was positive in the SAT assay (Table 2). Among the 13 NG samples, none was positive in the qPCR assay, while 46.15% (6/13) was positive in the SAT assay (Table 2). Among the 10 UU samples, none was positive in the qPCR assay, while 80% (8/10) was positive in the SAT assay (Table 2). These results indicated that the SAT assay had higher sensitivities than the qPCR assay in the detection of CT, NG, and UU.

Table 2 Comparison of CT, NG, and UU results in samples with concentration less than 1×10^3 copies/ml

	SAT (+)	SAT (−)	Positive rate of SAT(%)	Positive rate of qPCR(%)	Accuracy rate (%)
CT					
qPCR (+)	4	0	57.14	28.57	71.43
qPCR (−)	4	6			
NG					
qPCR (+)	0	0	46.15	0	53.85
qPCR (−)	6	7			
UU					
qPCR (+)	0	0	80	0	20
qPCR (−)	8	2			

Discussion

Although the emergence and spread of sexually infectious pathogens remains a major global public health concern, severe diseases caused by CT and NG are curable with antibiotics [14]. Routine screening and test of cure (TOC) after treatments are mainstays of disease control. However, sexually transmitted diseases are frequently asymptomatic and the local pathogen concentrations are too low, which might increase the difficulty of diagnosis. The SAT assay is designed to amplify 16S rRNA which has a great number of copies in cells [12]. Thus, the advantage of the SAT assay might be helpful when patients are asymptomatic or pathogen concentrations are very low.

In this study, the SAT assay shows excellent agreement and higher sensitivity when compared with the qPCR assay. The SAT assay detects all bacteria strains (CT, NG, or UU) which are positive by the qPCR assay

Table 1 Comparison of CT, NG, and UU results in samples with concentration more than 1×10^3 copies/ml

	SAT (+)	SAT (−)	Sensitivity (%)	Specificity (%)	Accuracy rate (%)
CT					
qPCR (+)	19	0	100	100	100
qPCR (−)	0	10			
NG					
qPCR (+)	19	0	100	100	100
qPCR (−)	0	10			
UU					
qPCR (+)	19	0	100	100	100
qPCR (−)	0	9			

and there are no discrepant results when direct detection of clinical samples is performed. In addition, the assay can detect pathogens with low concentrations (less than 1×10^3 copies/ml) indicating a higher sensitivity. Our results are consistent with other studies where another rRNA-based assay (APTIMA, Hologic Inc) was compared with DNA-based assays [15–17].

TOC is recommended after initiation of treatment. Because traces of bacterial DNA can persist for prolonged periods after successful elimination of pathogens [18, 19] and only live metabolically active bacteria produce RNA, rRNA-based NAAT could potentially discriminate metabolically-active pathogens from dead ones so that RNA might be a better biomarker than DNA during surveillance of treatments. A previous study indicates that 95% of patients clear bacterial RNA at day 13 which is one day earlier than DNA [20]. These results suggest that rRNA-based NAAT could avoid potential overtreatment. Combination of its sensitivity and specificity, the SAT assay might be an ideal TOC tool during treatment.

Our results show the same results that rRNA-based NAATs appear to offer significantly higher sensitivity than DNA-based NAATs [15, 21]. Thus, current detections using DNA-based NAATs might underestimate the prevalence of sexually infectious pathogens and overestimated the effectiveness of anti-bacterial treatments.

Our study has three limitations. Firstly, it is performed at a single hospital which might limit the generalizability. Secondly, pathogen-positive samples with concentration less than 1×10^3 copies/ml used in this study are diluted from clinical samples due to less availability, which might bias the results. Thirdly, the sample size is small and further large size samples are needed to better understand the performance of the SAT assay. Nevertheless, excellent agreement and higher sensitivity of the SAT assay are warranted in this study.

Conclusions

This study demonstrates that the SAT assay has excellent agreements and higher sensitivities for CT, NG, and UU detection in urogenital swabs when compared with the qPCR assay. Thus, the SAT assay could be a better choice for screening, diagnosis, and surveillance of sexually transmitted diseases. However, considering high prevalence in healthy populations, UU screening is only recommended in symptomatic patients with suspected urogenital tract infections.

Abbreviations

CT: *Chlamydia trachomatis*; NAAT: Nucleic acid amplification test; NG: *Neisseria gonorrhoeae*; qPCR: Quantitative real-time polymerase chain reaction; SAT: Simultaneous amplification and testing; UU: *Ureaplasma urealyticum*

Acknowledgements

Not applicable.

Funding

None.

Authors' contributions

SC and YL designed the study. SC drafted and revised the manuscript. YL, XJ, and FY performed the experiments and analyzed the data. ZL extracted DNA/RNA from samples. All authors read and approved the final manuscript.

Consent for publication

Not applicable.

Competing interests

The authors declare that they have no competing interests.

Author details

[1]Department of Infection Control, Affiliated Hospital of Academy of Military Medical Sciences, Beijing, People's Republic of China. [2]Department of Laboratory Medicine, Affiliated Hospital of Academy of Military Medical Sciences, Beijing, People's Republic of China.

References

1. Frølund M, Lidbrink P, Wikström A, Cowan S, Ahrens P, Jensen JS. Urethritis-associated pathogens in urine from men with non-gonococcal urethritis: a case-control study. Acta Derm Venereol. 2016;96:689–94.
2. Zhang N, Wang R, Li X, Liu X, Tang Z, Liu Y. Are Ureaplasma spp. a cause of nongonococcal urethritis? A systematic review and meta-analysis. PLoS One. 2014;9:e113771.
3. Serra-Pladevall J, Caballero E, Roig G, Juvé R, Barbera MJ, Andreu A. Comparison between conventional culture and NAATs for the microbiological diagnosis in gonococcal infection. Diagn Microbiol Infect Dis. 2015;83:341–3.
4. Shipitsyna E, Guschin A, Maximova A, Tseslyuk M, Savicheva A, Sokolovsky E, Shipulin G, Domeika M, Unemo M. Comparison of microscopy, culture and in-house PCR and NASBA assays for diagnosis of Neisseria gonorrhoeae in Russia. APMIS. 2008;116:133–8.
5. Tabrizi SN, Unemo M, Limnios AE, Hogan TR, Hjelmevoll SO, Garland SM, Tapsall J. Evaluation of six commercial nucleic acid amplification tests for detection of Neisseria gonorrhoeae and other Neisseria species. J Clin Microbiol. 2011;49:3610–5.
6. Ursi D, Crucitti T, Smet H, Ieven M. Evaluation of the bio-rad dx CT/NG/MG® assay for simultaneous detection of chlamydia trachomatis, Neisseria gonorrhoeae and mycoplasma genitalium in urine. Eur J Clin Microbiol Infect Dis. 2016;35:1159–63.
7. Qing L, Song QX, Feng JL, Li HY, Liu G, Jiang HH. Prevalence of chlamydia trachomatis, Neisseria gonorrhoeae, mycoplasma genitalium and Ureaplasma urealyticum infections using a novel isothermal simultaneous RNA amplification testing method in infertile males. Ann Clin Microbiol Antimicrob. 2017;16:45.
8. Li W, Fang YH, Shen HQ, Yang DH, Shu Q, Shang SQ. Evaluation of a real-time method of simultaneous amplification and testing in diagnosis of mycoplasma pneumoniae infection in children with pneumonia. PLoS One. 2017;12:e0177842.
9. Chen Q, Hu Z, Zhang Q, Yu M. Development and evaluation of a real-time method for testing human enteroviruses and coxsackievirus A16. Diagn Microbiol Infect Dis. 2016;85:36–41.
10. Xu J, Cao L, Su L, Dong N, Yu M, Ju J. A new accurate assay for Coxsackievirus a 16 by fluorescence detection of isothermal RNA amplification. J Virol Methods. 2013;193:459–62.

11. Cui Z, Wang Y, Fang L, Zheng R, Huang X, Liu X, Zhang G, Rui D, Ju J, Hu Z. Novel real-time simultaneous amplification and testing method to accurately and rapidly detect Mycobacterium tuberculosis complex. J Clin Microbiol. 2012;50:646–50.
12. Mouton JW, Verkooyen R, van der Meijden WI, van Rijsoort-Vos TH, Goessens WH, Kluytmans JA, Deelen SD, Luijendijk A, Verbrugh HA. Detection of chlamydia trachomatis in male and female urine specimens by using the amplified chlamydia trachomatis test. J Clin Microbiol. 1997;35: 1369–72.
13. Chapin K, Andrea S. APTIMA® Trichomonas vaginalis, a transcription-mediated amplification assay for detection of Trichomonas vaginalis in urogenital specimens. Expert Rev Mol Diagn. 2011;11:679–88.
14. Workowski KA, Bolan GA. Sexually transmitted diseases treatment guidelines, 2015. MMWR Recomm Rep. 2015;64(RR-03):1–137.
15. de Barbeyrac B, Géniaux M, Hocké C, Dupon M, Bébéar C. Detection of chlamydia trachomatis in symptomatic and asymptomatic populations with urogenital specimens by AMP CT (gen-probe incorporated) compared to others commercially available amplification assays. Diagn Microbiol Infect Dis. 2000;37:181–5.
16. Ferrero DV, Meyers HN, Schultz DE, Willis SA. Performance of the gen-probe AMPLIFIED chlamydia trachomatis assay in detecting chlamydia trachomatis in endocervical and urine specimens from women and urethral and urine specimens from men attending sexually transmitted disease and family planning clinics. J Clin Microbiol. 1998;36:3230–3.
17. Yang JL, Schachter J, Moncada J, Habte D, Zerihun M, House JI, Zhou Z, Hong KC, Maxey K, Gaynor BD, Lietman TM. Comparison of an rRNA-based and DNA-based nucleic acid amplification test for the detection of chlamydia trachomatis in trachoma. Br J Ophthalmol. 2007;91:293–5.
18. Workowski KA, Lampe MF, Wong KG, Watts MB, Stamm WE. Long-term eradication of chlamydia trachomatis genital infection after antimicrobial therapy. Evidence against persistent infection. JAMA. 1993;270:2071–5.
19. Cangelosi GA, Meschke JS. Dead or alive: molecular assessment of microbial viability. Appl Environ Microbiol. 2014;80:5884–91.
20. Wind CM, Schim van der Loeff MF, Unemo M, Schuurman R, van Dam AP, de Vries HJ. Time to clearance of chlamydia trachomatis RNA and DNA after treatment in patients coinfected with Neisseria gonorrhoeae - a prospective cohort study. BMC Infect Dis. 2016;16:554.
21. Chernesky M, Jang D, Luinstra K, Chong S, Smieja M, Cai W, Hayhoe B, Portillo E, Macritchie C, Main C, Ewert R. High analytical sensitivity and low rates of inhibition may contribute to detection of chlamydia trachomatis in significantly more women by the APTIMA combo 2 assay. J Clin Microbiol. 2006;44:400–5.

Permissions

All chapters in this book were first published in ID, by BioMed Central; hereby published with permission under the Creative Commons Attribution License or equivalent. Every chapter published in this book has been scrutinized by our experts. Their significance has been extensively debated. The topics covered herein carry significant findings which will fuel the growth of the discipline. They may even be implemented as practical applications or may be referred to as a beginning point for another development.

The contributors of this book come from diverse backgrounds, making this book a truly international effort. This book will bring forth new frontiers with its revolutionizing research information and detailed analysis of the nascent developments around the world.

We would like to thank all the contributing authors for lending their expertise to make the book truly unique. They have played a crucial role in the development of this book. Without their invaluable contributions this book wouldn't have been possible. They have made vital efforts to compile up to date information on the varied aspects of this subject to make this book a valuable addition to the collection of many professionals and students.

This book was conceptualized with the vision of imparting up-to-date information and advanced data in this field. To ensure the same, a matchless editorial board was set up. Every individual on the board went through rigorous rounds of assessment to prove their worth. After which they invested a large part of their time researching and compiling the most relevant data for our readers.

The editorial board has been involved in producing this book since its inception. They have spent rigorous hours researching and exploring the diverse topics which have resulted in the successful publishing of this book. They have passed on their knowledge of decades through this book. To expedite this challenging task, the publisher supported the team at every step. A small team of assistant editors was also appointed to further simplify the editing procedure and attain best results for the readers.

Apart from the editorial board, the designing team has also invested a significant amount of their time in understanding the subject and creating the most relevant covers. They scrutinized every image to scout for the most suitable representation of the subject and create an appropriate cover for the book.

The publishing team has been an ardent support to the editorial, designing and production team. Their endless efforts to recruit the best for this project, has resulted in the accomplishment of this book. They are a veteran in the field of academics and their pool of knowledge is as vast as their experience in printing. Their expertise and guidance has proved useful at every step. Their uncompromising quality standards have made this book an exceptional effort. Their encouragement from time to time has been an inspiration for everyone.

The publisher and the editorial board hope that this book will prove to be a valuable piece of knowledge for researchers, students, practitioners and scholars across the globe.

List of Contributors

N. Fournet
Epidemiology and Surveillance Unit, Centre for Infectious Diseases Control, National Institute for Public Health and the Environment (RIVM), 3720 BA Bilthoven, The Netherlands
European Programme for Intervention Epidemiology Training (EPIET), European Centre for Disease Prevention and Control (ECDC), Stockholm, Sweden

F. D. H. Koedijk
Epidemiology and Surveillance Unit, Centre for Infectious Diseases Control, National Institute for Public Health and the Environment (RIVM), 3720 BA Bilthoven, The NetherlandsPublic Health Service Twente, Enschede, The Netherlands

A. P. van Leeuwen, M. S. van Rooijen and M. G. van Veen
Public Health Service Amsterdam, Amsterdam, The Netherlands

M. A. B. van der Sande
Epidemiology and Surveillance Unit, Centre for Infectious Diseases Control, National Institute for Public Health and the Environment (RIVM), 3720 BA Bilthoven, The NetherlandsJulius Centre for Health Sciences and Primary Care, University Medical Centre Utrecht, Utrecht, The Netherlands

Maartje Visser, Fleur van Aar and Janneke C. M. Heijne
National Institute for Public Health and the Environment, 3720, BA, Bilthoven, the Netherlands

Femke D. H. Koedijk and Carolina J. G. Kampman
Public Health Service Twente, postbus 1400, 7500, BK, Enschede, the Netherlands

Jekaterina Jevtuševskaja, Liis Andresen, Katrin Krõlov and Tiia Grellier
University of Tartu, Institute of Technology Laboratory of Molecular Biotechnology, Nooruse 1, Tartu 50411, Estonia

Julia Uusna
University of Tartu, Institute of Technology Laboratory of Molecular Biotechnology, Nooruse 1, Tartu 50411, Estonia
SelfD Technologie GmbH, Leipzig, Germany

Made Laanpere
The Tartu University Hospital's Women's Clinic and Tartu Sexual Health Clinic, Tartu Estonia

Indrek Tulp
SelfD Technologie GmbH, Leipzig, Germany
University of Tartu, Institute of Chemistry, Tartu, Estonia

Ülo Langel
University of Tartu, Institute of Technology Laboratory of Molecular Biotechnology, Nooruse 1, Tartu 50411, Estonia
Stockholm University, Stockholm, Sweden

Menne Bartelsman
Department of Infectious Diseases, STI Outpatient Clinic, Public Health Service of Amsterdam (GGD Amsterdam), Weesperplein 1, 1018, XA, Amsterdam, The Netherlands

Maarten F. Schim van der Loeff
Center for Infection and Immunology Amsterdam (CINIMA), Academic Medical Center (AMC), University of Amsterdam, Amsterdam, The Netherlands
Department of Research, Public Health Service of Amsterdam (GGD Amsterdam), Nieuwe Achtergracht 100, 1018, WT, Amsterdam, The Netherlands

Henry J. C. de Vries
Department of Infectious Diseases, STI Outpatient Clinic, Public Health Service of Amsterdam (GGD Amsterdam), Weesperplein 1, 1018, XA, Amsterdam, The Netherlands
Center for Infection and Immunology Amsterdam (CINIMA), Academic Medical Center (AMC), University of Amsterdam, Amsterdam, The Netherlands
Department of Dermatology, Academic Medical Center (AMC), University of Amsterdam, Amsterdam, The Netherlands

Jannie J. van der Helm
Department of Infectious Diseases, STI Outpatient Clinic, Public Health Service of Amsterdam (GGD Amsterdam), Weesperplein 1, 1018, XA, Amsterdam, The Netherlands
Department of Research, Public Health Service of Amsterdam (GGD Amsterdam), Nieuwe Achtergracht 100, 1018, WT, Amsterdam, The Netherlands

Leslie O. A. Sabajo
Dermatological Service, Ministry of Health Suriname, Tourtonnelaan 5, Paramaribo, Suriname

Fa-Xing Jiang and Qian Lan
Department of Dermatology, Anhui Provincial Hospital, Hefei 230001, China

Wen-Jing Le and Xiao-Hong Su
STD clinic, Institute of Dermatology, Chinese Academy of Medical Sciences & Peking Union Medical College, Nanjing 210042, China

S. Menon and S. H. Stansfield
Institute of Health and Biomedical Innovation, Queensland University of Technology, Brisbane, Australia

M. Walsh, A. A. Righarts and P. C. Hill
Centre for International Health, University of Otago, Dunedin, New Zealand

E. Hope and L. Auvaa
National University of Samoa, Apia, Samoa

L. Isaia
National Health Service Laboratory Division, Apia, Samoa

T. Niupulusu
Samoa Family Health Association, Apia, Samoa

S. V. A. Temese
Centre for Samoan Studies, National University of Samoa, Apia, Samoa

L. Iosefa-Siitia and M. F. Motu
Samoa National Council of Churches, Apia, Samoa

S. A. Tapelu
Samoa AIDS Foundation, Apia, Samoa

T. Suaalii-Sauni
Victoria University of Wellington, Wellington, New Zealand

P. Timms
Faculty of Science, Health, Education and Engineering, University of the Sunshine Coast, Maroochydore, Australia

W. M. Huston
Institute of Health and Biomedical Innovation, Queensland University of Technology, Brisbane, Australia
School of Life Sciences, Faculty of Science, University of Technology Sydney, Broadway, Sydney, NSW, Australia
School of Life Sciences, University of Technology Sydney, Broadway, Sydney, NSW 2007, Australia

Susanne Buder and Eva Guhl and Peter K. Kohl
German Consiliary Laboratory for Gonococci, Department of Dermatology and Venerology, Vivantes Hospital Berlin, Berlin, Germany

Klaus Jansen, Anna Loenenbach, Andrea Sailer and Viviane Bremer
Department for Infectious Disease Epidemiology, Robert Koch Institute, Berlin, Germany

Sandra Dudareva
Department for Infectious Disease Epidemiology, Robert Koch Institute, Berlin, Germany
Charité University Medicine Berlin, Berlin, Germany

Sergejs Nikisins
Department for Infectious Disease Epidemiology, Robert Koch Institute, Berlin, Germany
Department of Infectious Diseases, Robert Koch Institute, Berlin, Germany
European Public Health Microbiology Training (EUPHEM) programme, European Centre for Disease Prevention and Control (ECDC), Stockholm, Sweden

Vincent J. Cornelisse, Marcus Y. Chen, Catriona S. Bradshaw, Clare Bellhouse, Christopher K Fairley and Eric P. F. Chow
Melbourne Sexual Health Centre, Alfred Health, 580 Swanston St, Carlton, Melbourne, VIC 3052, Australia
Central Clinical School, Faculty of Medicine, Nursing and Health Sciences, Monash University, Melbourne, Australia

Jane S Hocking and Henrietta Williams
Melbourne Sexual Health Centre, Alfred Health, 580 Swanston St, Carlton, Melbourne, VIC 3052, Australia
Melbourne School of Population and Global Health, University of Melbourne, Melbourne, Australia

Christopher J. Sherman
Melbourne School of Population and Global Health, University of Melbourne, Melbourne, Australia

Lei Zhang
Melbourne Sexual Health Centre, Alfred Health, 580 Swanston St, Carlton, Melbourne, VIC 3052, Australia
The Kirby Institute, The University of New South Wales, Sydney, Australia

Young Ah Kim
Department of Laboratory Medicine, National Health Insurance Service Ilsan Hospital, Baekseok-dong 1232, Ilsandong-gu, Goyang 10444, South Korea

Kyungwon Lee
Department of Laboratory Medicine, Yonsei University College of Medicine, 50-1 Yonsei-ro, Seodaemun-gu, Seoul 03722, South Korea
Research Institute of Bacterial Resistance, Yonsei University College of Medicine, Seoul, South Korea

Jae Eun Chung
Department of Obstetrics and Gynecology, National Health Insurance Service Ilsan Hospital, Baekseok-dong 1232, Ilsandong-gu, Goyang 10444, South Korea

Emily Bond, Donghao Lu, Eva Herweijer, Lisen Arnheim-Dahlström, Pär Sparén and Fang Fang
Department of Medical Epidemiology and Biostatistics, Karolinska Institutet, Nobels väg 12A, Stockholm 17177, Sweden

Karin Sundström
Department of Laboratory Medicine, Karolinska Institutet, H5, Division of Pathology, Karolinska Universitetssjukhuset Huddinge, Stockholm 14186, Sweden

Unnur Valdimarsdóttir
Department of Medical Epidemiology and Biostatistics, Karolinska Institutet, Nobels väg 12A, Stockholm 17177, Sweden
Center of Public Health Sciences, Faculty of Medicine, University of Iceland, Stapi v/Hringbraut, 101 Reykjavik, Iceland
Department of Epidemiology, Harvard School of Public Health, 677 Huntington Avenue, Boston, MA 02115, USA

Katja Fall
Department of Medical Epidemiology and Biostatistics, Karolinska Institutet, Nobels väg 12A, Stockholm 17177, Sweden
Clinical Epidemiology and Biostatistics, School of Medical Sciences, Örebro University, Örebro, Sweden

Bart Versteeg
Public Health Laboratory, Cluster Infectious Diseases, Public Health Service Amsterdam, Amsterdam, The Netherlands

Sylvia M. Bruisten
Public Health Laboratory, Cluster Infectious Diseases, Public Health Service Amsterdam, Amsterdam, The Netherlands
Center for Infection and Immunity Amsterdam (CINIMA), Academic Medical Center, University of Amsterdam, Amsterdam, The Netherlands

Arie van der Ende and Yvonne Pannekoek
Center for Infection and Immunity Amsterdam (CINIMA), Academic Medical Center, University of Amsterdam, Amsterdam, The Netherlands
Department of Medical Microbiology, Academic Medical Center, Amsterdam, The Netherlands

Sherri Pals, Chunfu Yang, Joy Chang, Maroya Spalding Walters, Naomi Bock, Larry Westerman and Carlos Toledo
Division of Global HIV/AIDS and Tuberculosis, US Centers for Disease Control, Atlanta, GA, USA

Elijah Odoyo-June
Division of Global HIV/AIDS and Tuberculosis, US Centers for Disease Control, Kisumu, Kenya

Walter Jaoko
Department of Medical Microbiology, University of Nairobi, Nairobi, Kenya

Robert C. Bailey
Division of Epidemiology and Biostatistics, University of Illinois Chicago School of Public Health, Chicago, IL, USA

Stephanie M. Davis
Division of Global HIV/AIDS and Tuberculosis, US Centers for Disease Control, Atlanta, GA, USA
Division of Global HIV and TB, HIV Prevention Branch US Centers for Disease Control and Prevention, 1600 Clifton Rd. NE Mail Stop E-04, Atlanta, GA 30329, USA

Carolien M. Wind
STI Outpatient Clinic, Department of Infectious Diseases, Public Health Service Amsterdam, 1000 CE Amsterdam, The Netherlands
Department of Dermatology, Academic Medical Center, University of Amsterdam, Amsterdam, The Netherlands

Maarten F. Schim van der Loeff
Department of Infectious Diseases, Public Health Service Amsterdam, The Netherlands
Center for Infection and Immunity Amsterdam, Academic Medical Center, University of Amsterdam, Amsterdam, The Netherlands

Henry J. C. de Vries
STI Outpatient Clinic, Department of Infectious Diseases, Public Health Service Amsterdam, 1000 CE Amsterdam, The Netherlands
Department of Dermatology, Academic Medical Center, University of Amsterdam, Amsterdam, The Netherlands
Center for Infection and Immunity Amsterdam, Academic Medical Center, University of Amsterdam, Amsterdam, The Netherlands

Magnus Unemo
WHO Collaborating Centre for Gonorrhoea and Other STIs, National Reference Laboratory for Pathogenic Neisseria, Department of Laboratory Medicine, Microbiology, Örebro University, SE-701 85 Örebro, Sweden

Rob Schuurman
Department of Medical Microbiology, University Medical Centre Utrecht, The Netherlands

Alje P. van Dam
Public Health Laboratory, Public Health Service Amsterdam, Amsterdam, The Netherlands
Department of Medical Microbiology, Onze Lieve Vrouwe Gasthuis General Hospital, Amsterdam, The Netherlands

Steven G. Badman, Lisa M. Vallely, Rebecca Guy, Handan Wand, Louise Causer, John Kaldor and Andrew Vallely
The Kirby Institute, University of New South Wales, Sydney, Australia

Pamela Toliman and William Pomat
Papua New Guinea Institute of Medical Research, Goroka, Papua New Guinea

Grace Kariwiga
Department of Obstetrics & Gynaecology, Alotau General Hospital, Milne Bay Province, Alotau, Papua New Guinea

Bomesina Lote
Alotau Urban Clinic, Alotau, Milne Bay Province, Papua New Guinea

Caroline Holmer
University of Technology, Sydney, Australia

Chris Morgan
The Burnet Institute, Melbourne, Australia

Stanley Luchters
The Burnet Institute, Melbourne, Australia
Melbourne School of Population and Global Health, University of Melbourne, Melbourne, VIC, Australia

Sepehr Tabrizi
Department of Microbiology and Infectious Diseases, The Royal Women's Hospital, Parkville, VIC, Australia

Suzanne M. Garland
Department of Microbiology and Infectious Diseases, The Royal Women's Hospital, Parkville, VIC, Australia
Department of Obstetrics and Gynaecology, University of Melbourne, Murdoch Children's Research Institute, Parkville, VIC, Australia

David Whiley
University of Queensland, Herston, QLD, Australia

Stephen J. Rogerson
Department of Medicine, University of Melbourne, Melbourne, Australia

Glen Mola
Department of Obstetrics & Gynaecology, School of Medicine and Health Sciences, University of Papua New Guinea, National Capital District, Papua New Guinea

Basil Donovan
The Kirby Institute, University of New South Wales, Sydney, Australia
Sydney Sexual Health Centre, Sydney, Australia

Sally B. Rose, Susan M. Garrett and Susan R. H. Pullon
Department of Primary Health Care and General Practice, University of Otago, Wellington, Wellington South 6242, New Zealand

James Stanley
Biostatistical Group, University of Otago, Wellington, Wellington South 6242, New Zealand

Kauser Jabeen, Pushpa Bhawan Mal, Erum Khan and Saeeda Chandio
Department of Pathology and Laboratory Medicine, Aga Khan University, Stadium Road, Karachi, Pakistan

Susanne Jacobsson and Magnus Unemo
WHO Collaborating Centre for Gonorrhoea and Other STIs, National Reference Laboratory for Pathogenic Neisseria, Department of Laboratory Medicine, Microbiology, Faculty of Medicine and Health, Örebro University, Örebro, Sweden

Alexandra Sarah Lang, Matthias an der Heiden, Klaus Jansen, Andrea Sailer and Viviane Bremer
Department for Infectious Disease Epidemiology, Robert Koch Institute, Berlin, Germany

Sandra Dudareva
Department for Infectious Disease Epidemiology, Robert Koch Institute, Berlin, Germany
Charité Universitätsmedizin Berlin Berlin, Germany

Brian Arturo Mondeja, Nadia Maria Rodríguez, Orestes Blanco and Carmen Fernández
Pedro Kourí Tropical Medicine Institute, La Habana, Cuba

Javier Couri
Pedro Kourí Tropical Medicine Institute, La Habana, Cuba
Faculty of Biology, University of Havana, La Habana, Cuba

Jørgen Skov Jensen
Statens Serum Institut, Research Unit for Reproductive Tract Microbiology, Artillerivej 5, DK-2300 Copenhagen S, Denmark

Kara Krista Osbak
HIV/STI Unit, Institute of Tropical Medicine, Antwerp, Belgium

Chris Kenyon
HIV/STI Unit, Institute of Tropical Medicine, Antwerp, Belgium
Division of Infectious Diseases and HIV Medicine, University of Cape Town, Anzio Road, Observatory, Cape Town 7700, South Afric

Tania Crucitti
HIV/STI Reference Laboratory, Institute of Tropical Medicine, Antwerp, Belgium

Luc Kestens
Immunology Unit, Institute of Tropical Medicine, Antwerp, Belgium
Department of Biomedical Sciences, University of Antwerp, Antwerp, Belgium

Siraj Hussen and Endale Tadesse
Department of Medical Laboratory Science, College of Medicine and Health Sciences, Hawassa University, Hawassa, Ethiopia

Demelash Wachamo
Department of Public Health, Hawassa College of Health Sciences, South Nations and Nationalities Peoples' Region, Hawassa, Ethiopia

Zemenu Yohannes
Department of Midwifery, College of Medicine and Health Sciences, Hawassa University, Hawassa, Ethiopia

Coumba Toure-Kane
Laboratory of Bacteriology and Virology of Aristide Le Dantec University Hospital, Dakar, Senegal

Moussa Sarr and Carlos Suarez
Westat, 1600 Research Blvd, WB 258, Rockville, MD 20850, USA

Christopher S. Murrill and Jacob Dee
Centers for Disease Control and Prevention, 1600 Clifton Road, Atlanta, USA

Ndeye Fatou Ngom-Faye
Division pour la Lutte Contre Le SIDA et les ISTs (DLSI), Dakar, Senegal

Pape Amadou Niang Diallo
Conseils National pour la Lutte Contre le SIDA (CNLS), Dakar, Senegal

Ousmane Diouf, Astou Gueye-Gaye, Abdou Salam Mbengue, Papa Ousmane Diaw, Massaer Gueye, Aminata Mboup and Souleymane Mboup
Laboratory of Bacteriology and Virology of Aristide Le Dantec University Hospital, Dakar, Senegal
IRESSEF: Institut de Recherche en Santé, de Surveillance Epidémiologique et de Formations, Arrondissement 4 Rue 2 D1, Pole Urbain de Diamniado, 7325 Dakar, BP, Senegal

Bahman Pourabbas, Zahra Rezaei, Mozhgan Shahian and Abdolvahab Alborzi
Professor Alborzi Clinical Microbiology Research Center, Shiraz University of Medical Sciences, Shiraz, Iran

Jalal Mardaneh
Departments of Microbiology, School of Medicine, Gonabad University of Medical Sciences, Gonabad, Iran

Amy Matser and Catharina J. Alberts
Department of Infectious Diseases, Public Health Service of Amsterdam (GGD Amsterdam), Nieuwe Achtergracht 100, 1018, WT, Amsterdam, The Netherlands

Sebastiaan H. Hulstein, Maria Prins and Maarten F. Schim van der Loeff
Department of Infectious Diseases, Public Health Service of Amsterdam (GGD Amsterdam), Nieuwe Achtergracht 100, 1018, WT, Amsterdam, The Netherlands
Department of Internal Medicine, Amsterdam Institute for Infection and Immunity (AI&II), Academic Medical Center, Meibergdreef 9, 1105, AZ, Amsterdam, The Netherlands

Marieke B. Snijder
Department of Public Health, Amsterdam Public Health Research Institute, Academic Medical Center, Meibergdreef 9, 1105, AZ, Amsterdam, The Netherlands
Department of Clinical Epidemiology, Biostatistics and Bioinformatics, Amsterdam Public Health Research Institute, Academic Medical Center, Meibergdreef 9, 1105, AZ, Amsterdam, The Netherlands

Martina Willhauck-Fleckenstein, Katrin Hufnagel and Tim Waterboer
Molecular Diagnostics of Oncogenic Infections Division, German Cancer Research Center (Deutsches Krebsforschungszentrum DKFZ), Im Neuenheimer Feld 280, 69120 Heidelberg, Germany

Henry J. C. de Vries and Henry J. C. de Vries
Department of Infectious Diseases, Public Health Service of Amsterdam (GGD Amsterdam), Nieuwe Achtergracht 100, 1018, WT, Amsterdam, The Netherlands
Department of Dermatology, Academic Medical Center, Meibergdreef 9, 1105, AZ, Amsterdam, The Netherlands

Sabrina Bakeera-Kitaka, Joseph Rujumba and Nicolette Nabukeera-Barungi
Department of Paediatrics and Child Health, School of Medicine, Makerere University College of Health Sciences, Kampala, Uganda

Mariama Mustapha
Department of Paediatrics and Child Health, School of Medicine, Makerere University College of Health Sciences, Kampala, Uganda
Ministry of Health and Sanitation, Freetown, Sierra Leone

Victor Musiime
Department of Paediatrics and Child Health, School of Medicine, Makerere University College of Health Sciences, Kampala, Uganda
Joint Clinical Research Centre, Kampala, Uganda

Li-Gang Yang, Xiao-Hui Zhang, Pei-Zhen Zhao, Zheng-Yu Chen, Wu-Jian Ke, Xu-Qi Ren, Liu-Yuan Wang and Wei-Ying Chen
Department of Sexually Transmitted Diseases, Dermatology Hospital, Southern Medical University, Guangzhou 510091, China
Guangdong Provincial Dermatology Hospital, Guangzhou 510091, China

Joseph D. Tucker
Department of Sexually Transmitted Diseases, Dermatology Hospital, Southern Medical University, Guangzhou 510091, China
Guangdong Provincial Dermatology Hospital, Guangzhou 510091, China
Institute for Global Health and Infectious Diseases, University of North Carolina at Chapel Hill, Raleigh, USA
Faculty of Infectious and Tropical Diseases, London School of Hygiene and Tropical Medicine, London, UK

Pengcheng Huai
Shandong Provincial Hospital for Skin Disease, Shandong University, Jinan, China
Shandong Provincial Institute of Dermatology and Venereology, Shandong Academy of Medical Sciences, 27397 Jingshi Road, Jinan 250022, China
Department of Epidemiology, School of Public Health, Shandong University, Jinan, China

Furong Li, Zhen Li, Tongsheng Chu, Dianchang Liu and Jian Liu
Shandong Provincial Institute of Dermatology and Venereology, Shandong Academy of Medical Sciences, 27397 Jingshi Road, Jinan 250022, China

Aiqiang Xu
Department of Epidemiology, School of Public Health, Shandong University, Jinan, China
Shandong Center for Disease Control and Prevention, Jinan, China

Lele Sun, Xi'an Fu, Qing Pan, Gongqi Yu, Zemin Chai, Zihao Mi, Fangfang Bao, Honglei Wang, Bingni Zhou, Chuan Wang, Yonghu Sun, Guiye Niu, Yuan Zhang, Fanghui Fu, Xiaoqiao Lang, Xiaoling Wang, Hui Zhao, Daina Liu, Hong Liu and Furen Zhang
Shandong Provincial Institute of Dermatology and Venereology, Shandong Academy of Medical Sciences, 27397 Jingshi Road, Jinan 250022, China
Shandong Provincial Key Laboratory for Dermatovenereology, Jinan, China

Angela Kaida, Patricia Smith, Laura Cotton, Kalysha Closson and Mark Brockman
Faculty of Health Sciences, Simon Fraser University, Blusson Hall Rm 10522, 8888 University Drive, Burnaby B.C. V5A 1S6, Canada

Janan J. Dietrich and Fatima Laher
Perinatal HIV Research Unit (PHRU), Faculty of Health Sciences, University of the Witwatersrand, Johannesburg, South Africa

Mags Beksinska, Manjeetha Jaggernath and Jenni A. Smit
Maternal Adolescent and Child Health (MatCH) Research Unit (MRU), Faculty of Health Sciences, University of the Witwatersrand, Durban, South Africa

Megan Bardsley
London School of Hygiene and Tropical Medicine, London, UK

Pooja Chitneni
Harvard combined Infectious Diseases Fellowship, Boston, MA, USA

David A. Lewis
Centre for HIV and STIs, National Institute for Communicable Diseases, Johannesburg, South Africa
Faculty of Medicine and Health & Marie Bashir Institute for Infectious Diseases and Biosecurity, University of Sydney, Sydney, Australia

Thumbi Ndung'u
HIV Pathogenesis Programme and Africa Health Research Institute, University of KwaZulu-Natal, Durban, South Africa
Ragon Institute of Massachusetts General Hospital, Massachusetts Institute of Technology and Harvard University, Cambridge, MA, USA
Max Planck Institute for Infection Biology, Berlin, Germany

Glenda Gray
Perinatal HIV Research Unit (PHRU), Faculty of Health Sciences, University of the Witwatersrand, Johannesburg, South Africa
South African Medical Research Council, Cape Town, South Africa

Yuying Liang and Shuiping Chen
Department of Infection Control, Affiliated Hospital of Academy of Military Medical Sciences, Beijing, People's Republic of China

Xin Jin, Fang Yuan and Zhanjia Li
Department of Laboratory Medicine, Affiliated Hospital of Academy of Military Medical Sciences, Beijing, People's Republic of China

Index

www.ingramcontent.com/pod-product-compliance
Lightning Source LLC
Chambersburg PA
CBHW081214180926
51613CB00003B/235
* 9 7 8 1 6 3 9 2 7 2 3 2 7 *